Treatment of Benign Prostatic Hyperplasia: Modern Alternative to Transurethral Resection of the Prostate

Bilal Chughtai • Alexis E. Te
Steven A. Kaplan
Editors

Treatment of Benign Prostatic Hyperplasia: Modern Alternative to Transurethral Resection of the Prostate

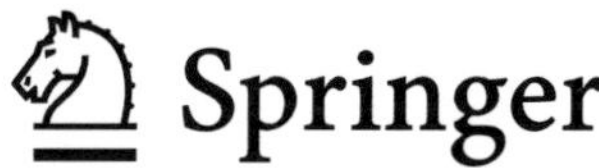

Editors
Bilal Chughtai
Department of Urology
Weill Cornell Medical College
New York, NY, USA

Alexis E. Te
Department of Urology
Weill Cornell Medical College
New York, NY, USA

Steven A. Kaplan
Department of Urology
Weill Cornell Medical College
New York, NY, USA

ISBN 978-1-4939-1586-6 ISBN 978-1-4939-1587-3 (eBook)
DOI 10.1007/978-1-4939-1587-3
Springer New York Heidelberg Dordrecht London

Library of Congress Control Number: 2014949781

Printed on acid-free paper

Springer is part of Springer Science+Business Media (www.springer.com)

Preface

The development and enhancement of treatments for male voiding dysfunction and benign prostatic hyperplasia over the last decade has led to improvement in the care of men who suffer from this condition. This book speaks of the novel and varied ways of approaching this bothersome and extremely common condition. The chapters of this book have been authored by some of the top experts on lower urinary tract symptoms of men secondary to benign prostatic hyperplasia. The authors who have contributed these chapters represent some of the most progressive and forward thinking in their techniques and approaches to these patients and disorders.

One of the important learning points of this book is that there are several correct approaches to dealing with this disease process; not necessarily is one approach better than another. Some of the techniques described here represent a tool, and the operator determines which tool is best for the specific anatomy that is being approached. In some ways this may seem contradictory, but the purpose is more to allow the reader to understand the breadth of the topic at hand.

This book represents a state-of-the-art and contemporary approach to this disease state. We hope this book provides the framework to help build and create excellence in helping our patients.

New York, NY, USA

Bilal Chughtai, M.D.
Alexis E. Te, M.D.
Steven Kaplan, M.D.

Contents

Contributors

David M. Albala, M.D. Urology, Associated Medical Professionals of NY/ Crouse Hospital, Syracuse, NY, USA

Ilija Aleksic, M.D. Urology, Associated Medical Professionals of NY, Syracuse, NY, USA

Adnan Ali, M.B.B.S. Department of Urology, Icahn School of Medicine at Mount Sinai, Mount Sinai Hospital, New York, NY, USA

Alexander Bachmann, M.D. Department of Urology, University Hospital Basel, Basel, Switzerland

Gina M. Badalato, M.D. Department of Urology, Columbia University Medical Center, New York, NY, USA

Aaron M. Bernie, M.D., M.P.H. Department of Urology, Weill Cornell, New York Presbyterian Hospital, New York, NY, USA

Naeem Bhojani, M.D., FRCSC Urology Department, School of Medicine, University of Montreal, Montreal, QC, Canada

Jeffrey D. Branch, M.D. Department of Urology, Loyola University Chicago, Loyola University Medical Center, Maywood, IL, USA

Bilal Chughtai, M.D. Department of Urology, Weill Cornell Medical College, New York, NY, USA

Doreen E. Chung, M.D., FRCSC Section of Urology, Department of Surgery, University of Chicago Medical Center and Mount Sinai Hospital, Chicago, IL, USA

Claire Dunphy, B.A. Department of Urology, Weill Cornell Medical College, New York, NY, USA

Peter J. Gilling, M.D. (Otago), FRACS Department of Urology, Tauranga Hospital, Tauranga, New Zealand

Ricardo R. Gonzalez, M.D. Department of Urology, Baylor College of Medicine; Houston Metro Urology, Houston Methodist Hospital, Houston, TX, USA

Pierre-Alain Hueber, M.D., Ph.D. Section of Urology, Department of Surgery, Centre Hospitalier de l'Université de Montréal, CHUM, Montreal, QC, Canada

Arman Adam Kahokehr, M.B.Ch.B., Ph.D. Department of Urology, Tauranga Hospital, Bay of Plenty District Health Board, Tauranga, New Zealand

Steven A. Kaplan, M.D. Department of Urology, Weill Cornell Medical College, New York, NY, USA

Bethany A. Kearns, M.D. Department of Urology, Loyola University Chicago, Loyola University Medical Center, Maywood, IL, USA

Rajeev Kumar, M.Ch. Department of Urology, All India Institute of Medical Science, New Delhi, India

Richard Lee, M.D., M.B.A. Urology and Public Health, Weill Cornell Medical College, New York Presbyterian Hospital, New York, NY, USA

Lori B. Lerner, M.D. Section of Urology, VA Boston Healthcare System, Boston University School of Medicine, Hingham, MA, USA

Department of Urology, Boston University School of Medicine, Boston, MA, USA

Victor Lizarraga, M.D. Department of Urology, Baylor College of Medicine, Houston, TX, USA

Rao S. Mandalapu, M.D. Department of Urology, Icahn School of Medicine at Mount Sinai, Mount Sinai Hospital, New York, NY, USA

Ciara S. Marley, M.A., M.D. Department of Urology, Columbia University Medical Center, New York, NY, USA

Vladimir Mouraviev, M.D. Clinical Research, Urology, Associated Medical Professionals of NY, Syracuse, NY, USA

Tony Nimeh, M.D. Department of Urology, VA Boston Healthcare System, West Roxbury, MA, USA

Roger Valdivieso O'Donova, M.D. Urology Department, University of Montreal Hospital Center (CHUM), Laval, QC, Canada

Michael A. Palese, M.D. Urology Department, The Mount Sinai Medical Center, New York, NY, USA

Joseph J. Pariser, M.D. Section of Urology, Department of Surgery, University of Chicago Medical Center, Chicago, IL, USA

Sailaja Pisipati, M.D., FRCS (Urol) Department of Urology, Icahn School of Medicine at Mount Sinai, Mount Sinai Hospital, New York, NY, USA

Malte Rieken, M.D. Department of Urology, University Hospital Basel, Basel, Switzerland

Matthew P. Rutman, M.D. Department of Urology, Columbia University College of Physicians and Surgeons, New York, NY, USA

Jaspreet S. Sandhu, M.D. Department of Surgery/Urology, Memorial Sloan-Kettering Cancer Center, New York, NY, USA

Grace B. Delos Santos, M.D. Department of Urology, Loyola University Chicago, Loyola University Medical Center, Maywood, IL, USA

Alexander M. Sarkisian, M.S. Department of Urology, Weill Cornell Medical College, New York, NY, USA

Joseph Shirk, M.D. Department of Urology, David Geffen School of Medicine at University of California-Los Angeles, Los Angeles, CA, USA

Jonathan Shoag, M.D. Department of Urology, Weill Cornell Medical College, New York Presbyterian Hospital, New York, NY, USA

Michael Shy, M.D., Ph.D. Department of Urology, Baylor College of Medicine, Houston, TX, USA

Alexander C. Small, M.D. Department of Urology, New York Presbyterian Hospital, Columbia University Medical Center, New York, NY, USA

Shahin Tabatabaei, M.D. Department of Urology, Harvard Medical School, Massachusetts General Hospital, Boston, MA, USA

Saman Shafaat Talab, M.D. Department of Urology, Harvard Medical School, Massachusetts General Hospital, Boston, MA, USA

Alexis E. Te, M.D. Department of Urology, Weill Cornell Medical College, New York, NY, USA

Ashutosh K. Tewari, M.B.B.S., M.Ch. Department of Urology, Icahn School of Medicine at Mount Sinai, Mount Sinai Hospital, New York, NY, USA

Quoc-Dien Trinh, M.D. Surgery Department, Brigham and Women's Hospital, Boston, MA, USA

Henry H. Woo, M.B.B.S., FRACS (Urol) Sydney Adventist Hospital Clinical School, University of Sydney, Wahroonga, NSW, Australia

Kevin C. Zorn, M.D. Robotic Surgery, Section of Urology, University of Montreal Hospital Center (CHUM), Montreal, QC, Canada

1 Introduction

Bilal Chughtai, Claire Dunphy, Alexis E. Te, and Steven A. Kaplan

History of TURP

The modern TURP originated from an apparatus constructed by McCarthy in 1932, which had an oblique lens system cystoscope with a tungsten loop for resection [1]. Technological advances in the 1970s allowed for the development of the Hopkins rod lens system as well as fiber-optic lighting systems, which allowed for significant improvements in visualization [2]. After the use of video became an invaluable instructional tool for the education of urologists in the 1980s, additional developments in the use of video cameras greatly improved surgical visualization. Advances in electrical generators have likewise enhanced the surgical process by allowing for more precision and efficiency during resection. Higher-power generators allow for improved vaporization and appropriate coagulation and desiccation of tissue during the procedure. This has led to the TURP being known as the gold standard to relieve LUTS secondary to BPH, making it one of the most commonly performed procedures by urologists.

B. Chughtai, M.D. (✉) • C. Dunphy, B.A.
A.E. Te, M.D. • S.A. Kaplan, M.D.
Department of Urology, Weill Cornell Medical College, 425 East 61st Street, 12th Floor, New York, NY, USA
e-mail: bic9008@med.cornell.edu; cld3002@med.cornell.edu; Aet2005@med.cornell.edu; kaplans@med.cornell.edu

Indications for Surgical Intervention for Bladder Outlet Obstruction (BOO)

Absolute indications for surgical intervention for BOO have included refractory urinary retention, azotemia secondary to bladder outlet obstruction, gross hematuria from the prostate, and bladder stone formation, but the most common indication for TURP is relief of symptoms secondary to outlet obstruction.

A previous study found that 81 % of patients who underwent TURP from 1991 to 1998 had lower urinary tract symptoms only. The five most common indications were urinary retention (15 %), recurrent prostatitis (10 %), gross hematuria (4 %), and bladder stones (6 %) [3].

A contrasting transurethral prostatectomy outcomes study reported by Mebust and colleagues in 1989, which included men from 13 operating centers from 1978 to 1987, found lower urinary tract symptoms alone in 30 % of men at TURP. They found that 27 % of men had recurrent retention, 12 % suffered from recurrent prostatitis, 12 % underwent TURP for hematuria, and 3 % for bladder stones [4]. Less than a decade later, the indications for TURP shifted toward improving symptoms and quality of life.

As subjective decisions about quality of life should be made collaboratively by patient and physician, the Agency for Health Care Policy and Research created clinical guidelines to aid

B. Chughtai et al. (eds.), *Treatment of Benign Prostatic Hyperplasia: Modern Alternative to Transurethral Resection of the Prostate*, DOI 10.1007/978-1-4939-1587-3_1,

urologists and patients in the decision-making process [5]. Generally, patients with minimal symptoms (i.e., an AUA symptom score less than seven or a urinary flow rate greater than 15 mL/s) should be counseled to undergo watchful waiting. Men with higher symptom scores (greater than seven) or impaired urinary flow (flow rate less than 15 mL/s) with symptoms are to be considered for intervention, after discussing possible therapeutic benefits and risks. Those with the most severe pre-operative voiding symptoms report the greatest postoperative improvements after TURP [6].

This book presents an up-to-date review of modern techniques used to treat benign prostatic hyperplasia. This review spans both office and operating room techniques, including both electrosurgical and laser-based methods. Among these are photoselective laser vaporization of the prostate (PVP), holmium laser enucleation/ablation of the prostate (HoLEP/HoLAP), and bipolar electrovaporization of the prostate (bipolar EVP/bipolar TURP). A comprehensive review of therapies currently being developed is also included. All techniques are presented in a balanced fashion with a focus on modern literature.

References

1. Nesbit RM. A history of transurethral prostatectomy. Rev Mex Urol. 1975;35:349–62.
2. Fitzpatrick JF, Mebust WK. Minimally invasive and endoscopic management of benign prostatic hyperplasia. In: Walsh PC, Retik AB, Vaughan Jr ED, Wein A, editors. Campbell's urology, vol. 2. 8th ed. Philadelphia: Saunders; 2003. p. 1379–422.
3. Borboroglu PG, Kane CJ, Ward JF, Roberts JL, Sands JP. Immediate and postoperative complications of transurethral prostatectomy in the 1990s. J Urol. 1999;162:1307–10.
4. Mebust WK, Holtgrewe HL, Cockett ATK, Peters PC, Committee W. Transurethral prostatectomy: immediate and postoperative complication. A cooperative study of 13 participating institutions evaluating 3,885 patients. J Urol. 1989;141:243–7.
5. McConell J, Barry M, Bruskewitz R, et al. In: Services AFH, editor. Benign prostatic hyperplasia: diagnosis and treatment, Clinical practice guidelines no. 8. AHCPR publication 94–0582. Rockville: U.S. Department of Health and Human Services; 1994.
6. Greene LF, Holcumb GR. Transurethral resection in special situations. In: Greene LF, Segura JW, editors. Transurethral surgery. Philadelphia: WB Saunders; 1979. p. 216.

2 Principles of Electrocautery-Based Techniques

Alexander M. Sarkisian, Aaron M. Bernie, and Richard Lee

Introduction

Electrosurgery was first described in great detail by A.J. McLean, who provided histological analysis and interpretation of the healing process in various animal tissues subjected to electrosurgery [1]. McLean also extensively studied principles regarding current density and heat transfer governing the effects of electrical current on tissue [1]. Since its initial description, electrosurgery has evolved into a widely used technology that allows surgeons to obtain a surgical effect such as cutting or coagulation by applying a high-frequency electrical current to a target tissue [1, 2]. This chapter will focus on the technical aspects of several electrosurgical techniques used in the treatment of BPH.

A.M. Sarkisian, M.S.
Department of Urology, Weill Cornell Medical College, New York, NY, USA

A.M. Bernie, M.D., M.P.H. (✉)
Department of Urology, Weill Cornell, New York Presbyterian Hospital, 525 East 68th Street, Box 94, New York, NY 10032, USA
e-mail: amb9064@nyp.org

R. Lee, M.D., M.B.A.
Urology and Public Health, Weill Cornell Medical College, New York Presbyterian Hospital, New York, NY, USA

Basic Principles

The core principles of electrosurgery revolve around the fact that human tissue introduced into an incomplete circuit will conduct current, therefore closing the circuit and resulting in heating of the tissue [3–5]. In an electrical circuit, current generated in an electrosurgical generator flows from a positive (active) electrode to a negative (return) electrode to form a complete circuit [4]. The amount of heat produced increases with increased current density, tissue resistance, and time as described by the following modification of Joule's Law (Eq. 2.1) [5].

$$\text{Energy} = \left(\frac{\text{current}}{\text{cross-sectional area}}\right)^2 \times \text{resistance} \times \text{time} \tag{2.1}$$

A small surface on an active electrode leads to a current density sufficient to cause the desired tissue effect in a short amount of time, while a larger electrode would require a stronger current or more time to achieve the same degree of heating [2, 5]. In fact, the given effect on the tissue largely depends on the rate of temperature rise in tissue that can be varied by adjusting the settings of the electrosurgical generator [4, 5].

Cutting of tissue may be achieved by the application of a high-current, low-voltage continuous wave form causing a quick increase in tissue temperature [4]. Rapid rise in tissue temperature leads to the vaporization of tissue

B. Chughtai et al. (eds.), *Treatment of Benign Prostatic Hyperplasia: Modern Alternative to Transurethral Resection of the Prostate*, DOI 10.1007/978-1-4939-1587-3_2,

water and subsequent fragmentation [1, 4]. Coagulation can be achieved by using a wave form that is dampened, therefore delivered in short interrupted bursts with current-free intervals between the bursts [2, 4]. The slow temperature rise achieved by the dampened current leads to coagulation by thermal denaturizing of the tissue and with further time desiccation may subsequently occur [1, 4]. Various "blend" settings often exist on modern electrosurgical generators that can achieve a combination of cutting and coagulation by producing variations of dampened currents based on the surgeon's preference and desired outcome. Fulguration is a technique using a high-voltage interrupted current in which the active electrode is held a few millimeters away from tissue and passed over in a sweeping motion as sparks bridging the air gap lead to broad and superficial coagulation [2, 6]. As these tissue effects are a result of tissue heating, they can all be achieved with both monopolar and bipolar configurations.

Electrosurgical generators typically produce currents at a frequency ranging from 0.3 to 5 MHz for safety reasons [2]. At lower frequencies near or less than 100 kHz, electrical currents can cause neuromuscular stimulation resulting in muscle contraction and adverse effects in the patient [2]. At higher-range frequencies near 5 MHz or greater, the current can be more difficult to contain, and leak becomes a threat to the safety of both the patient and operator [2]. The output frequency of a given electrosurgical generator is typically a variable inherent to the device and manufacturer's specifications and is not adjusted by the user [7].

Fundamentals of Monopolar Endoscopic Techniques

Monopolar endoscopic techniques feature an active resection electrode typically in the form of a loop, a large dispersive pad located on the patient that acts as the return electrode and a continuous irrigating resectoscope [4]. The ideal irrigating fluid in monopolar procedures should be clear in color, chemically inert, and electrolyte free to avoid dispersion of current away from the targeted tissue, similar in osmolality to serum and able to be detected by the surgeon when absorbed into the intravascular compartment [8]. Classically, glycine has represented the irrigation fluid of choice in monopolar transurethral resection of the prostate (TURP) although mannitol, sorbitol, and glucose-based solutions are also used as alternatives [8–11]. The most commonly used irrigating fluid, 1.5 % glycine, is hypotonic to serum and has been known to cause TUR syndrome in a small portion of patients after TURP. Maintenance of body temperature is also an issue with continuous irrigation; therefore, pre-warming or continuous warming of irrigation solutions is helpful to avoid large perioperative decreases in body temperature and the potential adverse effects associated with hypothermia [12, 13].

TURP, initially developed as a monopolar technique, utilizes monopolar current to resect hypertrophied prostatic tissue through a variety of resection strategies. Monopolar transurethral electrovaporization of the prostate (TUVP) is a modification of the standard TURP; the first peer-reviewed study demonstrating its safety and efficacy was published by Kaplan and Te in 1994. A separate prospective, randomized controlled trial which compared TUVP to TURP in 150 men demonstrated improvements in the international prostate symptom score (IPSS), quality of life questionnaire (QoL), symptom problem index (SPI), and BPH impact index (BII) after TUVP which were comparable with TURP and endured at 10 years of follow-up [14]. With adjustment in the power and equipment, TUVP enables a surgeon to achieve a combination of vaporization, desiccation, and coagulation of prostate tissue using standard TURP equipment fitted with a grooved roller electrode [9, 15]. Electrovaporization is generally accomplished at a cutting current that is approximately 25 % higher power and a slower resection speed than the standard TURP [15]. As the roller electrode is moved along the surface of the prostate, cutting is achieved at the leading edge by the high current density that rapidly heats tissue leading to vaporization, while coagulation is produced at the trailing edge by a more diffuse current [15]. The difference in current density is based on the principle that electricity flows via the path of least resistance, and as the tissue is vaporized, the underlying tissue experiences a certain degree of desiccation and therefore has a reduced conductance to current. Advantages to the simultaneous vaporization and coagulation include reduced blood loss, less fluid absorption, and reduced incidence of TUR syndrome [16, 17]. Monopolar transurethral electrovapor resection of the prostate (TUVRP) is similar to TUVP with the exception of using a thick loop to perform the vaporization at depth, which allows for the resection of "prostate chips" which may be sent for histological analysis, if desired.

Fundamentals of Bipolar Techniques

In contrast to monopolar techniques, bipolar electrosurgery features both active and return electrodes built into the instrument a small distance apart from each other [18]. This allows current to pass through the target tissue and return to the return electrode in the resectoscope, negating the need for a dispersive pad on the patient [4, 5, 18]. Additionally, resection can be carried out in a saline medium, which removes the risk of TUR syndrome and dilutional hyponatremia [7, 18, 19]. While the risk for TUR syndrome is theoretically reduced, one must still be cautious in patients with cardiac comorbidities, as the risk for fluid overload does exist with isotonic saline use [7].

The estimated depth of penetration for bipolar techniques is 0.5–1 mm, compared to an estimated 3–5 mm for monopolar techniques [20, 21]. The lower voltage and reduced depth of penetration result in reduced damage to surrounding tissues, which in principle reduces the risk of postoperative erectile dysfunction or adjacent organ damage [7, 20]. Bipolar setups have been used to perform bipolar TURP (B-TURP) which has shown to be an effective method of prostate resection and also can achieve vaporization of prostatic tissue while providing favorable hemostatic results [18, 22, 23]. Table 2.1 provides a detailed comparison of the differences between bipolar and monopolar technology.

Table 2.1 Side-by-side comparison of features of monopolar and bipolar transurethral resection of the prostate

	Monopolar TURP	Bipolar TURP
Irrigation solutions	Glycine, mannitol, sorbitol, glucose	Normal saline
Requires return pad on patient?	Yes	No
Approximate depth of coagulative necrosis	3–5 mm	0.5–1 mm
Can obtain prostate chips for histologic analysis?	Yes	Yes

Plasma kinetic vaporization of the prostate (PKVP) is an additional bipolar modality that utilizes radiofrequency energy in an electroconductive irrigation medium to create an ionized plasma layer to vaporize prostate adenoma [18, 19, 24]. A bipolar configuration may also be used to perform a TUVP or TUVRP.

Conclusion

Advancements in electrosurgical techniques have certainly had a significant impact on the practice of surgery. To achieve desired outcomes and protect patient safety, the operator must be aware of the technology and its appropriate use. In the electrosurgical management of BPH, the surgeon must choose from a wide range of techniques with the same goal in mind. Selection of the desired technique and technology may depend on several factors including patient characteristics, availability of equipment, operator experience, and preference. It is important to keep up to date with the body of available technologies to ensure that the chosen method will allow for the best possible outcome and patient safety profile.

References

1. McLean A. The Bovie electrosurgical current generator: some underlying principles and results. Arch Surg. 1929;18(4):1863–73. doi:10.1001/archsurg.1929.01140130965064.
2. Taheri A, Mansoori P, Sandoval LF, Feldman SR, Pearce D, Williford PM. Electrosurgery: Part I.

Basics and principles. J Am Acad Dermatol. 2014;70(4):591 e591–591 e514. doi:10.1016/j.jaad.2013.09.056.
3. Morris ML. Electrosurgery in the gastroenterology suite: principles, practice, and safety. Gastroenterol Nurs. 2006;29(2):126–32. Quiz 132–124.
4. Jones CM, Pierre KB, Nicoud IB, Stain SC, Melvin 3rd WV. Electrosurgery. Curr Surg. 2006;63(6):458–63. doi:10.1016/j.cursur.2006.06.017.
5. Massarweh NN, Cosgriff N, Slakey DP. Electrosurgery: history, principles, and current and future uses. J Am Coll Surg. 2006;202(3):520–30. doi:10.1016/j.jamcollsurg.2005.11.017.
6. Wang K, Advincula AP. "Current thoughts" in electrosurgery. Int J Gynecol Obstet. 2007;97(3):245–50. doi:10.1016/j.ijgo.2007.03.001.
7. Smith D, Khoubehi B, Patel A. Bipolar electrosurgery for benign prostatic hyperplasia: transurethral electrovaporization and resection of the prostate. Curr Opin Urol. 2005;15(2):95–100.
8. Collins JW, MacDermott S, Bradbrook RA, Keeley FX, Timoney AG. A comparison of the effect of 1.5 % glycine and 5 % glucose irrigants on plasma serum physiology and the incidence of transurethral resection syndrome during prostate resection. BJU Int. 2005;96(3):368–72. doi:10.1111/j.1464-410X.2005.05633.x.
9. Akgul KT, Ayyildiz A, Nuhoglu B, Caydere M, Ustun H, Germiyanoglu C. Comparison of transurethral prostate resection and plasmakinetic prostate resection according to cautery artefacts in tissue specimens. Int Urol Nephrol. 2007;39(4):1091–6. doi:10.1007/s11255-007-9174-1.
10. Dawkins GPC, Miller RA. Sorbitol-mannitol solution for urological electrosurgical resection – a safer fluid than glycine 1.5 %. Eur Urol. 1999;36(2):99–102. doi:10.1159/000067978.
11. Hahn RG. Irrigating fluids in endoscopic surgery. Br J Urol. 1997;79(5):669–80. doi:10.1046/j.1464-410X.1997.00150.x.
12. Pit MJ, Tegelaar RJ, Venema PL. Isothermic irrigation during transurethral resection of the prostate: effects on peri-operative hypothermia, blood loss, resection time and patient satisfaction. Br J Urol. 1996;78(1):99–103. doi:10.1046/j.1464-410X.1996.04819.x.
13. Jin YH, Tian JH, Sun M, Yang KH. A systematic review of randomised controlled trials of the effects of warmed irrigation fluid on core body temperature during endoscopic surgeries. J Clin Nurs. 2011;20(3–4):305–16. doi:10.1111/j.1365-2702.2010.03484.x.
14. Hoekstra RJ, van Melick HHE, Kok ET, Bosch JLHR. A 10-year follow-up after transurethral resection of the prostate, contact laser prostatectomy and electrovaporization in men with benign prostatic hyperplasia; long-term results of a randomized controlled trial. BJU Int. 2010;106(6):822–6. doi:10.1111/j.1464-410X.2010.09229.x.
15. Kaplan SA, Te AE. Transurethral electrovaporization of the prostate: a novel method for treating men with benign prostatic hyperplasia. Urology. 1995;45(4):566–72. doi:10.1016/s0090-4295(99)80044-2.
16. Hammadeh MY, Madaan S, Hines J, Philp T. 5-year outcome of a prospective randomized trial to compare transurethral electrovaporization of the prostate and standard transurethral resection. Urology. 2003;61(6):1166–71.
17. Hammadeh MY, Philp T. Transurethral electrovaporization of the prostate (TUVP) is effective, safe and durable. Prostate Cancer Prostatic Dis. 2003;6(2):121–6. doi:10.1038/sj.pcan.4500654.
18. Wendt-Nordahl G, Hacker A, Reich O, Djavan B, Alken P, Michel MS. The Vista system: a new bipolar resection device for endourological procedures: comparison with conventional resectoscope. Eur Urol. 2004;46(5):586–90. doi:10.1016/j.eururo.2004.07.018.
19. Rassweiler J, Teber D, Kuntz R, Hofmann R. Complications of transurethral resection of the prostate (TURP)–incidence, management, and prevention. Eur Urol. 2006;50(5):969–79. doi:10.1016/j.eururo.2005.12.042. Discussion 980.
20. Sinanoglu O, Ekici S, Tatar MN, Turan G, Keles A, Erdem Z. Postoperative outcomes of plasmakinetic transurethral resection of the prostate compared to monopolar transurethral resection of the prostate in patients with comorbidities. Urology. 2012;80(2):402–6. doi:10.1016/j.urology.2012.02.029.
21. Botto H, Lebret T, Barre P, Orsoni JL, Herve JM, Lugagne PM. Electrovaporization of the prostate with the Gyrus device. J Endourol/Endourol Soc. 2001;15(3):313–6. doi:10.1089/089277901750161917.
22. Starkman JS, Santucci RA. Comparison of bipolar transurethral resection of the prostate with standard transurethral prostatectomy: shorter stay, earlier catheter removal and fewer complications. BJU Int. 2005;95(1):69–71. doi:10.1111/j.1464-410X.2005.05253.x.
23. Bach T, Herrmann TR, Cellarius C, Geavlete B, Gross AJ, Jecu M. Bipolar resection of the bladder and prostate–initial experience with a newly developed regular sized loop resectoscope. J Med Life. 2009;2(4):443–6.
24. Dincel C, Samli MM, Guler C, Demirbas M, Karalar M. Plasma kinetic vaporization of the prostate: clinical evaluation of a new technique. J Endourol/Endourol Soc. 2004;18(3):293–8. doi:10.1089/089277904773582921.

3 Monopolar TURP

Jeffrey D. Branch, Grace B. Delos Santos, and Bethany A. Kearns

Introduction

Endoscopic resection of the prostate was borne from a need to improve upon the highly morbid procedure of open prostatectomy, which conferred a mortality rate of 20–30 % [1]. In their 1932 editorial, Caulk and Wiseman outlined the necessary components for a procedure such as TURP to be the successor of open prostatectomy, namely, "simplicity of operative technique, applicability, freedom from complications and disabling sequelae, a negligible mortality rate, and above all uniformly satisfactory and lasting results." Even the evolution of TURP in the first quarter of the twentieth century was tempered by editorial discussions. Miley B. Wesson, AUA president from 1934 to 1935, cautioned urologists not to be swept up in the band wagon of cystoscopic resection but instead stating that large hypertrophies "can be removed much quicker and with less shock by open prostatectomy" [2]. This sentiment is much the opposite today, with open prostatectomy being performed much less often than transurethral resection. Herman Kretschmer, a strong proponent of transurethral resection, observed in 1936 that there were three different points of view toward selection of cases for resection: the first group who took up TURP with enthusiasm and who believed that surgical prostatectomy had been completely replaced, the second group who believed that surgical prostatectomy remained the method of choice, and the third group who believed that both TURP and surgical prostatectomy had their place in the urologist's armamentarium [3]. In this chapter we will discuss the early days of monopolar TURP and its evolution to what we see today as the "gold standard" for endoscopic management of bladder outlet obstruction (BOO) secondary to BPH. The technique for monopolar TURP will be discussed in detail, as well as short term and long term outcomes. Monopolar TURP remained the gold standard for several decades, with various modifications to address adverse events such as bleeding complications and transurethral resection (TUR) syndrome. Just as TURP challenged open prostatectomy, new modalities have been introduced to address its shortcomings.

History

From its pre-twentieth century days, surgical treatment of BPH has undergone gradual refinement. Figure 3.1 shows a timeline of the development of endoscopic equipment and medical therapies for BPH. Early accounts showed surgical excision of the median portion of the prostate,

J.D. Branch, M.D. (✉) • G.B. Delos Santos, M.D.
B.A. Kearns, M.D.
Department of Urology, Loyola University Chicago, Loyola University Medical Center,
2160 S. First Ave., Maywood, IL 60153, USA
e-mail: jbranch@lumc.edu

B. Chughtai et al. (eds.), *Treatment of Benign Prostatic Hyperplasia: Modern Alternative to Transurethral Resection of the Prostate*, DOI 10.1007/978-1-4939-1587-3_3,

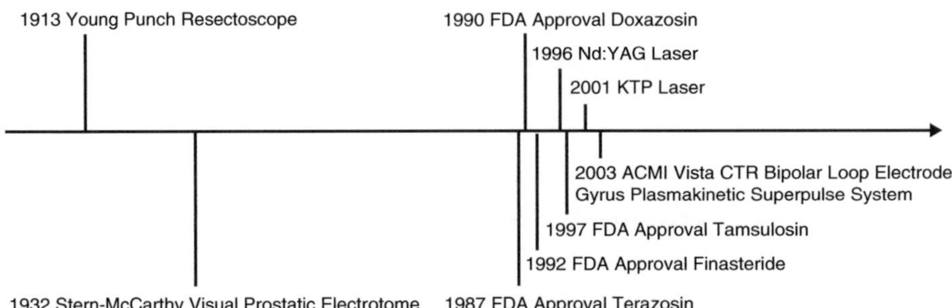

Fig. 3.1 Timeline of the development of endoscopic equipment and medical therapies for BPH

often called the prostatic bar, either suprapubically via an incision or perineally. In addition to these direct-vision procedures, various instruments were introduced per urethra in a blind fashion in order to create a prostatic channel. In 1913 Hugh Hampton Young introduced the punch resectoscope which had the advantage of direct visualization of the tissue to be excised through the cystoscopic sheath [4]. In 1910 Edwin Beer introduced the application of high-frequency current via an insulated copper wire through a cystoscope with the purpose of cauterizing a symptomatic inoperable bladder tumor [5]. Maximilian Stern in 1926 described the transurethral resectoscope with the application of bipolar energy through a tungsten loop [6]. And John Francis McCarthy modified the resectoscope into the apparatus largely as we know it today [7].

Monopolar TURP Versus Open Prostatectomy

Traditional indications for performing open prostatectomy in the modern era were for glands over 100 g and when concomitant procedures were needed, including cystolithotomy and bladder diverticulectomy, though some endoscopists have challenged this size constraint by tackling larger glands. Consequently there have not been many contemporary series which compare monopolar TURP to open prostatectomy. A 1990s series from Italy featured a cohort with a median prostate volume of 70 cm^3. Their early complications include bleeding requiring blood transfusion (8.2 %), sepsis (8.6 %), urinary incontinence (3.7 %), and death (0.06 %). Bladder neck stricture occurred in 4.8 %, and reinterventions during a follow-up period of 2 years, primarily due to bladder neck stenosis, accounted for 3.6 % of patients [8]. In a small randomized trial comparing transvesical prostatectomy to monopolar TURP for glands larger than 80 g, the operative time between the two groups was not significantly different, but the resected tissue weight (69.7 g vs. 116.8 g) favored transvesical prostatectomy, while the postoperative irrigation time and admission time favored TURP. Complication rates were not significantly different between the two groups [9].

Changes in Practices

Monopolar TURP usage has declined worldwide since the 1990s. An analysis at one institution in the United Kingdom showed a 31.6 % decrease in the number of monopolar TURPs from 1990 to 2000, as well as more cases performed for urinary retention on an older cohort of patients [10]. Yu et al. analyzed the total number of BPH procedures claimed through Medicare, the US federally administered health insurance for patients over 65 years old, from the years 1999 through 2005 [11]. They found a 44 % increase in the total number of procedures performed for BPH but a steady decrease in TURP by approximately 5 % annually. Procedures such as microwave therapy, transurethral needle ablation, transurethral laser coagulation, or laser vaporization constituted the remainder. Elliott et al. also conducted a Medicare database analysis from the years 2000 to 2008 and found a decline in the number of TURP procedures done annually per 100,000 persons [12]. Although TURP remained the most commonly performed procedure, in aggregate thermotherapy and laser modalities were implemented more frequently. The factors that determined whether patients underwent TURP versus laser prostatectomy included age and health status, but surgeon preference has also been determined to be a major contributor to the decline in TURP usage [13].

Surgeon training may have an effect as well on which procedure is ultimately performed. In a study by Lowrance et al., case logs submitted by urologists applying for certification or recertification for the American Board of Urology from 2004 to 2010 showed an increase in the number of endoscopic laser vaporization or enucleation procedures performed [14]. On the other hand, older surgeons were not as likely to perform laser procedures.

The number of TURPs performed by resident training programs parallels this trend. Several factors have been proposed to explain the trend, including patient preference for new and highly advertised procedures, increased use of medical therapy and acceptance of medical therapy as a first-line therapy, and learning curve for surgeons. In a study based on a review of ACGME case logs from 2001 to 2007, the number of electrosurgical TURPs performed has declined despite a stable number of graduating residents [15]. The number of TURPs logged decreased from 58 per resident in 2001 to 43 per resident in 2007. In contrast, the number of laser procedures performed rose, beginning in 2004, from 2 to 3 per resident in years previous to 13.5 in 2007. In a prospective cohort study from 2008, the authors showed that a surgeon who had performed greater than 50 TURPs was able to resect four times more tissue than those that had performed less than 50 TURPs [16]. Given the variable emphasis of TURP in training programs, surgeon unfamiliarity with the procedure may ultimately translate into a decline in comparative efficacy. In general this has yet to be observed in the literature.

Technique

The classic description of the monopolar TURP technique was published by Nesbit in 1943, and a four-step lobar anatomic approach to resections was characterized by Mauermayer and modified by Hartung and May in 2002 [17–19]. The monopolar TURP loop allows the surgeon to cut and coagulate tissue with an electrical current that passes through a hypoosmotic irrigant within the patient from the active electrode on the resectoscope loop to a grounding pad attached to the patient. Obstructing periurethral tissue, often referred to as adenoma, is removed within the accepted boundaries of resection.

The technique described further here is a synopsis of monopolar TURP technique at our institution, and the authors acknowledge that the approach to the procedure may vary. Generally, spinal anesthesia can be chosen to allow for early recognition of mental status changes that are the hallmark of hyponatremia and TUR syndrome. The patient is placed in dorsal lithotomy position with padded stirrups and then prepped and draped in typical sterile fashion. Preoperative antibiotics are administered prior to resection; this is especially important in patients with indwelling catheters. Equipment typically includes a 24 or 26 French resectoscope sheath which allows for continuous flow irrigation and a monopolar loop. The irrigant is a hypotonic solution, such a glycine or mannitol, which conducts current. Ideally, continuous flow irrigation is available, with the option to add a continuous pump to the irrigation circuit. A continuous flow setup improves visualization with vascular glands and contributes to low pressure irrigation and decreased absorption of irrigant. The case begins with endoscopic inspection to characterize lobar anatomy and identify the critical proximal (ureteral orifices) and distal (verumontanum) landmarks. Many urologists begin resection at the proximal portion of the middle lobe at the 6 o'clock position to create a working space and enhance irrigation, taking care to avoid resection of the ureteral orifices. Attention is then turned to the lateral lobes. Resection should not occur distal to the level of the verumontanum to minimize the complication of injury to the rhabdosphincter. Tissue removal can be carried to the level of the prostatic capsule, identified by its distinct appearance. Apical tissue alongside the verumontanum should be resected carefully after the lateral lobes have been taken down. Variations in lobar anatomy, including an enlarged median lobe or intravesical median lobe or extensive lateral lobe tissue, can make cases challenging. The surgeon should document and monitor the time of resection to minimize absorption of hypotonic irrigant. Arterial branches enter the prostate at the 5 and 7 o'clock positions of the lateral lobes. Extra cautery may be required in these areas. Additionally, incising the bladder neck at the 5 and 7 o'clock positions may prevent postoperative bladder neck contracture. At the completion of the procedure and after hemostasis is felt to be adequate, the resected tissue is irrigated from the bladder lumen and typically sent to pathology for analysis. A large catheter, at least 20 Fr, is placed after the operation, and balloon is inflated with 20–30 cc of fluid. An inflated catheter balloon and catheter traction can tamponade prostatic bleeding. Continuous bladder irrigation with isotonic saline is usually necessary.

Outcomes

Monopolar TURP is the endoscopic procedure for BOO with the longest follow-up data available to guide decision making and counseling for patients about potential benefits and complications. Level I evidence shows the superiority of monopolar TURP compared to watchful waiting [20]. Furthermore, medical therapy has had a significant influence on those men that ultimately undergo surgery for BPH and LUTS. In addition, long term data from both prospective cohort series and randomized, comparative head-to-head surgical trials has consistently reinforced the efficacy and durability of the procedure and established TURP as the gold standard to which other endoscopic BOO procedures are compared. Several prospective cohort series, published just prior to the introduction of bipolar TURP, validate the efficacy and improved complication rates of TURP in the modern era [21]. The outcomes of monopolar TURP are a testament to endoscopic surgical therapy for BPH.

Monopolar TURP Versus Watchful Waiting

The control, non-treatment arms of large trials of men with BPH and LUTS have provided insight into the natural history of the condition and allowed us to define progression of disease [23]. It is generally accepted that as men age, urinary maximum flow decreases and prostate size typically increases, but for some men, treatment is delayed or not recommended [24]. Noninvasive methods of managing BPH include watchful waiting, endorsed in the AUA guidelines as recommended for men with minimal symptoms, and minimal QOL assessments [25].

Randomized trials demonstrate that monopolar TURP for symptoms related to BPH leads to improved quality of life compared to watchful waiting [20]. In the 1990s the Veteran Affairs Cooperative Study Group on Transurethral Resection of the Prostate studied transurethral surgery compared to watchful waiting [26, 27]. In a multicenter, randomized trial of TURP versus watchful waiting for men with moderate symptoms attributed to BPH with a 3-year follow-up, it was found that treatment failures were significantly higher in the watchful waiting group than in those who underwent surgery. Treatment failures were defined as death, urinary retention, post-void residual (PVR) volumes greater than 350 cc, formation of bladder stones, new incontinence, high symptom score, or doubling of serum creatinine. The most common treatment failures included retention, elevated PVRs, or high symptom scores. Additionally, 24 % of those randomized to the watchful waiting group had surgery sometime during the 3-year follow-up period. This was most often due to a defined treatment failure event or the patient request for surgery. Surgery was associated with improved peak flow rate and improved symptoms. This study confirms that post op complication rates are low and that TURP does not often lead to incontinence and/or impotence as previously thought [26].

Monopolar TURP and Medical Therapy

The introduction and evolution of medical therapy has changed the landscape of BPH treatment and the profile of the patient that ultimately undergo a BOO procedure such as monopolar TURP. Because most men present first to their primary care physicians with symptoms, medical therapy – namely, α-blockers and 5α-reductase inhibitors alone or in combination – is typically the first-line treatment for men with BPH [16]. Current analysis of prescribing activity by Izard et al. shows both widespread adoption of α-blockers, a gradual adoption of 5α-reductase inhibitors, and combination treatments by internists and family physicians [28]. Additional medications have FDA approval for LUTS, including anticholinergic medications and more recently PDE-5 inhibitors and β-receptor agonists.

Since the introduction of medications for BPH, the number of patients previously treated with medical therapy prior to undergoing TURP has steadily increased. In a retrospective review, authors estimated that in 2008 at their center, 87 % of patients undergoing TURP had been previously treated with medical therapy for BPH [28]. This is in stark contrast to the 36 % of men in 1998. Thus, the indications for TURP have evolved to include failure of medical management. Furthermore, medical management contributes to a higher proportion of patients undergoing TURP because of urinary retention. This has shown to be a risk factor for poorer outcomes after TURP than if patients were not in urinary retention at the time of surgery. Blanchard et al. found that patients with urinary symptoms refractory to α-blockers had poorer responses to TURP than patients who were α-blocker naïve [29]. In a study by Flanigan et al., patients who underwent immediate TURP showed greater improvement in symptom score and peak flow rate than those who delayed TURP by 5 years [27]. Further considerations include the overall age and health of the patients after years of medical therapy, which may compromise the efficacy of the procedure. Seemingly, the bladder has a relatively poorer functional status after many years of obstruction which may ultimately lead to worse surgical outcomes [28].

Finally, cost and necessity of follow-up should be discussed with patients prior to initiating initial therapy for BPH. Surgery typically incurs higher upfront expenses, but medical management costs can ultimately exceed surgery due to the necessity of lifelong therapy and follow-up. TURP requires minimal follow-up and is therefore also an attractive option for the nonadherent patient.

Monopolar TURP as the Gold Standard

The traditional or monopolar TURP has an exclusive position, with such a wealth of data which validates both the short and long term efficacy of resection of prostate tissue as a treatment for men with BPH and LUTS. Newer, competing technologies retain the surgical goal of creating a TURP-like defect within the prostate to reduce symptoms and improve flow. Furthermore, researchers and industry acknowledge the standard that TURP carries by performing and funding head-to-head randomized trials versus TURP. The perioperative, short term objective outcomes typically measured in these trials include improvements in AUA or IPSS, QoL/bother scores, flow rate (Qmax) improvements, and decreases in PVR. Long term outcomes include reoperation rate for repeat resection due to return of symptoms and relief from medical therapy.

Systematic meta-analyses are published of preoperative measurements versus 1-year postoperative outcomes. Improvements in symptom scores (28 vs. 4) and Qmax flow rate (4 cc/s vs. 28 cc/s) were uniformly present and highly statistically significant. Data for analysis was collected at the

1-year endpoint of randomized controlled trials with a TURP arm, published prior to introduction of bipolar TURP [21, 22].

Long Term Outcomes

Over the years, worldwide advances in technique, equipment, and intraoperative monitoring have decreased short and long term complication rates and confirmed the durable nature of monopolar TURP. A retrospective review of 30 years of TURP performed at a single institution demonstrated that the rate of perioperative UTI has decreased substantially (from 25 % in 1970s to 6 % in 1999) due to the routine use of perioperative antibiotics and treatment of preoperative bacteriuria [30]. The rate of subsequent resections has decreased from 8 % in the 1970s to 1 % in 1999. The rate of postoperative urethral stricture and bladder neck contracture has remained stable over the years at 6 %. Long term follow-up in another prospective cohort trial shows 9 % reoperation rate at 6 years and 16 % reoperation rate at 12 years, with reoperations including either transurethral resection of bladder neck or repeat TURP [31]. Additionally, mean quality of life measures improved postoperatively and remained durable at 6 and 12 years. In this study, no variable had reached or surpassed its baseline postoperative value at 12 years follow-up, which attests to the long term efficacy and sustainability of monopolar TURP.

Competing Technologies

Despite the improvements in complication rates, bipolar-loop TURP and electrovaporization done with isotonic irrigation solution widely contributed to the decrease in surgical volumes of monopolar TURP performed in the United States. Additionally, increasing numbers of laser vaporizations and enucleation techniques have resulted in a decline in the popularity of monopolar TURP [32]. Medicare claims data shows TURP rates have decreased by 5 % per year from 1999 to 2005, while laser procedures increase by 60 % per year. The reported benefits of laser procedures include decreased reliance on inpatient hospital monitoring, shorter catheterization time, and ability to perform surgery on anticoagulated patients.

Validation of the efficacy and potential benefits of newer technologies has traditionally been with trials comparing these procedures to TURP. Further discussion of comparable technologies is detailed in later chapters of this textbook and includes a review of published head-to-head, randomized controlled trials of newer modalities versus monopolar TURP. Intraoperative factors that are considered include operative time and blood loss. Long term outcomes that are measured include reoperation rate and relief from medical therapy. The careful reviewer should clarify whether monopolar, bipolar, or both resection techniques are compared with newer technologies in modern studies.

Complications

While TURP was initially developed as a less invasive alternative to open prostatectomy, it has its own unique set of complications. Classification systems for standardization of complications reporting allows for ease of communication in scientific manuscripts. The Clavien classification system (CCS) is one such tool that is applicable to all surgical procedures and can be adapted for endoscopic procedures such as TURP. Table 3.1 shows the system, which is divided into grades based on escalating intervention [33].

Retrospective studies of patients who underwent monopolar TURP for BPH reported the

Table 3.1 Clavien classification system

I	Any deviation from the normal postoperative course that does not require any intervention, including pharmacological, surgical, or radiological
II	Pharmacological intervention or blood transfusion
III	Surgical, endoscopic, or radiological intervention
IV	Life-threatening complications requiring ICU management
V	Death

complication rates by Clavien grade [34, 35]. As expected, the majority of complications were grade I and II (59.1 % and 29.5 %, respectively), and higher-grade complications (III and IV) were uncommon. Bedside catheter irrigations were included in grade I. Most studies find the mortality rate of TURP to be 2.5 % [36]. The use of this system or one similar can certainly promote ease of communication but may need adjustments or subclassifications based on the type of complications encountered after endoscopic prostate-reducing surgery. For example, a prospective study designed specifically to validate a modified version of the CCS in terms of its applicability to TURP explicitly organized TURP-specific complications. The authors proposed that transient hematuria, acute urinary retention, and UTI be considered grade I; hematuria requiring blood transfusion or UTI with bacteremia grade II; extraperitoneal fluid collection grade III; and finally myocardial infarction, respiratory distress, and TUR syndrome as grade IV. These authors concluded that TURP is a procedure whose complications can mostly be categorized into low Clavien grades [37].

Bleeding

When defining blood loss as a complication, one should take into consideration intraoperative blood loss, transfusion risk during the procedure or hospitalization, bleeding requiring reoperative intervention, and delayed bleeding complications. In several early series which evaluated blood loss for TURP, gland size and resection time were risk factors for postoperative bleeding [38]. The risk of bleeding increased in patients whose prostate size surpassed 45–60 g and in those that had a resection time longer than 90 min. In many studies, this bleeding was specifically noted to be intraoperative bleeding rather than postoperative bleeding [36]. Other studies, however, show that neither the weight of resected tissue nor resection time significantly contributes to postoperative bleeding [39].

One important patient-related factor which increases the risk of bleeding is anticoagulant and antiplatelet medication. This concerns must be balanced with the potential risk of thromboembolic events while withholding therapy when preparing for surgery. Many urologists considered anticoagulation to be an absolute contraindication to performing TURP. As such there have been many small studies which have evaluated the safety of performing TURP on anticoagulation and antiplatelet therapy [40]. Interestingly, these studies showed that patients who were on aspirin preoperatively had increased blood loss postoperatively, regardless of whether it was held prior to the procedure or continued through the procedure, when compared to those who did not have a history of aspirin use. Alternatively, hospital stay and time to catheter removal were significantly shorter in those patients that had held aspirin preoperatively. In accordance with other surgical literature, patients that stopped aspirin preoperatively had significantly higher incidences of cardiovascular and cerebrovascular events [41]. Of note, this was seen only in groups that used aspirin for secondary prevention. These adverse events usually occurred 8–10 days after cessation of therapy.

There have been several studies that investigated the use of 5α-reductase inhibitors in preventing bleeding complications of TURP. Pastore et al. showed that dutasteride use significantly decreased the rate of perioperative bleeding [42]. This group compared hemoglobin concentrations both before and after surgery and found a statistically significant difference for patients on dutasteride therapy than those who were not. Similar results have been seen with finasteride as well [43].

TUR Syndrome

TUR syndrome is the term used to describe the neurological and cardiovascular events caused by absorption of large amounts of hypotonic solution used for irrigant. Symptoms include altered mental status, nausea, vomiting, hypertension, bradycardia, and visual abnormalities. Absorption occurs from the prostatic vessels or periprostatic and perivesical space [44]. It has been found in some studies that up to 20 ml/min of irrigant is absorbed by the patient [45]. There are uncertainties in whether this syndrome is caused by absorptive hyponatremia or ammonium intoxication caused by the conversion of glycine to ammonium in the liver.

Water was traditionally used as an irrigant for monopolar TURP; however, this was found to cause hemolysis of red blood cells. This led to the use of glycine as an irrigant which did not lead to hemolysis but still lead to TUR syndrome in 2–10 % of cases [44]. Other hypotonic solutions, such as mannitol and sorbitol, were not found to be superior in preventing TUR syndrome. Additionally, sorbitol specifically leads to complications of lactic acidosis related to sorbitol metabolism [46]. In an effort to quantify fluid absorption, agents such as ethanol were added to irrigant fluid. However, this maneuver did not translate into decreased rates of TUR syndrome.

An additional safety maneuver aimed at minimizing the incidence of TUR syndrome was to limit the resection time to less than 1 h. However, this did not reliably decrease the incidence of TUR syndrome [44]. Interestingly, instituting a resection time of 1 h remains dogma for many surgeons who perform monopolar TURP. Other reported maneuvers to decrease the risk of TUR syndrome include limiting the height of the irrigation fluid to 60 cm above the patient and using a continuous flow mechanism to limit intravesical pressure during resection. Other, less common tactics include intraprostatic vasopressin injection. Still, even with these measures, the incidence of clinically significant TUR syndrome in the modern age remains around 2 % [47]. Despite much attention paid toward prevention, most studies have found that TUR syndrome can be effectively treated with diuretics and electrolyte monitoring [36].

Mortality and Other Complications

In addition to TUR syndrome, other postoperative complications from TURP include failure to void, need for surgical revision, clot retention, and UTI. A prospective cohort study from Germany published in 2008 showed that rates of these postoperative complications and deaths were also related to the amount of prostatic tissue resected [38]. Rates of death and bleeding which requires transfusion increased when greater than 60 g of tissue was resected, whereas failure to void after surgery and UTI did not seem to be dependent on this factor. Other studies show that age also contributes to the incidence of postoperative complications [36]. Specifically, patients greater than 80 years old had a significantly higher rate of these post op complications, and this did not correlate with preoperative medical comorbidities. Resection time or size of the adenoma was not associated with other complications of TURP. Retrospective analyses of TURP show decreased mortality (2.5 % in 1962 and 0.10 % in 2008) and decreased rates of blood transfusion (3.9 % in 1969 to 2.9 % in 2008) [38].

Long Term Complications

Late complications of TURP include bladder neck contracture (0.3–9.2 %), urethral stricture (2–10 %), persistent urgency (2.2 % as compared to early, transient urge incontinence 30–40 %), stress incontinence (<0.5 %), and the need for retreatment due to regrowth of prostatic adenoma (3–14.5 %) [48–50]. One prospective study highlighted that most bladder neck contractures occurred after resection of glands weighing less than 20 g [51].

Future Considerations

The impetus for development of newer endoscopic modalities to treat BPH came from the need to improve upon the complications of monopolar TURP while not sacrificing efficacy of the procedure. Certainly in the early developments of monopolar TURP, a great improvement was seen as a result of the evolution and refinement of general endoscopic equipment. Lighting improved with the fiber optic cord [52]. The camera eased urologic training as both resident trainee and mentor shared the same view [53]. After this initial time period, the complication rates for monopolar TURP appeared to plateau.

The movement toward bipolar energy sources aimed to decrease this risk even further. While some studies claim that bipolar TURP eliminates the risk of TUR syndrome, others show that it is solely dilutional hyponatremia that is eliminated [47]. Bipolar TURP is typically associated with less total fluid absorption than monopolar TURP considering the same resection time. Even with bipolar TURP, large fluid shifts can lead to significant cardiovascular and pulmonary events, especially if a patient has a preoperative health factors which predispose them to such events. Some groups theorize that the decrease in fluid absorption may be a result of a decrease in capsular perforation rather than the use of isotonic irrigant [54]. Subsequently, typical risk factors for TUR syndrome such as increased length of surgery did not negatively impact the rate of TUR syndrome in bipolar TURP cohorts [55].

Laser TURP has several characteristics that make it appealing to the urologic surgeon, including shallow learning curve and less observed bleeding complications compared to monopolar TURP, as discussed above. Studies show that short term complication rates can favor laser therapies. One randomized controlled trial showed that catheter time, length of hospital stay, adverse events and complications, and overall cost was less for laser vaporization when compared to traditional TURP. However, follow-up was only 12 months which is significantly shorter than studies with long term follow-up for TURP [56].

Long term complications such as bladder neck contracture and reoperation rates will need to be closely monitored for competing procedures. Unlike TURP, data is lacking from high-quality randomized controlled trials to examine long term efficacy and complications for many techniques being used in the modern era of surgical therapy for BPH.

References

1. Caulk JR, Wiseman JL. Transurethral resection of prostatic obstructions. Can Med Assoc J. 1932; 27(1):23–8.
2. Thompson GJ. Transurethral prostatic resection: a general estimate and a special study of twenty physician-patients. Cal West Med. 1934;40(1):1–6.
3. Kretschmer HL. Transurethral resection. Ann Surg. 1936;104(5):917–33.
4. Young HH. A new procedure (punch operation) for small prostatic bars and contracture of the prostatic orifice. JAMA. 1913;60(4):253–7.
5. Beer E. Removal of neoplasms of the urinary bladder. A new method, employing high frequency (oudin) currents through a catheterizing cystoscope. JAMA. 1910;54(22):1768–9.
6. Stern M. Resection of obstructions at the vesical orifice. New instruments and a new method. JAMA. 1926;87(21):1726–30.
7. McCarthy J. A new apparatus for endoscopic plastic surgery of the prostate, diathermia and excision of vesical growths. J Urol. 1931;26:695–6.
8. Serretta V, Morgia G, Fondacaro L, Curto G, Lo bianco A, Pirritano D, et al. Open prostatectomy for benign prostatic enlargement in southern Europe in the late 1990s: a contemporary series of 1800 interventions. Urology. 2002;60(4):623–7.
9. Ou R, You M, Tang P, Chen H, Deng X, Xie K. A randomized trial of transvesical prostatectomy versus transurethral resection of the prostate for prostate greater than 80 mL. Urology. 2010;76(4):958–61.
10. Wilson JR, Urwin GH, Stower MJ. The changing practice of transurethral prostatectomy: a comparison of cases performed in 1990 and 2000. Ann R Coll Surg Engl. 2004;86(6):428–31.
11. Yu X, Elliott SP, Wilt TJ, McBean AM. Practice patterns in benign prostatic hyperplasia surgical therapy: the dramatic increase in minimally invasive technologies. J Urol. 2008;180(1):241–5.
12. Malaeb BS, Yu X, McBean AM, Elliott SP. National trends in surgical therapy for benign prostatic hyperplasia in the United States 2000–2008. Urology. 2012; 79(5):1111–6.
13. Schroeck FR, Hollingsworth JM, Kaufman SR, Hollenbeck BK, Wei JT. Population based trends in the surgical treatment of benign prostatic hyperplasia. J Urol. 2012;188(5):1837–41.
14. Lowrance WT, Southwick A, Maschino AC, Sandhu JS. Contemporary practice patterns of endoscopic surgical management for benign prostatic hyperplasia among urologist in the United States. J Urol. 2013; 189(5):1811–6.
15. Sandhu JS, Jaffe WI, Chung DE, Kaplan SA, Te AE. Decreasing electrosurgical transurethral resection of the prostate surgical volume during graduate medical education training is associated with increased surgical adverse events. J Urol. 2010; 183(4):1515–9.
16. Cury J, Coelho RF, Bruschini H, Srougi M. Is the ability to perform transurethral resection of the prostate influenced by the surgeon's previous experience? Clinics. 2008;63(3):315–20.
17. Nesbit RM, Flocks RH. Transurethral prostatectomy. Ann Arbor: Thomas; 1943.
18. Mauermayer W, Kirschner M, Zenker R. Transurethrale operationen. Berlin: Springer; 1981.
19. Hartung R, May F. Die transurethraleElektroresektion der Prostata. Akt Urol. 2002;33:469–82.

20. Barry MJ, Mulley Jr AG, Fowler FJ, Wennberg JW. Watchful waiting vs immediate transurethral resection for symptomatic prostatism. The importance of patients' preferences. JAMA. 1988;259(20):3010–7.
21. Lourenco T, Pickard R, Vale L, Grant A, Fraser C, MacLennan G, et al. Alternative approaches to endoscopic ablation for benign enlargement of the prostate: systematic review of randomised controlled trials. BMJ. 2008;337:a449.
22. Lourenco T, Pickard R, Vale L, Grant A, Fraser C, MacLennan G, et al. Minimally invasive treatments for benign prostatic enlargement: systematic review of randomized controlled trials. BMJ. 2008;337:a1662.
23. McConnell JD, Roehrborn CG, Bautista OM, Andriole Jr GL, Dixon CM, Kusek JW, et al. The long-term effect of doxazosin, finasteride, and combination therapy on the clinical progression of benign prostatic hyperplasia. N Engl J Med. 2003; 349(25):2387–98.
24. Kirby RS. The natural history of benign prostatic hyperplasia: what have we learned in the last decade? Urology. 2000;56(5 Suppl 1):3–6.
25. McVary KT, Roehrborn C, Avins AL, Barry MJ, Bruskewitz RC, Donnell RF, et al. American urological association guideline: management of benign prostatic hyperplasia. J Urol. 2011;185(5):1793–803.
26. Wasson JH, Reda DJ, Bruskewitz RC, Elinson J, Keller AM, Henderson WG. A comparison of transurethral surgery with watchful waiting for moderate symptoms of benign prostatic hyperplasia. The Veterans Affairs Cooperative Study Group on transurethral resection of the prostate. N Engl J Med. 1995;332(2):75–9.
27. Flanigan RC, Reda DJ, Wasson JH, Anderson RJ, Abdellatif M, Bruskewitz RC. 5-year outcome of surgical resection and watchful waiting for men with moderately symptomatic benign prostatic hyperplasia: a Department of Veterans Affairs Cooperative Study. J Urol. 1988;160(1):12–6.
28. Izard J, Nickel JC. Impact of medical therapy on transurethral resection of the prostate: two decades of change. BJU Int. 2011;108(1):89–93.
29. Blanchard K, Hananel A, Rutchik S, Sullivan J. Transurethral resection of the prostate: failure patterns and surgical outcomes in patients with symptoms refractory to alpha-antagonists. South Med J. 2000;93(12):1192–6.
30. Lim KB, Wong MY, Foo KT. Transurethral resection of prostate (TURP) through the decades-a comparison of results over the last thirty years in a single institution in Asia. Ann Acad Med Singapore. 2004;33(6):775–9.
31. Mishriki SF, Grimsley SJ, Nabi G, Martindale A, Cohen NP. Improved quality of life and enhanced satisfaction after TURP: prospective 12-year follow-up study. Urology. 2008;72(2):322–6.
32. Sandhu JS, Ng CK, Gonzalez RR, Kaplan SA, Te AE. Photoselective laser vaporization prostatectomy in men receiving anticoagulants. J Endourol. 2005; 19(10):1196–8.
33. Dindo D, Demartines N, Clavien PA. Classification of surgical complications: a new proposal with evaluation in a cohort of 6336 patients and results of a survey. Ann Surg. 2004;240(2):205–13.
34. Mamoulakis C, Efthimiou I, Kazoulis S, Christoulakis I, Sofras F. The modified Clavien classification system: a standardized platform for reporting complications in transurethral resection of the prostate. World J Urol. 2011;29(2):205–10.
35. Mitropoulos D, Artibani W, Graefen M, Remzi M, Roupret M, Truss M, et al. Reporting and grading of complications after urologic surgical procedures: an ad hoc EAU guidelines panel assessment and recommendations. Eur Urol. 2012;61(2):341–9.
36. Mebust WK, Holtgrewe HL, Cockett AT, Peters PC. Transurethral prostatectomy: immediate and postoperative complications. A cooperative study of 13 participating institutions evaluating 3,885 patients. J Urol. 2002;167(2 Pt 2):999–1003.
37. DeNunzio C, Lombardo R, Autorino R, Cicione A, Cindolo L, Damiano R, et al. Contemporary monopolar and bipolar transurethral resection of the prostate: prospective assessment of complications using the Clavien system. Int Urol Nephrol. 2013;45(4):951–9.
38. Reich O, Gratzke C, Bachmann A, Seitz M, Schlenker B, Hermanek P, et al. Morbidity, mortality and early outcome of transurethral resection of the prostate: a prospective multicenter evaluation of 10,654 patients. J Urol. 2008;180(1):246–9.
39. Shrestha BM, Prasopshanti K, Matanhelia SS, Peeling WB. Blood loss during and after transurethral resection of prostate: a prospective study. Kathmandu Univ Med J. 2008;6(23):329–34.
40. Wenders M, Wenzel O, Nitzke T, Popken G. Perioperative platelet inhibition in transurethral interventions: TURP/TURB. Int Braz J Urol. 2012; 38((5):606–10.
41. Taylor K, Filgate R, Guo DY, Macneil F. A retrospective study to assess the morbidity associated with transurethral prostatectomy in patients on antiplatelet or anticoagulant drugs. BJU Int. 2011;108 Suppl 2: 45–50.
42. Pastore AL, Mariani S, Barese F, Palleschi G, Valentni AM, Pacini L, et al. Transurethral resection of prostate and the role of pharmacological treatment with dutasteride in decreasing surgical blood loss. J Endourol. 2013;27(1):68–70.
43. Donohue JF, Sharma H, Abraham R, Natalwala S, Thomas DR, Foster MC. Transurethral prostate resection and bleeding: a randomized, placebo controlled trial of role of finasteride for decreasing operative blood loss. J Urol. 2002;168(5):2024–6.
44. Collins JW, Macdermott S, Bradbrook RA, Keeley Jr FX, Timoney AG. Is using ethanol-glycine irrigating fluid monitoring and "good surgical practice" enough to prevent harmful absorption during transurethral resection of the prostate? BJU Int. 2006;97(6): 1247–51.

45. Fitzpatrick JM. Minimally invasive and endoscopic management of benign prostatic hyperplasia. In: Wein AJ, editor. Campbell-Walsh urology. Philadelphia: Elsevier Saunders; 2011. p. 2684.
46. Trepanier CA, Lessard MR, Brochu J, Turcotte G. Another feature of TURP syndrome: hyperglycaemia and lactic acidosis caused by massive absorption of sorbitol. Br J Anaesth. 2001;87(2):316–9.
47. Issa MM, Young MR, Bullock AR, Bouet R, Petros JA. Dilutional hyponatremia of TURP syndrome: a historical event in the 21st century. Urology. 2004; 64(2):298–301.
48. Ahyai SA, Gilling P, Kaplan SA, Kuntz RM, Madersbacher S, Montorsi F, et al. Meta-analysis of functional outcomes and complications following transurethral procedures for lower urinary tract symptoms resulting from benign prostatic enlargement. Eur Urol. 2010;58(3):348–97.
49. Kallenberg F, Hossack TA, Woo HH. Long-term followup after electrocautery transurethral resection of the prostate for benign prostatic hyperplasia. Adv Urol. 2011;2011:359478.
50. Rassweiler J, Teber D, Kuntz R, Hofmann R. Complications of transurethral resection of the prostate (TURP)-incidence, management, and prevention. Eur Urol. 2006;505:969–79.
51. Lee YH, Chiu AW, Huang JK. Comprehensive study of bladder neck contracture after transurethral resection of prostate. Urology. 2005;65(3):498–503.
52. Wallace FJ. Fiber optic endoscopy. J Urol. 1963; 90:324–34.
53. Nouira Y, Kbaier I, Attyaoui F, Horchani A. How did the endoscopic video camera change our practice in transurethral resection of the prostate? A retrospective study of 200 cases. J Endourol. 2002;16(10):763–5.
54. Chen Q, Zhang L, Fan QL, Zhou J, Peng YB, Wang Z. Bipolar transurethral resection in saline vs transitional monopolar resection of the prostate: results of a randomized trial with a 2 year follow up. BJU Int. 2010;106(9):1339–43.
55. Mamoulakis C, Schulze M, Skolarikos A, Alivizatos G, Scarpa RM, Rasweiler JJ, et al. Midterm results from an international multicentre randomised controlled trial comparing bipolar with monopolar transurethral resection of the prostate. Eur Urol. 2013; 64(4):667–76.
56. Douchier-Hayes DM, Van Appledorn S, Bugeja P, Crowe H, Challacombe B, Costello AJ. A randomized trial of photoselective vaporization of the prostate using the 80-W potassium-titanyl-phosphate laser vs transurethral prostatectomy, with a 1-year follow up. BJU Int. 2010;105(7):964–9.

4 Bipolar TURP

Rajeev Kumar and Jaspreet S. Sandhu

Introduction

Bipolar transurethral resection of the prostate (BiTURP) is a technical modification of the standard monopolar TURP. The procedure aims at endoscopic removal of the enlarged prostate in order to treat lower urinary tract symptoms (LUTS) secondary to benign prostatic hyperplasia (BPH). Monopolar TURP is widely considered the reference standard surgical treatment for BPH [1]. However, certain limitations of monopolar TURP have resulted in a constant attempt at finding newer treatment modalities which would provide similar efficacy without the limitations. The most important problem is the need for a non-isotonic irrigant fluid during the resection. Absorption-associated problems such as dilutional hyponatremia and the "TUR syndrome" are directly proportional to the resection time. Minimizing resection time limits the size of gland that can be treated. The other complications of monopolar TURP that need to be addressed are bleeding and management of patients on anticoagulants [2].

R. Kumar, M.Ch.
Department of Urology, All India Institute of Medical Science, New Delhi, India

J.S. Sandhu, M.D. (✉)
Department of Surgery/Urology,
Memorial Sloan-Kettering Cancer Center,
1275 York Avenue, New York, NY 10065, USA
e-mail: sandhuj@mskcc.org

Monopolar TURP is based on the principle of an electrocautery where current generated at the active electrode (the resection loop) travels through the tissue of contact (the prostate adenoma) and out through a neutralizing earth plate kept in contact with the patient. The high current generated at the point of contact cuts the tissue as the loop is moved along it. Fluid is required to keep the vision clear and dissipate the heat generated. This fluid must not be electrically conductive as it would then dissipate the current generated by the active electrode and decrease its cutting effect on the tissue. However, all such fluids (glycine, dextrose, sterile water) are hypotonic. Resection of tissue opens up vascular channels, and the irrigant fluid can be absorbed up to a rate of approximately 30 mL per minute. Resection times of around 1 h mean that almost 2 L of hypotonic fluid can be absorbed and can result in dilutional hyponatremia, particularly in the elderly BPH population which may have limited renal and cardiac reserve. Newer modalities for the surgical management of BPH aim to minimize these risks, including bipolar TURP, laser resection, vaporization, and thermotherapy.

Bipolar Technology

The development of a bipolar loop allows the use of isotonic saline during surgery. It is a design modification where the loop or the resectoscope contains both the active and return electrodes in

B. Chughtai et al. (eds.), *Treatment of Benign Prostatic Hyperplasia: Modern Alternative to Transurethral Resection of the Prostate*, DOI 10.1007/978-1-4939-1587-3_4,

close proximity to each other. The current generated has to pass through only a short distance between these electrodes, and this allows the use of saline as an irrigant. The short distance for bipolar circuits results in lower voltages being required to generate current, similar to a monopolar electrode. The lower voltages result in decreased tissue damage and charring. Theoretically, this has two advantages. First, the resection is sharper and cleaner, and, second, there is less damage to underlying vessels which results in lower immediate and later bleeding. Additional potential advantages are lower postoperative irritative symptoms due to less tissue charring and reduced spread of current and damage to adjacent tissue including the sphincter, urethra, and cavernosal nerves.

Bipolar technology evolved from prostatic vaporization techniques based on the monopolar platform [3]. These devices achieved higher currents and used broad electrodes to vaporize tissue at the cut edge of the resection. Vaporization differs from resection in that former does not provide any tissue for histopathology and is generally slower. It also results in postoperative sloughing of necrotic tissue. The more common, current use of bipolar TURP is to perform a resection similar to the standard TURP whereby prostatic adenoma is resected as chips and immediately evacuated.

Performance of BiTURP requires special surgical equipment. BiTURP relies on the creation of a "plasma corona" at the electrode, resulting in roughly 20 % of the tissue being vaporized, with the rest resected as prostate chips [4]. The electrocautery generator has to be capable of providing bipolar current for BiTURP through specialized circuits that are different from those used in traditional surgical bipolar devices. For older electrocautery generators, an external adapter allowed this conversion, while newer generators provide this as a standard feature. Current generators modulate voltage based on tissue impedance and therefore keep the current constant, allowing a smooth cut irrespective of the underlying tissue. The typical settings for the pure cutting current are high power (120–280 W), while settings for coagulation use lower power (60–120 W). All devices use a continuous flow resectoscope, usually of 26Fr diameter. The loop/resectoscope combination is designed to allow connection of both the active and return electrodes.

One of the first BiTURP devices, PK (PlasmaKinetic) system, was marketed by Gyrus/ACMI. This device has a dedicated current generator, connected to a proprietary surgical loop mounted on a resectoscope working element. Depending on the manufacturer, working elements in the resectoscope may differ. Like the PK system, the TURiS system by Olympus Corporation (Tokyo, Japan) is paired to a specific generator.

Some manufacturers (Karl Storz, Tuttlingen, Germany; Richard Wolf) have combination loop/resectoscopes which can be connected to any electrocautery generator using cables; in other words, the generator and resectoscopes are not necessarily paired.

Another difference between these platforms is the location of the return electrode. Proximity between the active and return electrodes allows higher current generation over a smaller voltage. In the PK system, the return electrode is on the loop itself and is separated from the cutting element by a few millimeters of insulation. For the Storz system, the return electrode is shaped like a loop and is placed opposite the active loop, while for the Wolf and TURiS systems, the inner sheath of the resectoscope works as the return electrode. Each manufacturer now has loops and electrodes of different thicknesses and shapes to allow resection, vaporization, and coagulation. Figures 4.1 and 4.2 show examples of Gyrus electrodes and the PK generator.

Surgical Technique

The basic difference in the surgical technique for BiTURP, as compared to a monopolar TURP, is the ability to operate for longer times without worrying about dilutional hyponatremia. All BiTURP devices use continuous irrigation, allowing uninterrupted surgery. The cutting electrode loop develops a "plasma corona" prior to the start of resection (Fig. 4.3). During resection, there may be increased impedance within the loop due to

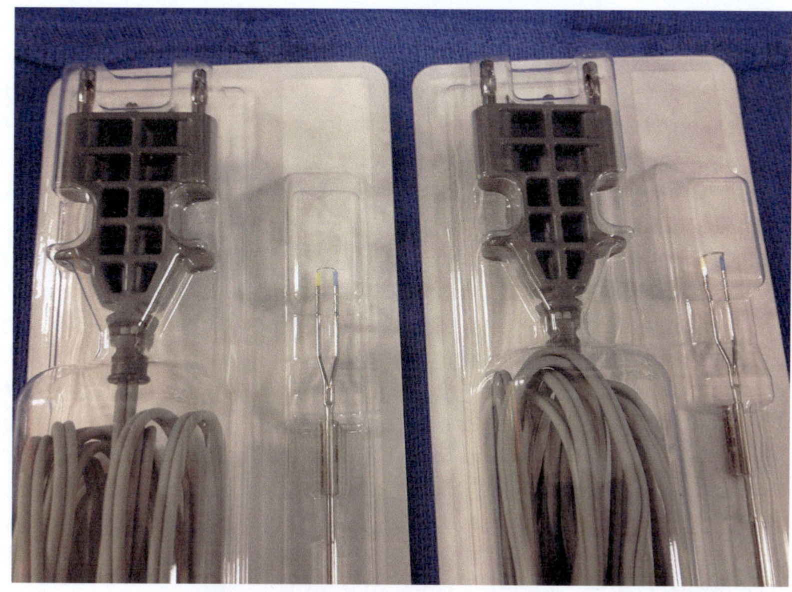

Fig. 4.1 The Gyrus PK SuperSect loop

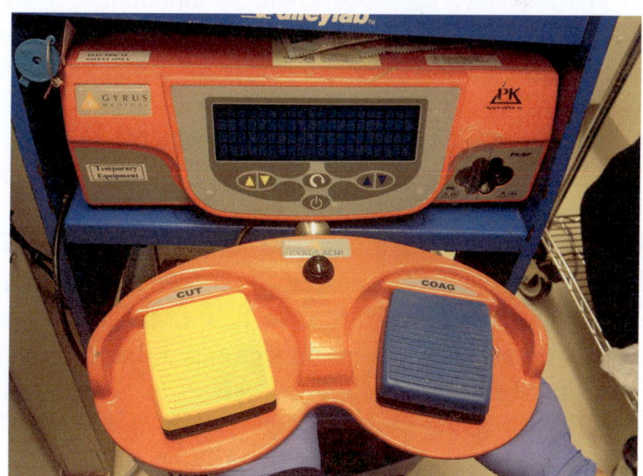

Fig. 4.2 Gyrus PK generator

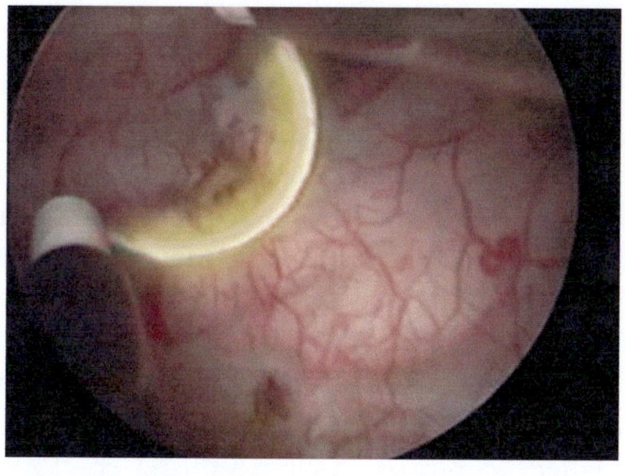

Fig. 4.3 The plasma corona firing in the bladder

accumulation of charred tissue on its surface. Activating the loop in the bladder without being in contact with any tissue often dislodges this accumulated tissue without the need to remove the loop and physically clean it. Coagulation does not rely on the formation of a corona and can be performed as for monopolar TURP.

Efficacy

In 2001, Botto et al. [5] published a pilot study of 42 patients who underwent electrovaporization of the prostate using saline bipolar electrocautery with the Gyrus PK system between 1998 and 1999. This was one of the first reports of BiTURP. Their 3-month follow-up data showed no significant postoperative bleeding with two strictures. The mean catheterization time was 1.4 days, and length of stay was 2.2 days. The IPSS decreased from 16 at baseline to 9, and peak flow rate increased from 7.9 to 19.7 mL/s.

The Gyrus PK system continued to be popular as one of the first devices, and Yang et al. [6] performed a randomized study comparing it with conventional monopolar TURP. Fifty-eight patients underwent BiTURP and 59 monopolar TURP. At 3 months, both groups reported significant improvements in IPSS (BiTURP: 10.8 from 20.9 at baseline; TURP: 11.1 from 21.6 at baseline) and peak flow rates (BiTURP: 17.1 mL/s from 10.4 mL/s; TURP: 14.8 mL/s from 10.9 mL/s). BiTURP results were equivalent to monopolar TURP with similar complications in the two groups except one TUR syndrome in the monopolar TURP group.

De Sio et al. [7] randomized 70 patients to Gyrus PK BiTURP or monopolar TURP groups and reported 12-month outcomes. They noted shorter operative and catheter times in the BiTURP group with similar 1-year outcome parameters including IPSS, peak flow rates, and residual urine. There were no significant differences in adverse events.

Addressing the issue of large glands where fluid absorption and prolonged resection times are a particular concern with monopolar TURP, Bhansali et al. [8] performed a randomized trial of 70 patients with prostate sizes greater than 60 g comparing Gyrus PK BiTURP to monopolar TURP. They reported significantly greater blood loss and larger changes in serum sodium in the monopolar group with similar length of stay and functional outcomes, suggesting that BiTURP may be safer in large volume prostates. Similarly, Seckiner et al. [9] reported decreased serum sodium in patients undergoing monopolar TURP including two patients exhibiting mild dilutional hyponatremia, unlike those in the BiTURP group.

The safety of BiTURP with the Gyrus PK system was further supported in a large study of 401 patients [10]. The authors reported no intraoperative complications, significant improvement in IPSS, and peak flow rates that were consistent at 3-year of follow-up.

Fagerstrom et al. [11] evaluated the newer Olympus TURisBiTURP system in a randomized trial. They reported on 185 patients and found lower blood loss in the BiTURP group. In another study on the same device, Ho et al. [12] compared 52 patients undergoing monopolar TURP with 48 undergoing BiTURP in a prospective randomized study. Similar to the findings with Gyrus PK studies, they reported significantly greater decrease in serum sodium in the monopolar group with two cases of clinically significant dilutional hyponatremia. The improvement in functional outcomes with IPSS and peak flow was similar in both groups.

In one of the larger prospective trials with the Olympus TURis device, Michielsen et al. [13] compared monopolar TURP in 120 patients with BiTURP in 118. There was no difference is the resected tissue weight, but longer operating time was observed for BiTURP. As in previous studies, the decrease in serum sodium was significantly greater for the monopolar TURP group with one case of TUR syndrome.

At least two systematic reviews and meta-analyses have also addressed the issue of efficacy with bipolar TURP. In 2009, Mamoulokis et al. [14] evaluated 16 randomized controlled trials including 1406 patients in a meta-analysis. Although the trial quality was low, the authors reported equivalent efficacy of both procedures at 12 months. They also reported significantly larger decrease in serum sodium and a significantly higher rate of TUR syndrome in patients undergoing monopolar TURP such that treating 50 patients with BiTURP resulted in one fewer case of TUR syndrome and treating 20 patients resulted in one fewer clot retention. There was no increase in urethral or other complications with BiTURP, and the data was more robust for Gyrus PlasmaKinetic than for TURiS.

More recently, Lee et al. [15] reported a meta-analysis of transurethral procedures for BPH and included 36 out of 784 randomized controlled trials identified for their high level of evidence.

BiTURP showed a significantly greater reduction in IPSS scores, improvement in maximum flow rates, decline in residual volume, and better satisfaction than monopolar TURP. This was associated with lower complications and lower catheterization time.

Morbidity/Complications

The series reviewed in the previous section suggest that BiTURP maybe safer than monopolar TURP in terms of serum sodium decrease and dilutional hyponatremia. This is consistent with the fact that BiTURP utilizes normal saline for irrigation, and fluid absorption should not cause hyponatremia. Some of these studies also showed lower blood loss, and the meta-analysis suggested significantly lower incidence of clot retention.

There has been a concern about higher incidence of urethral strictures with BiTURP, fueled by two studies that reported higher stricture rates in the BiTURP group [12, 16]. The use of continuous flow resectoscopes, which have larger outer diameters than single-flow scopes, was considered a factor; however, Michielsen et al. [13] who actually used smaller scopes for BiTURP reported that their longer operating times with the bipolar device may be the cause for strictures. The Olympus TURisBiTURP uses the resectoscope inner sheath as the return electrode, and "current leakage" from this sheath has been thought of as a potential problem [12]. However, in this report, the authors could not actually demonstrate any current leak. The high currents used in BiTURP (180–200 W) also generate fear of injuries and complications. This high current is used only in the initial few milliseconds of activation to allow formation of the plasma corona where after the devices automatically decrease the current generated.

The pooled analyses have not shown any increase in these complications [14, 15]. They, in fact, show comparable stricture and bladder neck contracture rates with BiTURP and monopolar TURP. These analyses also address the issue of blood loss. Both showed no worse outcomes with BiTURP, and one analyses actually showed lower clot retention rates with BiTURP. These findings are significant in light of the fact that there is a perception of increased intraoperative and postoperative blood loss with BiTURP. This partly stems from the visibly sharper cuts with the BiTURP device. While some studies have shown BiTURP to have a smaller zone of coagulation than monopolar TURP [17], others have reported contrary findings [18, 19].

Cost

The Urologic Diseases in America project estimated that over $1 billion was spent in the United States for the management of BPH, not including costs of medicines [3]. BiTURP requires newer generators and resection loops. This may increase the cost of surgery, particularly for institutions that already have a monopolar TURP setup. However, potentially shorter hospital stay and fewer postoperative complications may actually lower the costs. Further, the surgical technique does not require retraining. This is unlike laser prostatectomy, which has a long learning curve and associated costs. BiTURP may be an advantage in resident training due to the use of saline, allowing longer operating time without the risk of dilutional hyponatremia. Issa et al. [4] reported that despite an average operating time of 2 h and 22 min with BiTURP performed by residents under supervision, there was no significant hyponatremia in their patients. Similarly, Gilleran et al. [20] reported a series of 21 men who underwent Gyrus PK TURP in an academic setting. Even though the prostate size was small, the median resection time was 65 min. However, there was no significant decline in serum sodium, and no patient needed blood transfusions, leading the authors to state that BiTURP is a safe modality for resident education.

The number of prostate surgeries seems to be decreasing every year [21, 22]. The availability of multiple modalities of treatment will likely decrease the number of each procedure seen, assisted or performed by each resident. BiTURP, due to a commonality of technique with monopolar TURP, may allow proficiency in a single technique to address most clinical situations.

Conclusion

BiTURP seems to be a natural evolution of the monopolar TURP. It utilizes the same surgical technique with a set of equipment that may be safer for the patient. There is no new technique to learn, no increase in complications, and negligible increase, if any, in costs. The technology is still in evolution but already seems to be at least as good as the gold standard TURP.

References

1. Reich O, Gratzke C, Stief CG. Techniques and long-term results of surgical procedures for BPH. Eur Urol. 2006;49:970–8.
2. Reich O, Gratzke C, Bachmann A, Seitz M, Schlenker B, Hermanek P, Lack N, Stief CG. Urology Section of the Bavarian Working Group for Quality Assurance. Morbidity, mortality and early outcome of transurethral resection of the prostate: a prospective multicenter evaluation of 10,654 patients. J Urol. 2008;180:246–9.
3. Poulakis V, Dahm P, Witzsch U, et al. Transurethral electrovaporization vs transurethral resection for symptomatic prostatic obstruction: a meta-analysis. BJU Int. 2004;94:89–95.
4. Issa MM, Young MR, Bullock AR, et al. Dilutional hyponatremia of TURP syndrome: a historical event in the 21st century. Urology. 2004;64:298–301.
5. Botto H, Lebret T, Barré P, et al. Electrovaporization of the prostate with the Gyrus device. Eur Urol. 2001;15:313–6.
6. Yang S, Lin WC, Chang HK, et al. Gyrus plasmasect: is it better than monopolar transurethral resection of prostate? Urol Int. 2004;73:258–61.
7. de Sio M, Autorino R, Quarto G, et al. Gyrus bipolar versus standard monopolar transurethral resection of the prostate: a randomized prospective trial. Urology. 2006;67:69–72.
8. Bhansali M, Patankar S, Dobhada S, Khaladkar S. Management of large (>60 g) prostate gland: PlasmaKinetic Superpulse (bipolar) versus conventional (monopolar) transurethral resection of the prostate. J Endourol. 2009;23:141–5.
9. Seckiner I, Yesilli C, Akduman B, et al. A prospective randomized study for comparing bipolar plasmakinetic resection of the prostate with standard TURP. Urol Int. 2006;76:139–43.
10. Martis G, Cardi A, Massimo D, et al. Transurethral resection of prostate: technical progress and clinical experience using the bipolar Gyrus plasmakinetic tissue management system. Surg Endosc. 2008;22:2078–83.
11. Fagerström T, Nyman CR, Hahn RG. Bipolar transurethral resection of the prostate causes less bleeding than the monopolar technique: a single-centre randomized trial of 202 patients. BJU Int. 2010;105:1560–4.
12. Ho HS, Yip SK, Lim KB, et al. A prospective randomized study comparing monopolar and bipolar transurethral resection of prostate using transurethral resection in saline (TURIS) system. Eur Urol. 2007;52:517–22.
13. Michielsen DP, Debacker T, De Boe V, et al. Bipolar transurethral resection in saline – an alternative surgical treatment for bladder outlet obstruction? J Urol. 2007;178:2035–9.
14. Mamoulakis C, Ubbink DT, de la Rosette JJMCH. Bipolar versus monopolar transurethral resection of the prostate: a systematic review and meta-analysis of randomized controlled trials. Eur Urol. 2009;56:798–809.
15. Lee SW, Choi JB, Lee KS, Kim TH, Son H, Jung TY, Oh SJ, Jeong HJ, Bae JH, Lee YS, Kim JC. Transurethral procedures for lower urinary tract symptoms resulting from benign prostatic enlargement: a quality and meta-analysis. Int Neurourol J. 2013;17(2):59–66.
16. Tefekli A, Muslumanoglu AY, Baykal M, et al. A hybrid technique using bipolar energy in transurethral prostate surgery: a prospective, randomized comparison. J Urol. 2005;174:1339–43.
17. Wendt-Nordahl G, Häcker A, Fastenmeier K, et al. New bipolar resection device for transurethral resection of the prostate: first ex-vivo and in-vivo evaluation. J Endourol. 2005;19:1203–9.
18. Ko R, Tan AH, Chew BH, et al. Comparison of the thermal and histopathological effects of bipolar and monopolar electrosurgical resection of the prostate in a canine model. BJU Int. 2010;105:1314–7.
19. Huang X, Wang XH, Qu LJ, et al. Bipolar versus monopolar transurethral resection of prostate: pathologic study in canines. Urology. 2007;70:180–4.
20. Gilleran JP, Thaly RK, Chernoff AM. Rapid communication: bipolar PlasmaKinetic transurethral resection of the prostate: reliable training vehicle for today's urology residents. J Endourol. 2006;20:683–7.
21. Wei JT, Calhoun EA, Jacobsen SJ. Benign prostatic hyperplasia. In: Litwin MS, Saigal CS, editors. Urologic diseases in America. US Department of Health and Human Services, Public Health Service, National Institutes of Health, National Institute of Diabetes and Digestive and Kidney Diseases, NIH publication no. 07–5512. Washington, DC: US Government Publishing Office; 2007. p. 43–70.
22. Sandhu JS, Jaffe WI, Chung DE, et al. Decreasing electrosurgical transurethral resection of the prostate surgical volume during graduate medical education training is associated with increased surgical adverse events. J Urol. 2010;183:1515–9.

Plasma Kinetic Vaporization

5

Bilal Chughtai and Steven A. Kaplan

Introduction

Plasma kinetic button vaporization of the prostate (bPKVP) is an endoscopic technique that is an alternative to the traditional monopolar TURP (mTURP). Plasma kinetic technology uses radiofrequency energy to create an ionized plasma corona. This is accomplished via an axipolar electrode and electroconductive solution such as normal saline [1]. This axipolar vapo-resection electrode is in the shape of a mushroom or the so-called "button." It utilizes a radiofrequency range of 320–450 kHz, a voltage range of 350–450 V, and has a 200 W capability [1, 2]. The current passing over the ball-shaped button creates a plasma corona that vaporizes tissue while achieving hemostasis [3]. This high-energy output is transmitted locally thus vaporizing tissue in its immediate vicinity, with thermal injury extending <1 mm into deeper tissues. Since the axipolar electrode functions as both the working element and the return electrode, the risk of accidental skin burns is eliminated. This also provides decreased interference with cardiac pacemakers and decreased risk of stray currents causing an obturator reflex. Since normal saline is used as irrigation, it is hypothesized to prevent the development of TUR syndrome [1–4]. We discuss the outcomes and complications of the bPKVP system in men with lower urinary tract symptoms secondary to benign prostatic hyperplasia (BPH).

B. Chughtai, M.D. (✉) • S.A. Kaplan, M.D.
Department of Urology, Weill Cornell Medical College, 425 East 61st Street, 12th floor, New York, NY 10065, USA
e-mail: bic9008@med.cornell.edu; kaplans@med.cornell.edu

Early Experience with Monopolar Electrovaporization Technology

Prior to the introduction of bipolar technology, a similar alternative to mTURP using the PK system was electrovaporization of the prostate. Transurethral electrovaporization of the prostate (TEVP) employs high-energy cutting currents to resect the prostate while maintaining hemostasis and field visibility [5]. Similar to bPKVP, it decreases damage to surrounding tissue since the electrovaporization process is localized to tissue in close proximity to the electrode [6]. Altogether, it has been shown to have similar efficacy and results to mTURP in multiple large trials.

Kaplan et al. (1996) conducted an early study on TEVP on 114 patients with follow-up of 18 months [5]. At 18 months, there was a reduction of both AUA symptom score (−11.3, $p<0.01$) and peak urinary flow (Qmax, +9.6 mL/s, $p<0.001$) from preoperative values. PVR, measured at 0 and 12 months, showed no significant change (64.5 vs. 33.6 mL, $p=0.07$). Postoperative complications of TUR syndrome and significant blood loss requiring transfusion were not seen in

B. Chughtai et al. (eds.), *Treatment of Benign Prostatic Hyperplasia: Modern Alternative to Transurethral Resection of the Prostate*, DOI 10.1007/978-1-4939-1587-3_5,

any patients. The mean catheterization was 10.4 h, mean hospital stay of 0.9 days, and mean operative time of 47.8 min [5].

Kaplan et al. performed a prospective randomized trial comparing TEVP tomTURP in 64 men with lower urinary tract symptoms (LUTS) with follow-up of 12 months [6]. AUA symptom score at 12 months showed greater reduction in the TEVP group over the mTURP group (12.8 vs. 12.2, $p<0.02$). However, Qmax had better results in the mTURP group compared to TEVP (11.3 vs. 9.7 mL/s, $p<0.03$). There was no statistically significant difference in the change of PVR between the two groups (43.6 mL for TEVP vs. 34.2 mL for mTURP, $p=0.11$). Both catheterization time and total hospitalization time were less for the TEVP group compared to mTURP (catheterization: 12.9 vs. 67.4 h, $p<0.01$; hospitalization: 1.3 vs. 2.6 days, $p<0.03$). However, there was a shorter operative time seen in the mTURP group than the TEVP (34.6 vs. 47.6 min in TUVP, $p<0.01$). There was a significantly larger decrease in sodium levels with mTURP group (3.9 vs. 1.4 mEq/L, $p<0.03$) as well as more days of work lost (18.4 vs. 6.7 days, $p<0.02$). In the mTURP group, one patient developed TUR syndrome, and one patient required a blood transfusion compared to none in the TEVP group. There was no statistical difference in hematocrit decrease between the two groups (2.8 vs. 5.6 ml/dL, $p=0.50$) [6]. TEVP appears to have a similarly acceptable outcome profile in comparison to mTURP with fewer overall complications and was thus an early alternative for prostatic resection.

Results

There have been three large randomized trials comparing the results of bPKVP to mTURP. BPKVP has been shown to have significantly reduced operative times. Mean operative durations using mTURP were 50.4, 55.6, and 55 min in the three randomized trials in comparison to that of bPKVP of 35.1, 39.7, and 40.3 min, respectively (Table 5.1) [1–3]. Shorter operative time is likely due to several factors including the rapid hemostasis with plasma kinetics, the elimination of debris from the subjacent tissue, and the maintenance of visibility from reduced bleeding [1]. Postoperatively, bPKVP has both less catheterization time and overall hospitalization time compared to mTURP (Table 5.1). In the largest study by Geavlete et al. [2], these two outcomes were reduced by over half with catheterization time decreasing from 72.8 h with mTURP to 23.5 h with bPKVP and hospitalization decreasing from 4.2 to 1.9 days, respectively (Table 5.1) [2].

BPKVP resulted in greater improvements than mTURP in measures of bladder outlet obstruction. These include International Prostate Symptom Score (IPSS) and post-void residual (PVR). In the Geavlete et al. [2] trial, which had the longest follow-up of 18 months, there was a statistically greater decrease in IPSS in bPKVP compared to mTURP (24.2–8.3 mTURP vs. 24.3–5 bPKVP, $p=0.671$ pre-op, $p<0.0001$ at 18 months) (Table 5.1) [2]. They also found PVR has a significantly greater increase in bPKVP compared to mTURP (6.4–20.2 mTURP vs. 6.6–23.7 bPKVP, $p=0.528$ pre-op, $p<0.107$ at 18 months) (Table 5.1) [2]. While the mean decrease in Qmax was greater in bPKVP in all trials, this was not statistically significant (Table 5.1). Similarly, both bPKVP and mTURP showed a drop in PSA, and were not also statistically significant.

Complications

Gleavette et al. (2010) in a prospective randomized trial found mTURP to have a greater number of capsular perforations (7 of 80 ptsmTURP vs. 1 of 75 ptsbPKVP, $p=0.037$) [2]. Intraoperative hemoglobin decrease was less so in bPKVP in both trials reporting this (Table 5.1). This is likely due to the immediate hemostasis provided by the plasma kinetic technology.

The postoperative complications of PKVP include a statistically significant decreased rate of clot retention, TUR syndrome, hematuria, and rehospitalization for hemorrhage compared to mTURP. Gleavette et al. (2010) reported clot

Table 5.1 Outcomes and complications

Outcomes

Authors	Trial size	Follow-up	Mean operative time	Mean catheterization duration	Hospital stay	Change in IPSS	Change in Qmax (mL/s)	Change in PVR (mL)	Change in PSA (ng/mL)
Geavlete et al. [1]	80 mTURP	6 months	50.4 min mTURP	71.2 h mTURP	93.1 h mTURP	24.4 pre-op to 9.1 at 6 months post-op mTURP	6.3 pre-op to 19.3 at 6 months post-op mTURP	85.3 pre-op to 26 at 6 months post-op mTURP	1.85 pre-op to 0.8 at 6 months post-op mTURP
	75 PKVP		35.1 min PKVP	23.8 h PKVP	47.6 h PKVP	24.2 pre-op to 5 at 6 months PKVP	6.2 pre-op to 21.8 at 6 months PKVP	84.8 pre-op to 16 at 6 months PKVP	1.82 pre-op to 0.74 at 6 months PKVP
			($p=0.002$)	($p=0.002$)	($p=0.018$)	($p=0.595$ *pre* and 0.020 *post*)	($p=0.878$ *pre* and 0.018 *post*)	($p=0.712$ *pre* and 0.281 *post*)	($p=0.501$ *pre* and 0.499 *post*)
Geavlete et al. [2]	170 mTURP	18 months	55.6 min mTURP	72.8 h mTURP	4.2 days mTURP	24.2 pre-op to 8.3 at 18 months post-op mTURP	6.4 pre-op to 20.2 at 18 months post-op mTURP	88 pre-op to 33 at 18 months post-op mTURP	2.06 pre-op to 0.91 at 18 months post-op mTURP
	170 PKVP		39.7 min PKVP	23.5 h PKVP	1.9 days PKVP	24.3 pre-op to 5 at 18 months PKVP	6.6 pre-op to 23.7 at 18 months PKVP	91 pre-op to 29 at 18 months PKVP	1.95 pre-op to 0.87 at 18 months PKVP
			($p=0.0001$)	($p=0.0001$)	($p=0.0001$)	($p=0.671$ *pre* and 0.0001 *post*)	($p=0.053$ *pre* and 0.0001 *post*)	($p=0.528$ *pre* and 0.107 *post*)	($p=0.369$ *pre* and 0.651 *post*)
Karaman et al. [3]	37 mTURP	12 months	55 min mTURP	68 h mTURP	68 h mTURP	22 pre-op to 12 at 12 months post-op mTURP	6 pre-op to 15 at 12 months post-op mTURP	n/a	n/a
	38 PKVP		40.3 min PKVP	35 h PKVP	35 h PKVP	21 pre-op to 7 at 12 months PKVP	6 pre-op to 16 at 12 months PKVP		
			($p=0.001$)	($p=0.001$)	($p=0.001$)	($p<0.001$ *post*)	($p>0.05$ *post*)		
Reich et al. [4]	30 PKVP	6 months	61 ± 26 min	41 ± 35 h	n/a	20.8 pre-op to 8.1 at 6 months PKVP	6.6 pre-op to 18.1 at 6 months PKVP	165 pre-op to 38 at 6 months PKVP	n/a

Complications

Authors	Hemoglobin change (dL)	Clot retention	UTI	Urge incontinence	Urethral stricture	TUR syndrome	Hematuria	Rehospitalization for hemorrhage
Geavlete et al. [1]	1.5 mTURP	4 ptsmTURP	9 ptsmTURP	n/a	n/a	n/a	13 ptsmTURP	2 ptsmTURP
	0.6 PKVP	0 pts PKVP	6 pts PKVP				3 pts PKVP	0 pts PKVP
	($p=0.002$)	($p=0.029$)	($p=0.561$)				($p=0.012$)	($p=0.167$)
Geavlete et al. [2]	1.6 mTURP	7 ptsmTURP	6 ptsmTURP	4 ptsmTURP	9 ptsmTURP	3 ptsmTURP	26 ptsmTURP	6 ptsmTURP
	0.5 PKVP	1 pts PKVP	4 pts PKVP	1 pts PKVP	8 pts PKVP	0 pts PKVP	5 pts PKVP	1 pts PKVP
	($p=0.0001$)	($p=0.042$)	($p=0.841$)	($p=0.363$)	($p=0.768$)	($p=0.049$)	($p=0.0001$)	($p=0.04$)
Karaman et al. [3]	n/a	n/a	n/a	n/a	2 ptsmTURP	0 ptsmTURP	0 ptsmTURP	n/a
					2 pts PKVP	0 pts PKVP	0 pts PKVP	
Reich et al. [4]	n/a	0 pts PKVP	3 pts PKVP	1 pts PKVP	O pts PKVP	0 pts PKVP	0 pts PKVP	0 pts PKVP

retention occurred significantly less in bPKVP compared to mTURP (1 ptbPKVP vs. 7 ptsmTURP, $p=0.042$). Postoperative hematuria occurred far less in the bPKVP group (5 pts bPKVP vs. 26 ptsmTURP, $p=0.0001$). Rehospitalization for hemorrhage was slightly less in bPKVP than in mTURP (1 pts bPKVP vs. 6 pts mTURP, $p=0.04$) [2]. TUR syndrome was not seen in any patients who underwent bPKVP, which is due to the use of normal 0.9 % saline with plasma kinetics (Table 5.1). While not statistically significant, postoperative complications of UTIs and urge incontinence were seen in fewer patients in the bPKVP group in all studies (Table 5.1). As well, it appears that the incidence of erectile dysfunction in both procedures is similar (13 % bPKVP vs. 12 % mTURP) [3]. There were higher rates of dysuria and urinary frequency in bPKVP compared to mTURP, although neither was found to be statistically significant in any of the trials (Table 5.1).

Conclusions

bPKVP provides practitioners with shorter operative times with a similar complication profile. Patient hospitalization and catheterization time are less, and they have equivalent or better outcome measures (IPSS, Qmax, PVR, PSA) postoperatively. As well, bPKVP has fewer perioperative and postoperative complications and specifically avoids TUR syndrome. At the same time, there remain very few large trials comparing bPKVP to the "gold" standard of mTURP as well as other new modalities. bPKVP seems to provide similar safety and efficacy profile to mTURP in these early trials.

References

1. Geavlete B, Multescu R, Dragutescu M, et al. Transurethral resection (TUR) in saline plasma vaporization of the prostate vs standard TUR of the prostate: 'the better choice' in benign prostatic hyperplasia? BJU Int. 2010;106(11):1695–9.
2. Geavlete B, Georgescu D, Multescu R, et al. Bipolar plasma vaporization vs monopolar and bipolar TURP-A prospective, randomized, long-term comparison. Urology. 2011;78(4):930–5.
3. Karaman I, Kaya C, Ozturk M, et al. Comparison of transurethral vaporization using PlasmaKinetic™ energy and transurethral resection of prostate: 1-year follow-up. J Endourol. 2005;19(6):734–7.
4. Reich O, Schlenker B, Gratzke C, et al. Plasma vaporisation of the prostate: initial clinical results. Eur Urol. 2010;57(4):693–7.
5. Kaplan SA, Santarosa RP, Te AE. Transurethral electrovaporization of the prostate: one-year experience. Urology. 1996;48(6):876–81.
6. Kaplan SA, Laor E, Fatal M, Te AE. Transurethral resection of the prostate versus transurethral electrovaporization of the prostate: a blinded, prospective comparative study with 1-year followup. J Urol. 1998;159(2):454–8.

6 Basic Principles of Laser-Based Techniques

Malte Rieken and Alexander Bachmann

Laser Radiation

The term "laser" is an acronym and stands for "light amplification by stimulated emission of radiation." The light of a laser has a defined wavelength and direction. This light is generated by the stimulated emission of radiation by an excited laser medium. These laser media can be gas, glass, dye, or crystals. When the laser medium is excited (e.g., by photons of a flash lamp), some of the excitation photons are absorbed by the laser medium. This leads to an increased energy level of the laser medium ion, which is called excited state. When this excited state returns to the ground state, a photon of a characteristic wavelength is emitted. When this photon hits another excited state ion, the excited state ion returns to ground state and releases a photon of the same wavelength itself. This process is called "stimulated emission of radiation" [1].

The emitted wavelength of the laser is defined by the active components of the lasing medium. Different laser media are used to generate laser radiation. For the treatment of BPO, the following media are used (Table 6.1):

- Holmium:yttrium-aluminum-garnet (Ho:YAG)
- Thulium:YAG (Thu:YAG)
- Neodymium:YAG (Nd:YAG)
- Semiconductors

In holmium lasers, a Ho:YAG crystal serves as active medium, and the excitation source is a flash lamp. Because of the pulsed excitation, the laser generates light in pulses and not continuously. This is called pulsed-wave mode. In thulium lasers, the Thu:YAG crystal is excited by a laser diode, and the laser operates in continuous mode. For the so-called GreenLight laser, an arc lamp or a laser diode excites a Nd:YAG crystal. The light emitted from this source is passed though a potassium titanyl phosphate (KTP) or lithium triborate (LBO) crystal. This crystal doubles the frequency and halves the wavelength of the laser radiation. The laser operates in a quasi-continuous or continuous mode. In contrast to crystal-based lasers, in diode lasers a semiconductor structure serves as the active medium. Electrical current is used as excitation source and the semiconductor material defines the emitted wavelength. Diode lasers convert electrical into optical energy very efficiently so that they can be operated on a normal power plug [1].

Laser-Tissue Interaction

Laser-tissue interaction determines the suitability of a laser for a surgical procedure. The most commonly used laser-tissue reaction is the

M. Rieken, M.D. • A. Bachmann, M.D. (✉)
Department of Urology, University Hospital Basel, Spitalstrasse 21, Basel 4031, Switzerland
e-mail: malte.rieken@usb.ch; alexander.bachmann@usb.ch

B. Chughtai et al. (eds.), *Treatment of Benign Prostatic Hyperplasia: Modern Alternative to Transurethral Resection of the Prostate*, DOI 10.1007/978-1-4939-1587-3_6,

Table 6.1 Physical specifications of laser types used in the treatment of benign prostatic obstruction

Laser name	Active medium	Excitation source	Emitted wavelength (nm)
Holmium laser	Ho:YAG crystal	Flash lamp	2,100
Thulium laser	Thu:YAG crystal	Laser diode	2,000, 2,013
GreenLight laser	Nd:YAG crystal[a]	Arc lamp	532
		Laser diode	
Diode laser	Semiconductors	Electrical current	940, 980, 1,318, 1,470

[a]The light emitted by the Nd:YAG crystal is frequency doubled by a KTP or LBO crystal to generate the wavelength of 532 nm

photothermal effect [2]. Laser light is absorbed by tissue chromophores and transformed into heat. A chromophore is the part of a molecule responsible for its color; in prostate tissue the chromophores are intracellular water and hemoglobin of the red blood cells. Depending on the amount of heat generated by laser absorption, coagulation, vaporization, or carbonization of tissue occurs [3]. To predict the photothermal effect, the wavelength of the laser and the amount of target chromophore in the tissue are important. The absorption coefficients of water and hemoglobin differ strongly in the range of currently used lasers. At a wavelength of around 500 nm, hemoglobin has its maximum absorption coefficient, whereas water has its maximum around 2,200 nm. Tissue absorption defines the penetration depth of a laser. This is the depth at which 90 % of the laser beam is absorbed and transformed into heat. A high absorption coefficient results in a shallow penetration depth, whereas a low absorption coefficient leads to a high penetration depth.

An understanding of the mechanisms taking place when a laser beam enters the tissue is crucial when discussing various types of lasers in prostate surgery. The optical energy of a laser is transformed into thermal energy once the laser enters the tissue. The volume of the heated tissue correlates with the absorption of laser energy. When the temperature is high enough to denaturize proteins without reaching the boiling point, coagulation occurs. Heating of the tissue above the boiling point leads to vaporization. Usually, vaporization and coagulation occur with every laser type. Superficial tissue is heated above the boiling point, resulting in vaporization, whereas the underlying tissue layers are heated below the boiling point, which causes coagulation. A high absorption coefficient within the target tissue leads to a concentration of heat in superficial tissue layers. The superficial tissue is vaporized and only a small proportion of energy causes coagulation of deeper tissue. In contrast, a low absorption coefficient leads to the heating of a larger tissue volume below the boiling point, which results in a deep necrotic zone.

Laser Fibers

In endourology, laser energy is delivered to the tissue through thin and flexible fibers. In recent years, major advances in fiber design have been made. The general design of a laser fiber comprises a circular core and two or three adjacent layers. These layers cover the laser fiber, provide stability and integrity, and prevent leakage of radiation. The core of the laser fiber is almost exclusively made of silica. Depending on the wavelength the fiber should transmit, different qualities of silica material are required [3].

Various fiber types with different diameters have been developed. Independent of fiber type, energy is always delivered through the core of the fiber. The laser beam can either exit the laser fiber on the side of the tip (side firing) or straight at the tip (front firing). In side-firing fibers, the radiation is deflected towards the tissue in an oblique angle. By changing the distance between laser fiber and tissue, coagulation and vaporization can be achieved. Limitations of side-firing fibers are their higher costs and a limited life span. Furthermore, carbonization at the laser tip, leading to a loss in energy output, has been described [4, 5]. The energy of front-firing fibers is delivered straight at the tip. These fibers are

Table 6.2 Laser types and surgical techniques for lasers used in prostate surgery

Laser name	Target chromophore	Optical penetration depth (mm)	Surgical technique
Holmium laser	Water	0.5	Enucleation (HoLEP)
Thulium laser	Water	0.2	Vaporesection (ThuVARP)
			Enucleation (ThuLEP)
GreenLight laser	Hemoglobin	0.8	Vaporization (PVP)
Diode laser	Hemoglobin, water	0.5–5	Vaporization (DiVAP)
			Enucleation (DiLEP)

primarily used for tissue incision (resection, enucleation). Tissue is heated in a very small area only leading to vaporization of a small tissue volume. A variation of front-firing fibers is the coating of the fiber tip with quartz. The fiber does not emit a free beam. The irrigation fluid surrounding the fiber absorbs the laser radiation, which created a steam bubble. Tissue is heated and vaporized by this steam bubble and the heated fiber tip [1, 6].

Clinical Application of Lasers in Prostate Surgery

The techniques of laser prostatectomy can be dived into three basic principles (Table 6.2):

- Vaporization: ablation of the tissue from the prostatic urethra to the prostatic capsule
- Resection: excision of small pieces of tissue from the prostatic urethra to the prostatic capsule
- Enucleation: dissection of the prostatic adenoma from the surgical capsule and removal of adenoma tissue by resection or morcellation

Wavelength and fiber design determine the ideal surgical technique. For vaporization, a side-firing fiber with a wavelength within the absorption maximum of hemoglobin is ideal. This results in superficial vaporization of the perfused prostate and a thin rim of coagulated tissue. For enucleation, which mimics the technique of open prostatectomy, a front-firing fiber allows precise dissection of the adenoma from the surgical capsule. As damage of adjacent structures by deep coagulation has to be avoided, a wavelength with a shallow penetration depth is preferable.

Holmium:YAG Lasers

The radiation of the holmium laser is emitted by a front-firing fiber and has a wavelength of 2,100 nm, which is strongly absorbed by water. The penetration depth is around 0.5 mm. The laser operates in pulsed-wave mode; a stream bubble of irrigation fluid is generated with each laser pulse. In holmium laser enucleation of the prostate, the steam bubble is used to separate the adenoma tissue from the surgical capsule by tearing the tissue apart. Once the adenoma tissue is dissected, it is pushed into the bladder and removed by a morcellator.

Thulium:YAG Lasers

Thulium lasers operate in continuous-wave mode and come in two wavelengths: 2,000 and 2,013 nm. Although side-firing fibers are available, applications mainly include front-firing fibers for resection and enucleation. The laser energy is strongly absorbed in water, and the penetration depth in prostatic tissue is around 0.2 mm. Due to the high amount of tissue vaporization at this wavelength, the terms vaporesection and vapoecleation have also been used to describe the surgical techniques.

GreenLight Laser

The radiation of the GreenLight laser is emitted from a side-firing fiber and has a wavelength of 532 nm. The laser operates in quasi-continuous (f 80-W model) and continuous mode (120-W and 180-W models). As water has its absorption minimum and hemoglobin has a very high absorption coefficient at this wavelength, the laser is suitable for application in well-perfused organs like the prostate. The penetration depth is around 0.8 mm, which leads to a sufficient vaporization of superficial prostate tissue and a coagulation of underlying areas. The technique is also called photoselective vaporization of the prostate (PVP).

Diode Lasers

Diode lasers are available in various wavelengths and fiber designs. Currently used diode lasers emit at 940, 980, 1,318, and 1,470 nm in continuous-wave mode. As laser-tissue interaction depends on the wavelength, each laser has to be judged independently. The optical penetration depth in prostate tissue ranges from 0.5 to 5 mm. Front-firing lasers with shallow optical penetration are used for diode laser enucleation of the prostate, whereas laser with higher optical penetration depth is in use for diode laser vaporization of the prostate.

Summary

- Various laser types and techniques are available for laser prostatectomy.
- Wavelength is the most important determent of laser-tissue interaction.
- Heating of tissue by laser radiation results in coagulation and vaporization.
- Vaporization and enucleation are the primary surgical techniques for laser prostatectomy.
- Wavelength and fiber type vary between different techniques.

References

1. Bach T, et al. Laser treatment of benign prostatic obstruction: basics and physical differences. Eur Urol. 2012;61(2):317–25.
2. Welch AJ, Torres JH, Cheong WF. Laser physics and laser-tissue interaction. Tex Heart Inst J. 1989; 16(3):141–9.
3. Teichmann HO, Herrmann TR, Bach T. Technical aspects of lasers in urology. World J Urol. 2007;25(3): 221–5.
4. Hermanns T, et al. Laser fibre deterioration and loss of power output during photo-selective 80-w potassium-titanyl-phosphate laser vaporisation of the prostate. Eur Urol. 2009;55(3):679–85.
5. Hermanns T, et al. Lithium triborate laser vaporization of the prostate using the 120 W, high performance system laser: high performance all the way? J Urol. 2011;185(6):2241–7.
6. Shaker H, Alokda A, Mahmoud H. The Twister laser fiber degradation and tissue ablation capability during 980-nm high-power diode laser ablation of the prostate. A randomized study versus the standard side-firing fiber. Laser Med Sci. 2012;27(5): 959–63.

532 nm Laser Photoselective Vaporization of the Prostate

7

Michael Shy, Victor Lizarraga, and Ricardo R. Gonzalez

Introduction

In the 1990s, the introduction of surgical lasers was met with great enthusiasm by urologists. As we gained clinical experience, enthusiasm faltered as adverse effects and unpredictable results became apparent. Over the last 20 years, laser technology has continued to evolve, with many laser systems now available, and outcomes continuing to improve. Each of these systems has specific interactions with tissue, greatly affecting the outcome when used in surgery as well as the skills needed to perform laser procedures. To select the ideal laser for endoscopic surgery, one would prefer a system that would allow safe, controllable prostate tissue removal, with excellent hemostatic ability and minimal adverse symptoms. Of the systems available today, the modern 532 nm laser used for photoselective vaporization of the prostate may best fulfill these requirements.

M. Shy, M.D., Ph.D. (✉) • V. Lizarraga, M.D.
Department of Urology, Baylor College of Medicine, Houston, TX, USA
e-mail: shy@bcm.edu

R.R. Gonzalez, M.D.
Department of Urology, Baylor College of Medicine; Houston Metro Urology, Houston Methodist Hospital, Houston, TX, USA

Laser Physics

Laser, as commonly known, is an acronym for light amplification by stimulated emission of radiation. Laser systems employ three parts: a pump source, a gain medium, and an optical resonator. Simplistically, the pump source excites the gain medium. The excited gain medium releases light energy which is amplified by the optical resonator. Unique to laser light, the output is a beam of a single wavelength with all electromagnetic waves in phase. These properties of laser light determine how the laser interacts with target tissue.

Each target tissue will have an absorption length which is the distance over which approximately 2/3 of the laser energy is absorbed. The extinction length describes the distance over which about 90 % of the laser energy is absorbed and transformed into heat energy [1]. Thus, for a tissue with a long extinction length at a given wavelength, the effect of the laser energy is spread over a greater volume of tissue. At a wavelength with a short extinction length, the laser energy is transferred to a lesser volume of tissue (Fig. 7.1).

With energy transfer, tissue is heated rapidly. At temperatures above 60 °C, protein is denatured, and the tissue is coagulated. At temperatures around the boiling point of water (100 °C), vaporization occurs. Above 150 °C, tissue carbonization results [2]. For prostate ablative surgery, vaporization is the goal, as target tissue is completely removed from the operative field.

B. Chughtai et al. (eds.), *Treatment of Benign Prostatic Hyperplasia: Modern Alternative to Transurethral Resection of the Prostate*, DOI 10.1007/978-1-4939-1587-3_7,

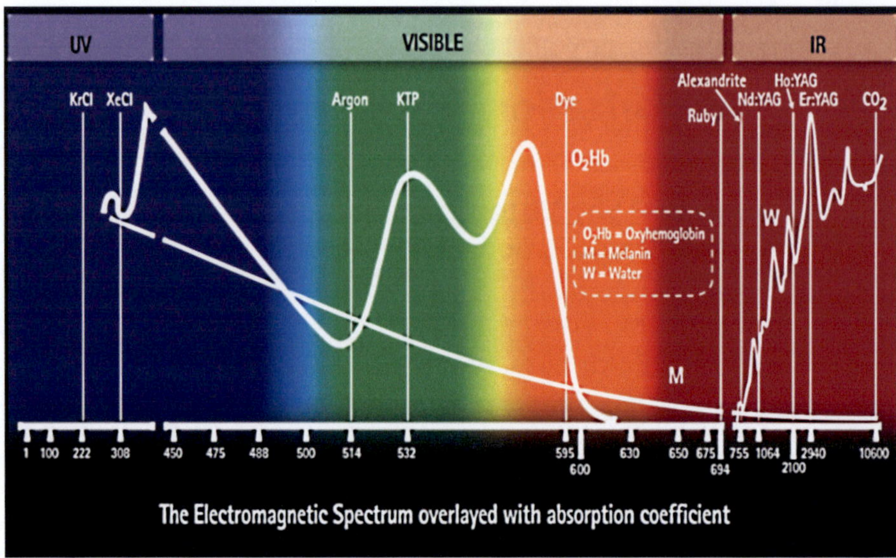

Fig. 7.1 Common lasers and the absorption coefficients with common chromophores (Courtesy of American Medical Systems)

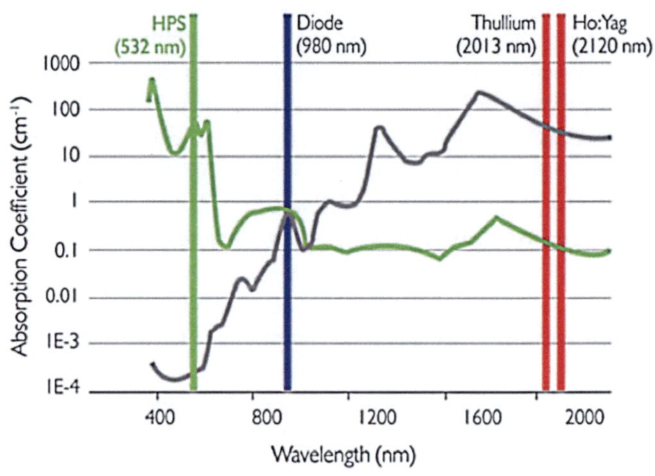

Fig. 7.2 The 532 nm laser (HPS – 120 W GreenLight system) demonstrates the ideal absorption coefficient for interaction with oxyhemoglobin and water (Courtesy of American Medical Systems)

There are multiple laser systems in use for ablative prostate surgery. They can be divided by wavelength into two groups: those in the visible spectrum (390–700 nm) and those in the infrared spectrum (700 nm–1 mm). The 532 nm wavelength lasers – characterized as green light – are alone in the visible spectrum group, and the remainder of lasers for use in the prostate is in the infrared spectrum. To better understand the differences between these lasers, let us consider the clinical response based on laser-tissue interactions by laser wavelength (Figs. 7.2, 7.3, and 7.4).

Evolution of the 532 nm Laser System in Urology

The 532 nm laser system has been continually improved over its existence in the last two decades. Initially developed by adapting a KTP crystal as a pass-through on the Nd:YAG system, the laser wavelength was halved, resulting in a laser which was visible as a green light at 532 nm. This wavelength is preferentially absorbed by hemoglobin molecules, making it ideal for lasing

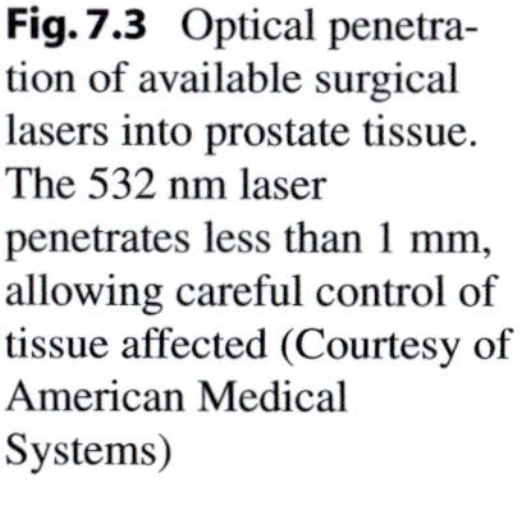

Fig. 7.3 Optical penetration of available surgical lasers into prostate tissue. The 532 nm laser penetrates less than 1 mm, allowing careful control of tissue affected (Courtesy of American Medical Systems)

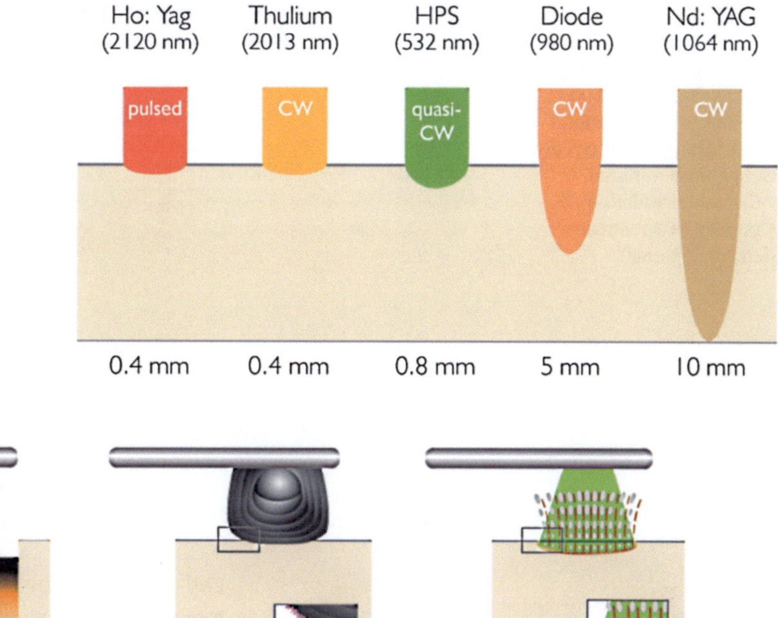

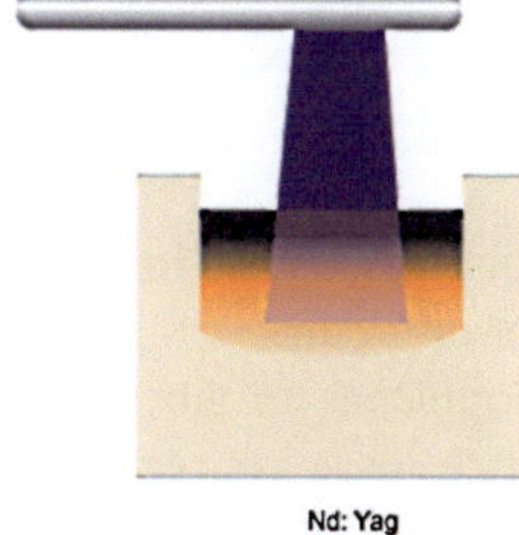

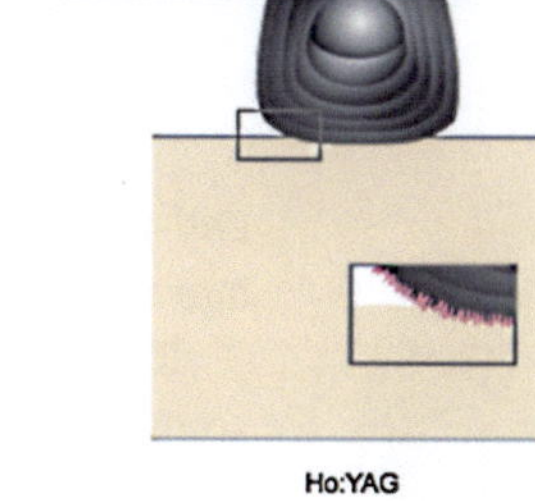

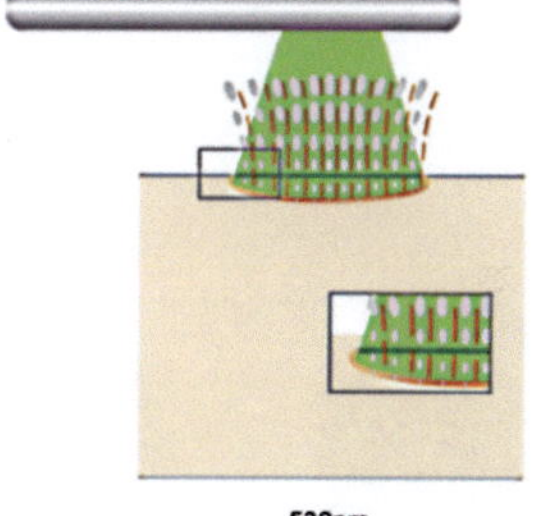

Fig. 7.4 A schematic demonstrating tissue effect of the Nd:YAG, Ho:YAG, and 532 nm lasers. The Nd:YAG typically causes superficial vaporization with a broad, deep zone of coagulation. The Ho:YAG system has a rapid decay of energy due to high absorption of the irrigant, with minimal energy reaching the target tissue, resulting in vaporization limited to the point of contact. The 532 nm laser causes controlled vaporization with a minimal rim of coagulation (Courtesy of American Medical Systems)

vascular tissue such as the prostate. After early enthusiasm with the Nd:YAG laser, prostate surgery was tempered by postoperative difficulties of protracted urinary retention and irritative voiding symptoms; modifications were sought to overcome these issues.

Early systems were low power, running at only 38 W. Vaporization of prostate tissue was feasible, albeit slow [3]. Improvement in laser design then produced a 60 W system which was initially tested successfully in dogs and human cadaveric prostates [4]. Human trials were performed in 1998 using a prototype 60 W system. This trial demonstrated that PVP was a viable, technically feasible technique. Patients tolerated the procedure well, without significant complication [5]. These early works did highlight one significant drawback, which was the slow rate of tissue vaporization in these early systems (Fig. 7.5).

The first commercially available KTP system sought to improve on the prototype by increasing power output. This system was launched with 80 W power source eventually known as GreenLight PV. This early system was greeted with much enthusiasm by the urologic community; however, long lasing times with relatively low tissue vaporization efficiency continued to limit widespread use. In 2006, after a significant redesign of the laser generator, a new higher-power system with 120 W output was launched. This new GreenLight HPS system eliminated the KTP crystal, instead using a LBO crystal adaptation to the Nd:YAG system. This produced a 532 nm laser with higher power than before. Additional benefits included a more focused beam (i.e., more collimated) and high power density. These all improved vaporization efficiency, which meant reducing laser times during PVP [6].

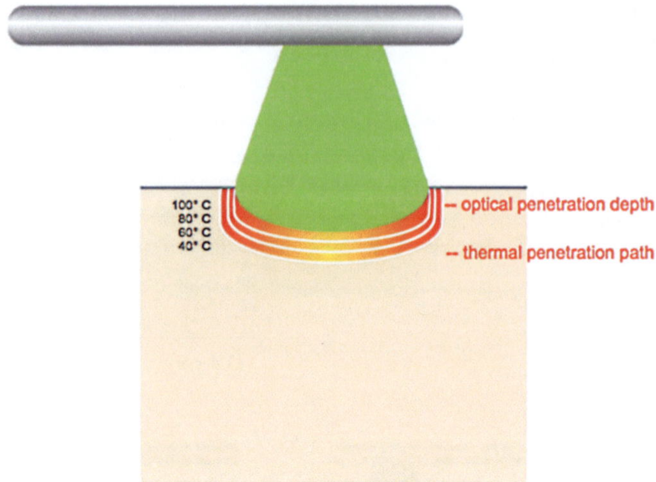

Fig. 7.5 Detail of tissue effect with use of 532 nm laser system. Surface tissue is rapidly heated to 100 °C resulting in vaporization. Temperature spread rapidly decays, with minimal collateral coagulation (Courtesy of American Medical Systems)

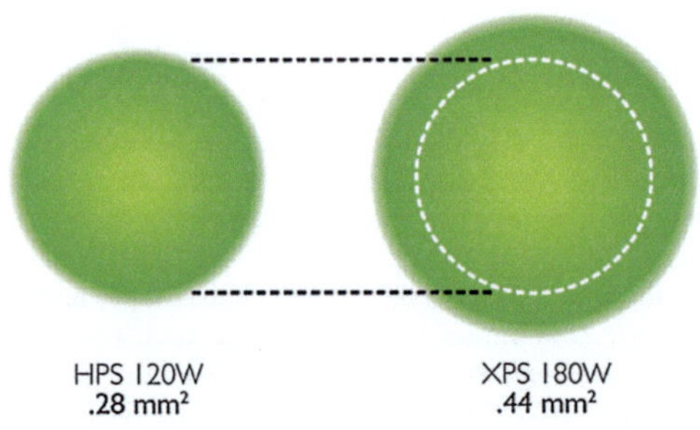

Fig. 7.6 The continued evolution of the 532 nm laser systems. XPS 180 W system by AMS demonstrating improvement in laser beam target size, further improving lasing efficiency (Courtesy of American Medical Systems)

In an effort to further improve the 532 nm photovaporization systems, the latest generation system from AMS increased power substantially. The GreenLight XPS system is able to generate 180 W of high-frequency pulses of laser energy into a wider beam, further improving vaporization efficiency while maintaining the same power density seen in the HPS (Figs. 7.6 and 7.7).

Fiber improvements have also been crucial in improving the efficiency of the photovaporization procedures. Early fibers were silica based with a 70° deflecting tip for side firing of the laser beam. Early fibers were limited by user wear during the case. If the fiber was brought into close contact with the lased tissue, the fiber tip would heat and fracture, causing degradation of the laser output and, more seriously, resulting in an end-firing fiber that may cause inadvertent damage to the bladder or urethra.

Recent developments in fiber design have sought to minimize these concerns. The MoXy fiber design was developed for use with the GreenLight XPS system. MoXy fibers are now available and have a metal-tipped cap to protect the fiber tip, as well as an active cooling system. Continuous irrigation is run through the fiber itself, minimizing the risk of overheating the fiber to its breaking temperature. A temperature monitoring system is integrated into the fiber, which is designed to automatically cease lasing if the fiber is overheating. These improvements all seek to minimize the dangers of fiber malfunction as well as limit the number of fibers needed per procedure, hopefully constraining costs associated with fiber usage (Fig. 7.8).

Today, the laser technology is available in the United States through American Medical Systems (Minnesota, USA). The GreenLight laser offers 532 nm laser systems for PVP in second-generation standard 120 W (HPS) and third-generation high-power 180 W (XPS) systems.

Surgical Technique and Preparation

The preparation of any patient for PVP of the prostate involves a thorough history and physical, per AUA guidelines [available on auanet.org].

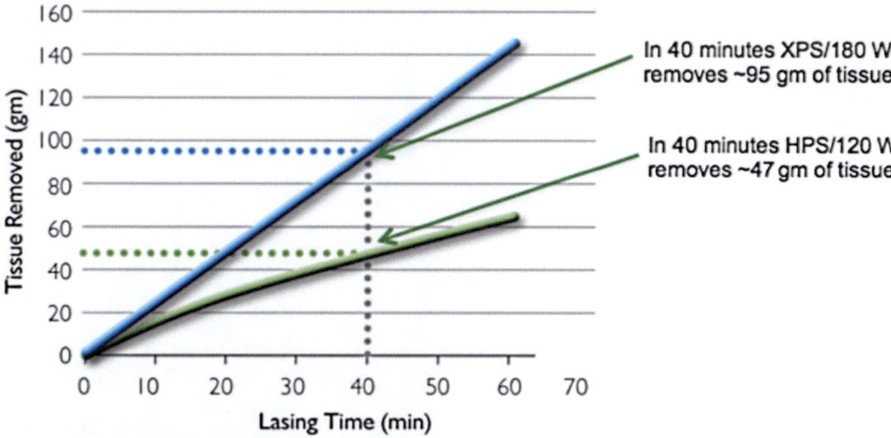

Fig. 7.7 In an in vitro model, high-powered 180 W 532 nm laser vaporization with MoXy fiber demonstrated excellent tissue ablation with improved efficiency compared to the 120 W HPS. *Blue line* 180 W XPS. *Green line* 120 W HPS (Courtesy of American Medical Systems)

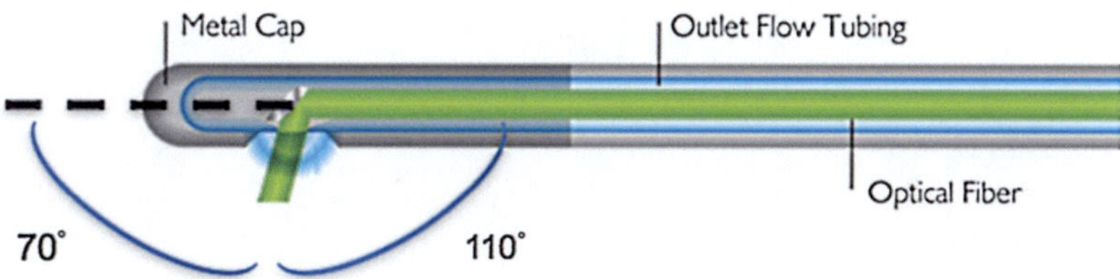

Fig. 7.8 The MoXy fiber by AMS for the 180 W XPS GreenLight laser. Fiber benefits include internal fiber irrigation for improved fiber cooling. Using this technology, fiber longevity is improved, allowing for single fiber per case utilization in most glands (Courtesy of American Medical Systems)

Close attention to voiding concerns, objectively assessed with a validated questionnaire, is encouraged. Digital rectal examination is performed to assess for prostate size and any abnormalities that would suggest a diagnosis of prostate cancer.

Transrectal ultrasound is recommended preoperatively to assess prostate size which may predict intraoperative parameters, such as surgical time and anesthetic duration. PSA level is recommended preoperatively. Suspicion for prostate cancer should be addressed by preoperative biopsy if indicated. Urinalysis and urine culture are obtained. Urinary tract infections are treated prior to surgical intervention.

A thorough discussion regarding risks and benefits is held with patient. The most common risks are hematuria requiring intervention, irritative urinary symptoms, urinary retention, and urinary tract infection. Retrograde ejaculation is a common occurrence, seen in >50 % of patients, and should be thoroughly discussed. Informed consent is obtained.

Anticoagulation is held if feasible; however, PVP can be carried out safely even in this setting by experienced surgeons. There are multiple studies describing PVP being performed safely in men on aspirin, clopidogrel, and warfarin [7, 8]. Recent analysis of complications of PVP on men anticoagulated with warfarin demonstrated a rate of significant postoperative hematuria requiring intervention of only 4 % [7].

Laser Safety

Laser use in the operating room is safe to both patient and operating room personnel as long as general safety principles are followed closely.

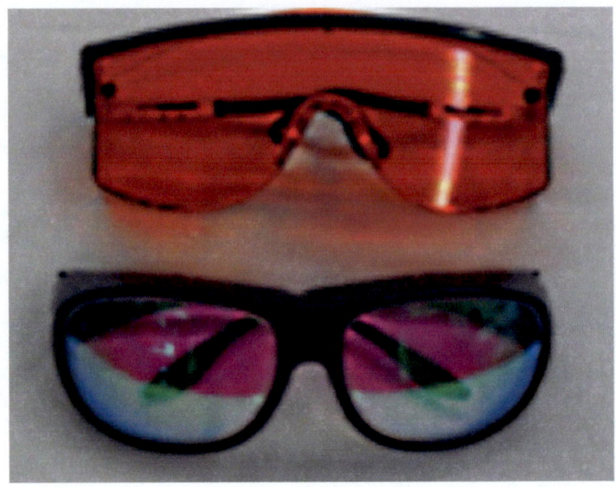

Fig. 7.9 Laser safety goggles for use with 532 nm laser systems (Courtesy of American Medical Systems)

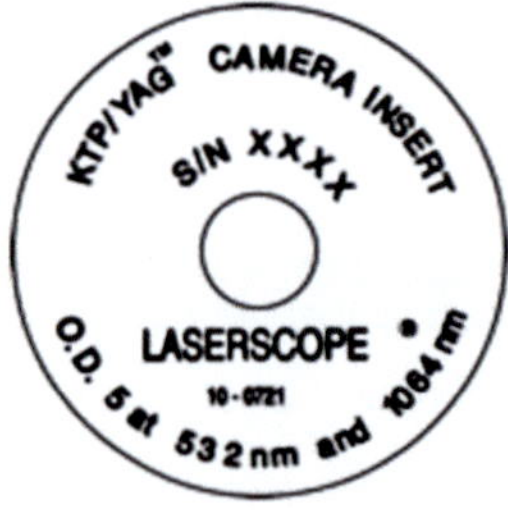

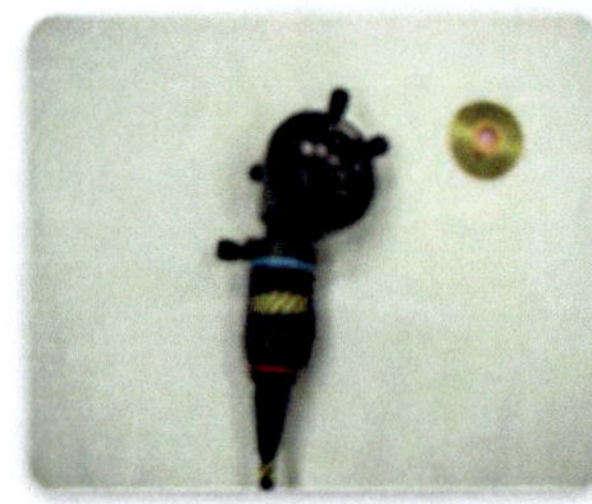

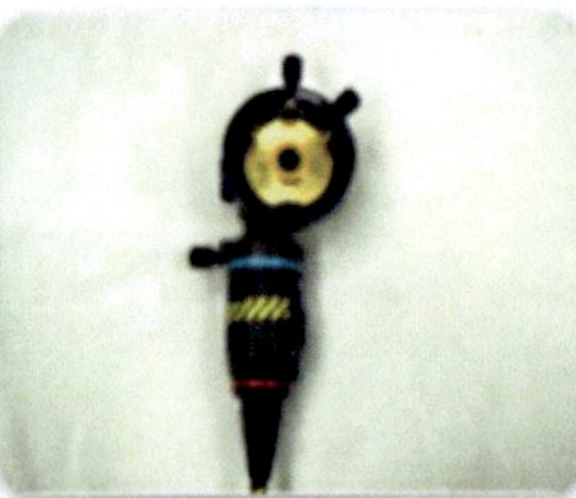

Fig. 7.10 The laser filter should be applied to camera element to prevent laser damage of digital camera equipment (Courtesy of American Medical Systems)

All lasers carry some inherent risks, including damage to the skin and eyes from direct laser exposure and potential for fire and electric shock. A team approach is key in preventing injury to all participants of any laser procedure.

The Occupational Safety and Health Administration (OSHA) published guidelines regarding safe laser use in the operating room. Recommendations include laser safety training for those involved in laser use, a defined laser use policy, and use of protective eyewear for all staff and patient. Local safety regulation regarding laser use should be identified and followed (Fig. 7.9).

Laser energy is carried in a fiber which has limits to the angulation it can withstand before fracture. On fracturing a fiber, laser energy may escape in an unintended direction. Appropriate handling of the laser fiber is paramount, to avoid undue angulation or damage to fiber coating. The use of protective eyewear specific to the wavelength of the laser being used is strongly recommended.

Standardized PVP Technique

Performance of safe, efficient photovaporization of the prostate is dependent on careful planning and preparation. The instruments required for PVP should be available and in good working condition before the start of the case.

A 24 Fr continuous-flow cystoscope is usually utilized. A 30° cystoscope is preferred. Camera head optics should be protected by a GreenLight filter applied between the scope and camera head, although some manufacturers integrate the filter into the lens itself (Fig. 7.10).

The patient is placed under general or spinal anesthesia per surgeon/anesthesiologist's

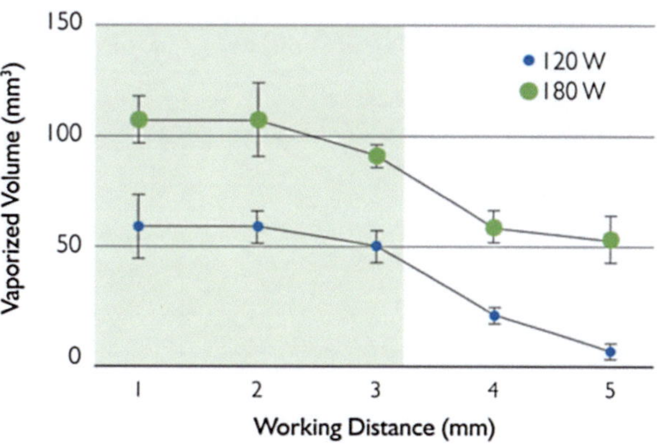

Fig. 7.11 Vaporized volume at given working distant using the GreenLight HPS (120 W) and XPS (180 W) laser systems (Courtesy of American Medical Systems)

preference. Patient is positioned in dorsal lithotomy. Surgical preparation and draping is done in the standard manner for retrograde endoscopic procedures.

Room temperature saline irrigation is hung and connected to irrigation tubing. If using the MoXy fiber, a second saline irrigant line should be connected to the MoXy fiber inflow port. A thorough inspection of the urethra and bladder is performed with close attention to the anatomical landmarks, including the verumontanum, bladder neck, and ureteral orifices. Careful technique is paramount to minimize mucosal disruption at this early stage. Any undue hemorrhage should be avoided to maximize visualization [9].

The ideal PVP technique utilizes maneuvers which are somewhat disparate from those utilized in standard TURP, where tissue ablation occurs with contact. Tissue vaporization during PVP occurs when laser energy is absorbed by hemoglobin within target tissue. The temperature of the hemoglobin increases dramatically causing the surrounding cellular water to boil, causing vapor bubbles to form. This disrupts the tissue structure causing vaporization. Hence, a noncontact approach is key in performing an efficient PVP. If contact with tissue occurs while laser is applied, heat is transferred from the lased tissue to the fiber tip, which increases the likelihood of tip degradation. Beyond a distance of 3 mm, vaporization efficiency decreases. Hence, an ideal working distance is between 1 and 2 mm from the tissue surface (i.e., near-contact technique).

The laser fiber is slowly swept across the tissue surface to be treated. Ideal sweep speed has been identified as <1 mm per second for maximal tissue vaporization in an experimental model [10]. A sweep angle of <30° appears to be the most efficient, with larger angles resulting in decreased tissue vaporization and increasing depth of coagulation [11] (Fig. 7.11).

Once anatomical landmarks have been confirmed, distal and proximal limits of resection may be marked with the coagulation low-energy setting. Resection at the bladder neck is commenced, being cognizant of the anatomical relationship of the ureteral orifices. Once the bladder neck is appropriately ablated, the floor is addressed. Techniques vary depending on surgeon's preference/patient anatomy. Sequentially, deeper troughs may be cut in the floor until the appropriate depth is achieved. Alternatively, a single deep trough may be made at 5 o'clock until capsule is encountered, and using this first cut as a depth guide, further resection continues from this point. The aiming beam should be clearly visible on the target tissue before applying laser energy. As the vaporization progresses distal to the bladder neck, energy may be increased to the maximal level to improve tissue removal.

Once the median lobe is resected in this manner, the lateral lobes are addressed sequentially. Starting inferiorly and advancing superiorly along the lateral lobes, vaporization is performed until a convex space is developed with lateral margins being the prostatic capsule.

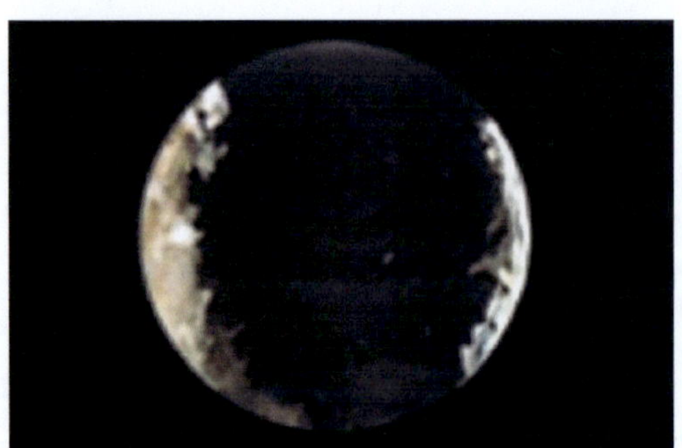

Fig. 7.12 Cystoscopic view of completed resection. Note absence of bleeding (Courtesy of American Medical Systems)

Special consideration must be given to the resection of large glands. In many cases, the lateral lobes are hypertrophic to the extent that they meet in the midline. This can severely limit the working space available, making it difficult to maintain a noncontact lasing position. Creating a small cavity – or "working channel" – using low power setting may be useful when starting a large gland. As with a TURP, a systematic approach is always recommended, and vaporization starting from the proximal to the distal prostate in an anterograde fashion is standard.

Troublesome bleeding can be encountered as the capsule is approached, especially at 5 and 7 o'clock positions. The coagulation mode on XPS system can readily control bleeding if utilized early and often. Bleeding should be controlled quickly, as an increase in red cells in the irrigant will limit laser transmission to the target tissue, making hemostasis more difficult as hemorrhage increases. Although uncommon, uncontrolled hemorrhage may require electrocauterization or conversion to TURP when surgeons are early in the learning curve [12]. Alternatively, one may place a urethral catheter under traction for a period after which resection is resumed or utilize a Bugbee electrode to directly coagulate bleeding tissue [9].

Once an adequate cavity has been created, the bladder and ureteral orifices are inspected. Any further bleeding points are sought out and coagulated. Once the surgeon is satisfied with the outcome, a 20 Fr Foley catheter is placed and left to gravity drainage (Fig. 7.12).

Typically, the catheter is left in place overnight. However, if there is no concern for continued bleeding nor any medical or anesthetic complicating issue, the catheter may be discontinued in as little as 4 h and the patient given a trial of void. Discharge on the day of surgery is reasonable if there are no significant comorbidities or significant bleeding requiring continuous irrigation.

Post-procedure care typically involves mild urinary analgesics with no strenuous activity.

A urethral catheter is used for bladder drainage and is typical discontinued after 24 h. Antibiotic therapy is at the discretion of the surgeon. Strenuous activity is usually limited for about 7 days.

Follow-up care should focus on voiding symptoms and include a post-void residual and flow estimation.

Outcomes

Early Efficacy Data

Since the development of 532 nm laser prostatectomy, there has been ever-growing evidence of its efficacy in treating lower urinary tract symptoms due to BPH. The mounting data supporting PVP comes in several forms: data pointing to its efficacy, safety, and, most particularly, its ability to be used in anticoagulated patients. One of the earliest large series was Te et al. who presented their results with the 80 W KTP in laser prostatectomy for 45 patients [13]. Significant improvements in AUA Symptom Index scores, QOL scores, Qmax, and PVR were seen for up to 12 months postoperatively. Mean AUA symptom scores declined from 24 to 1.8 at 12 months, mean QOL scores improved from 4.3 to 0.4, Qmax from 7.7 to 22.8 ml/s, and PVR volume from 114.2 to 7.2 ml. Mean prostate volume, as determined by ultrasound, decreased from 54.6 to 34.4 ml. Mean operative time was 36 min, and no patient required a blood transfusion. More than 30 % of patients were sent home without a catheter; those with postoperative catheters had them removed in a mean of 14 h. Reported morbidities were generally minor. 8 % of patients experienced mild-to-moderate dysuria lasting more than 10 days. Eight percent had transient hematuria, and 3 % had postoperative retention. Among the 56 men who were potent prior to the procedure, 27 % experienced retrograde ejaculation, but none of them experienced impotence.

The efficacy of the 80 W KTP was also shown with larger glands; Sandhu et al. detailed large prostate volume resection in 64 men with BPH possessing prostates with volumes of at least 60 ml who had failed medical therapy [14]. The mean preoperative volume was 101 ml with a mean operative time of 123 min. Postoperatively at 12-month follow-up, IPSS decreased from 18.4 to 6.7; Qmax increased from 7.9 ml/s to 18.9 ml/s, while PVR decreased from 189 ml to 109 ml. No transfusions were required and all patients were able to be discharged within 24 h. Given the larger gland size, an important outcome was that there was no evidence of postoperative hyponatremia.

Anticoagulated Patients

An important and unique safety aspect of the KTP laser is its use in anticoagulated patients at high risk for clinically significant bleeding. An early study looked at 24 anticoagulated patients with BPH treated with laser prostatectomy using the 80 W KTP laser [15]. Of these, eight were on warfarin, two on clopidogrel, and 14 on aspirin. Eight (33 %) of these patients had a previous myocardial infarction, seven (29 %) cerebrovascular disease, and seven (29 %) peripheral vascular disease. Postoperatively, there was no clinically significant hematuria nor any clot retention. No transfusions were required and there were no thromboembolic events. The only events were transient postoperative urinary retention in one patient requiring discharge with a catheter, two instances of retrograde ejaculation, and two postoperative urinary tract infections. Mean operative time was 101 min. Follow-up revealed a decrease in IPSS from 18.7 to 9.5 as well as an increase in Qmax from 9.0 to 20.1 ml/s at 12 months. PVR decreased from 134 to 69 ml at 1 month but was not statistically significant beyond that time point. In this study, all patients underwent PVP safely without any adverse thromboembolic or bleeding events.

Subsequently, larger studies have later confirmed the continued safety of the 532 nm laser in use in anticoagulated patients. Ruszat et al. studied their use of PVP laser prostatectomy in their series of 116 men: 36 receiving warfarin, 71 receiving aspirin, and 9 receiving clopidogrel [16]. No patients developed clinically significant intraoperative bleeding nor were there any that required postoperative blood transfusions. There were no instances of postoperative clot retention. Compared with their control group of 92 patients not receiving anticoagulation, their average postoperative decrease of hemoglobin was 8.6 % for patients on anticoagulation versus 8.8 % for the control. 11.2 % of patients receiving anticoagulation were discharged with catheters mainly for reasons of large initial prostate gland size (>80 ml). This was similar to the control group (12 %). As for functional outcomes, at 3, 6, 12, and 24 months postoperatively, improvement of the IPSS ranged from 60 % to 70 %, PVR improved from 80 % to 88 %, and average maximum urinary flow rate increased 116–140 %, respectively. Overall, postoperative complications were low and comparable to the control group.

Chung et al. followed up their earlier study by examining their cohort of 162 men on systemic anticoagulation who received PVP laser prostatectomy from 2002 to 2008 [17]. Within this group, 31 (19 %) were on warfarin, 101 (62 %) were on aspirin, 19 (12 %) were on clopidogrel, and 11 (7 %) were on 2 or more anticoagulants. Mean length of stay was 1.1 days. A total of 26 patients (16 %) were discharged home with a catheter. Significant improvements were seen in IPSS, Qmax, and PVR. Mean IPSS had improved from a baseline of 18 to 6 by 24 months postoperatively. Mean Qmax went from 8.3 ml per second preoperatively to 15 ml per second 1 month after surgery. This was sustained throughout postoperative follow-ups. Mean PVR improved from 124 ml at baseline to 75 ml by 2 years postoperatively. No patient required immediate blood transfusion. Two patients (1.2 %) were in urinary retention postoperatively, requiring catheterization. Postoperative urinary tract infection developed in four patients. There were six patients who need continuous bladder irrigation due to delayed bleeding, and three of these patients did subsequently need a transfusion. One patient required reoperation for fulguration of bleeding. In all, this is one of the larger series to date to report the safety of PVP laser prostatectomy in patients on systemic anticoagulation.

Contemporary Data

Within the past decade, with the development of the 120 W LBO laser, there have been increased undertakings to compare PVP with the gold standard TURP in a randomized setting. Indeed, there have been many randomized controlled trials (RCTs) undertaken to answer that question. Thangasamy et al. compiled all the RCTs that took place between 2002 and 2012 comparing the 80 W KTP laser or 120 W LBO laser with standard monopolar TURP [18]. Nine trials examined a total of 448 patients undergoing PVP and 441 undergoing TURP. As with previous studies, the overall data analysis showed that length of stay and catheterization times were significantly shorter in the PVP group, by 2.1 and 1.9 days, respectively. Operative time was shorter in the TURP group by 19.6 min, with fewer blood transfusions in the PVP group. There were no other significant differences in other perioperative complications. When comparing functional outcomes, there was no favorite either way. Six studies found no difference between the two groups, two favored TURP, and one favored PVP. Thus, while longer follow-up data is still needed, there seems to be no difference in the intermediate functional outcomes between PVP and TURP.

The GOLIATH Trial: 180 W LBO Laser PVP Versus TURP

The newest large-scale randomized multicenter prospective trial comparing the newest 180 W LBO laser technology with the gold standard TURP is the GOLIATH trial, of which the early results were announced at this year's annual meeting of the American Urological Association [19]. The GOLIATH study was designed to compare TURP and PVP with the 180 W LBO laser using a variety of symptomatic, functional, and safety outcome measures. The study evaluated 269 patients from 29 sites in 11 European countries based on 6-month post-procedural results. All adverse events were adjudicated and classified by an independent, blinded clinical events committee. Some of the important findings were an equivalency in safety, as evidenced by the number and rate of adverse events, and efficacy, as determined by IPSS (International Prostate Symptom Score) and Qmax (peak urinary flow rate). There was comparable prostate tissue volume and PSA (prostate-specific antigen) reduction in either modality. The study demonstrated superiority of the 180 W LBO laser in recovery times including shorter catheterization times, shorter hospital stay, and a faster return to a stable health status. There was a significantly lower rate of short-term re-intervention with the 180 W LBO laser and fewer bleeding and dysuria events with the 180 W LBO laser than TURP.

Cost

PVP has been shown to be favorable in cost when compared to TURP. When discussing costs, one should consider not only the expense of the capital equipment and disposable fibers and loops but also the institutional costs to provide perioperative care. In a published cost comparison of PVP and TURP at two institutions in the United States, the actual costs of PVP were lower than those associated with TURP [20]. In that study, both the direct (e.g., expenses specifically attributable to patient care service, including cost of the equipment and hospital stay) and indirect (e.g., support of clinical services like administration, medical records, and facility costs) were considered. Authors surmise that PVP costs are likely lower for two reasons. Firstly, PVP is more likely to be performed on an outpatient basis compared to TURP. Secondly, while significant complications are uncommon, those that prolong hospitalization (e.g., hyponatremia requiring intensive care monitoring) are more likely in the TURP group and add a significant expense.

For surgery to be cost-effective in the setting of symptomatic BPH, it should be effective and durable and minimize morbidity. The Goh and Gonzalez study above analyzed perioperative costs, which are only part of the cost burden carried by the patient and society [20]. The cost of follow-up procedures, loss of productivity, and long-term success were not reflected in that study, but economic modeling that takes those additional factors into account seems to support the finding that PVP is cost-effective compared to TURP [21, 22].

Conclusion

While the gold standard for surgical treatment of BPH remains TURP, its potential complications and side effects have led to continued search for safer and more efficacious treatment modalities. Over the past two decades, 532 nm wavelength laser vaporization has undergone an evolution from theory to practical application, becoming a safe and effective alternative to TURP. Laser prostatectomy, especially at 180 W, promises several advantages over TURP, including technical simplicity and the absence or minimization of complications such as intraoperative fluid absorption, bleeding, retrograde ejaculation, impotence, and incontinence. Laser prostatectomy can treat larger glands with less physiologic stress, thus allowing treatment of patients with more medical comorbidities, including those on active anticoagulation. The preponderance of outcomes data has demonstrated a shorter hospital stay and faster recovery with an improvement in lower urinary tract symptoms. Longer term follow-up in a randomized trial is necessary, but becoming available. Increasingly, practicing urologists are performing laser prostatectomies on patients with symptomatic BPH, and this trend is certain to continue.

References

1. Teichmann HO, Herrmann T, Bach T. Technical aspects of lasers in urology. World J Urol. 2007; 25(3):221–5.
2. Te A. The next generation in laser treatments and the role of the GreenLight high performance system laser. Rev Urol. 2006;8:24–30.
3. Kuntzman R, Malek R, Barrett D, Bostwick D. Potassium-titanyl-phosphate laser vaporization of the prostate: a comparative functional and pathologic study in canines. Urology. 1996;48:575–83.
4. Kuntzman R, Malek R, Barrett D, Bostwick D. High power (60W) potassium-titanyl-phosphate laser vaporization prostatectomy in living canines and in human and canine cadavers. Urology. 1997;49: 703–8.
5. Reza M, Barrett D, Kuntzman R. High-power potassium-titanyl-phosphate (KTP/532) laser vaporization prostatectomy: 24 hours later. Urology. 1998;51:254–6.
6. Malek RS. Greenlight photoselective 120-watt 532-nm lithium triborate laser vaporization prostatectomy in living canines. J Endourol. 2009;23(5):837–45.
7. Woo HH, Hossack T. Photoselective vaporization of the prostate with the 120-W lithium triborate laser in men taking coumadin. Urology. 2011;78(1):142–5.
8. Spernat DM, Hossack T, Woo H. Photoselective vaporization of the prostate in men taking clopidogrel. Urol Ann. 2011;3(2):93–5.
9. Zorn KC. GreenLight 180W XPS photovaporization of the prostate: how I do it. Can J Urol. 2011;18(5): 5918–26.
10. Kauffman EC, Kang HU, Choi B. The effect of laser-fiber sweeping speed on the efficiency of photoselective vaporization of the prostate in an ex vivo bovine model. J Endourol. 2009;23(9):1429–35.
11. Osterberg EC, Kauffman EC, Kang HW, Koullick E, Choi B. Optimal laser fiber rotational movement during photoselective vaporization of the prostate in a bovine ex-vivo animal model. J Endourol. 2011;25(7): 1209–15.
12. Ruszat R, Seitz M, Wyler S, Abe C, Rieken M. GreenLight laser vaporization of the prostate: single center experience and long term results after 500 procedures. Eur Urol. 2008;54:893–901.
13. Te A, Malloy TR, Stein BS, Ulchake JC, Nseyo UO, Mahmood AH, Malek RS. Photoselective vaporization of the prostate for the treatment of benign prostatic hyperplasia: 12-month results from the first United States multicenter prospective trial. J Urol. 2004;172:1404–8.
14. Sandhu JS, Ng C, VanderBrink BA, Egan E, Kaplan SA, Te AE. High power potassium-titanyl-phosphate (KTP) photoselective laser vaporization of the prostate (PVP) for the treatment of benign prostatic hyperplasia (BPH) in men with large prostates. Urology. 2004;64:1155–9.
15. Sandhu JS, Ng CK, Gonzalez RR, Kaplan SA, Te AE. Photoselective laser vaporization prostatectomy in anticoagulated men. J Endourol. 2004;18 Suppl 1:A3–246.
16. Ruszat R, Wyler S, Forster T, Reich O, Stief CG, Gasser TC, et al. Safety and effectiveness of photoselective vaporization of the prostate (PVP) in patients on ongoing oral anticoagulation. Eur Urol. 2007;51:1031–41.
17. Chung DE, Wysock JS, Lee RK, Melamed SR, Kaplan SK, Te AE. Outcomes and complications after 532 nm

laser prostatectomy in anticoagulated patients with benign prostatic hyperplasia. J Urol. 2011;186:977–81.
18. Thangasamy IA, Chalasani V, Bachmann A, Woo HH. Photoselective vaporisation of the prostate using 80-W and 120-W laser versus transurethral resection of the prostate for benign prostatic hyperplasia: a systematic review with meta-analysis from 2002 to 2012. Eur Urol. 2012;62:315–23.
19. Bachmann A, Tubaro A, Barber N, D'Ancona F, Muir G, Witzsch U, et al. A prospective multicenter randomized study comparing GreenLight XPS vaporization and transurethral resection of the prostate for the treatment of benign prostatic hyperplasia (GOLIATH). Abstract presented at the annual meeting of the American Urological Association, San Diego, 2013.
20. Goh AC, Gonzalez RR. Photoselective laser vaporization of the prostate versus transurethral prostate resection: a cost analysis. J Urol. 2010;183(4):1469–73.
21. Stovsky MD, Griffiths RI, Duff SB. A clinical outcomes and cost analysis comparing photoselective vaporization of the prostate to alternative minimally invasive therapies and transurethral prostate resection for the treatment of benign prostatic hyperplasia. J Urol. 2006;176:1500.
22. Ruszat R, Sulser T, Seifert HH, Wyler S, Forster T, Leippold T, Bachmann A. Photoselective vaporization versus transurethral electroresection of the prostate: a comparing cost analysis. Eur Urol. 2006;Suppl 5(2):271.

8 532 nm Laser Enucleation/Resection Techniques

Jonathan Shoag, Bilal Chughtai, and Alexis E. Te

Introduction

The use of lasers to treat symptomatic benign prostatic hypertrophy (BPH) was first described in the early 1990s and has grown in popularity over the past two decades [1–3]. Laser techniques have become widely accepted as an alternative to traditional transurethral resection of the prostate using electrocautery [1, 2]. Two predominant techniques for laser resection have emerged: photoselective vaporization of the prostate (PVP) and laser enucleation of the prostate. PVP, where the laser was initially applied, is a purely ablative approach whereby prostate tissue is systematically vaporized. Several perceived limitations of this approach, particularly when applied to patients with large prostates, led to the development of laser enucleation techniques. These limitations include the degradation of fiber integrity over time, which often necessitates the use of several fibers for larger prostates, and the longer operative times required to vaporize larger prostates [4].

Laser enucleation addresses the above problems. Laser enucleation techniques are able to apply the primary advantages of lasers over electrocautery to very large prostates, where these advantages are most important. These include the laser's excellent hemostatic properties and reduced risk of TUR syndrome stemming from the use of saline rather than glycine. Laser enucleation has no size limitations and therefore allows patients who would otherwise undergo open simple prostatectomy to receive the benefits of a minimally invasive procedure. There have been three primary modalities for laser enucleation described: holmium laser enucleation of the prostate (HoLEP), thulium laser enucleation (TmLEP), and enucleation using GreenLight™ lasers (American Medical Systems, Inc., Minnetonka, MN). The use of the GreenLight system for prostate enucleation is the topic of this chapter [5–8].

The GreenLight Laser

Initial studies in the early 1990s using lasers for prostate resection used a 1,064 nm neodymium:yttrium-aluminum-garnet (Nd:YAG) laser. While providing excellent hemostasis and coagulation, tissue was not efficiently vaporized and postoperative irritation and sloughing were common. It was found that halving the wavelength to 532 nm using a potassium-titanyl-phosphate

J. Shoag, M.D.
Department of Urology, Weill Cornell Medical College, New York Presbyterian Hospital, New York, NY, USA

B. Chughtai, M.D. (✉) • A.E. Te, M.D.
Department of Urology, Weill Cornell Medical College, 425 East 61st Street, 12th floor, New York, NY 10065, USA
e-mail: bic9008@med.cornell.edu; Aet2005@med.cornell.edu

B. Chughtai et al. (eds.), *Treatment of Benign Prostatic Hyperplasia: Modern Alternative to Transurethral Resection of the Prostate*, DOI 10.1007/978-1-4939-1587-3_8,

(KTP) crystal resulted in selective absorption by hemoglobin and a short optical penetration. These properties allow the 532-nm laser to vaporize only a superficial layer of prostatic tissue with a penetration depth of 0.8 mm with only a small (1–2 mm) rim of coagulation [9]. This GreenLight laser (so named because of its visible wavelength) has grown tremendously in popularity since its introduction in 2003. The initial system was equipped with a 60 W KTP crystal, which was then increased to 80 W. In 2006 the HPS (high-power system) incorporating an LBO (lithium triborate) crystal, which emits a beam at the same 532 nm wavelength, with a maximum power output of 120 W was launched. This system has recently been updated to the XPS model, which allows up to 180 W of power. This increase in power has been combined with developments such as a side-firing laser fiber, liquid-cooled irrigation channel, and pulsed coagulation mode [10–14].

Despite their potential advantages, holmium and thulium enucleation techniques have been slowly adopted. This is at least partially due to the need of a tissue morcellator, as well as the need for other specialized equipment [15]. Enucleation using the GreenLight laser as initially described by Brunken et al. used the same procedure used for HoLEP [16]. However, the techniques described here (TLEP or Seoul) allow for enucleation using the GreenLight laser that does not require the use of a tissue morcellator. Another major advantage of GreenLight systems is that they are more readily available to urologists given their widespread use for PVP.

TLEP Technique

The transurethral laser enucleation of the prostate (TLEP) technique consists of first creating a midline groove though the median lobe at the 6 o'clock position to the level of the trigone. Vaporization is not performed as traditionally defined with large sweeping motions. Instead, quick sweeping motions and proximal-distal movement of the fiber are used to create a groove. Efficient vaporization is confirmed by the appearance of bubbles.

Once the midline groove is created, a lateral groove on the 5 o'clock side of the median lobe is created. This groove is aimed lateral to the ipsilateral ureteral orifice and again deepened to the level of the trigone. The tissue in between the two grooves is next vaporized using larger sweeps, starting from the apex, or the most distal aspect, of the tissue. Care is taken to ensure the ureteral orifices are identified and the laser is targeted away from them when treating the bladder neck area. Small fragments of prostate tissue are detached (enucleated) and swept into the bladder by irrigation. These fragments are removed by an Ellik evacuator at the end of the case. A similar procedure is then performed on the contralateral 7 o'clock side.

Attention is next turned to the lateral lobes. A groove is created as previously described at the 11 o'clock position, and the right lateral lobe is subsequently vaporized until the groove at the floor of the prostate is encountered. Care is taken to limit lateral torque on the cystoscope to prevent prostatic perforation. The same technique is then performed on the opposite side with the starting groove at 1 o'clock. Once both lateral lobes have been vaporized/enucleated, the anterior prostate is vaporized and attention is turned toward the apex. With the cystoscope positioned at the verumontanum, apical tissue is vaporized. Care is taken not to position the fiber with the backside facing the verumontanum because the small amount of backscatter that occurs during PVP can injure the ejaculatory ducts when they are in close proximity.

Hemostasis is confirmed at the end of the case, and any remaining tissue in the bladder is removed. In most cases, a 22 or 24Fr three-way catheter is inserted. Continuous bladder irrigation is not usually needed, and often the catheter can be removed in the recovery room.

The TLEP technique may also be particularly useful for treating large glands, especially for the less experienced surgeon. With the traditional PVP technique, the anatomic landmarks can be lost early in the case with large glands. Bleeding combined with inadequate irrigation flow can also degrade visualization and efficient laser vaporization. Use of the TLEP technique first creates a resection landmark through use of deep grooves to the surgical capsule. This ensures complete vaporization of the transition zone without risking capsular perforation. Large intravesical or middle lobes are also treated more safely by creation of the lateral grooves, which allow the median lobe to be treated by aiming the laser from laterally to medially away from the ureteral orifice without having to aim toward the trigone. This is thought to decrease the forward scatter of the laser, thereby lessening the risk of injury to the ureteral orifices as well as trigone [4].

TLEP Versus PVP

A study comparing outcomes in TLEP vs. PVP using the 80 W GreenLight KTP laser was recently performed by Elterman and colleagues which retrospectively compared the rates of complications and outcomes (including IPSS, quality of life, Qmax, and PVR) between the two techniques [4]. Aside from a higher median prostate volume in the 97 patients undergoing TLEP (83 cc) than the 170 undergoing PVP (63 cc), baseline characteristics were similar between the two groups. This study found that TLEP required longer laser times (90 vs. 50 min), had lower volume lased per unit time than PVP (0.92 vs. 1.26 cc/min), and required more fibers (media 2.5 vs. 2.0). While QOL and Qmax were the same between groups, TLEP resulted in lower postoperative IPSS (9 vs. 5), and a decrease in PVR was statistically significant in the TLEP group but not in the PVP group.

Seoul Technique

Son et al. reported on the use of the 120 W GreenLight™ HPS laser [8]. Using the "Seoul technique," the median lobe is first vaporized-resected after the bladder neck is demarcated at the 5 and 7 o'clock positions. Lateral lobes are then vaporized-resected after two semicircular lines are made back to the level of the verumontanum. In their study, Son et al. reported on 104 men with prostate volumes greater than 40 mL who were grouped between standard vaporization alone ($n=40$) vs. the Seoul technique ($n=64$). IPSS, QoL, Qmax, and PVR were all significantly improved compared to baseline in both groups at 1, 3, 6, and 12 months ($p<0.05$). The Seoul technique group, however, had greater volume reduction per unit operative time (mL/min) (0.44 +/− 0.15 vs. 0.36 +/− 0.21, $p=0.31$), per lasing time (mL/min) (0.97 +/− 0.48 vs. 0.68 +/− 0.38, $p=0.001$), and per laser energy (mL/kJ) (0.25 +/− 0.15 vs. 0.19 +/− 0.14, $p=0.27$). In addition, two prostate cancers were detected in this group using the prostatic tissue obtained from the resection.

Summary

Over the past two decades, urologists have developed numerous techniques to treat LUTS in men with BPH. Currently available data suggests that enucleation using the GreenLight laser is equivalent to PVP. GreenLight enucleation appears to have the same advantages of holmium or thulium enucleation and is likely more readily available and does not require a tissue morcellator. While further randomized studies will be necessary to elucidate the advantages of these various techniques, GreenLight enucleation will likely remain a competitive alternative for the treatment of LUTS.

References

1. Ahyai SA, et al. Meta-analysis of functional outcomes and complications following transurethral procedures for lower urinary tract symptoms resulting from benign prostatic enlargement. Eur Urol. 2010;58(3):384–97.
2. Burke N, et al. Systematic review and meta-analysis of transurethral resection of the prostate versus minimally invasive procedures for the treatment of benign prostatic obstruction. Urology. 2010;75(5):1015–22.
3. Yu X, et al. Practice patterns in benign prostatic hyperplasia surgical therapy: the dramatic increase in minimally invasive technologies. J Urol. 2008;180(1):241–5. Discussion 245.
4. Elterman DS, et al. Comparison of techniques for transurethral laser prostatectomy: standard photoselective vaporization of the prostate versus transurethral laser enucleation of the prostate. J Endourol. 2013;27(6):751–5.

5. Kumar SM. Rapid communication: holmium laser ablation of large prostate glands: an endourologic alternative to open prostatectomy. J Endourol. 2007; 21(6):659–62.
6. Suardi N, et al. Holmium laser enucleation of the prostate and holmium laser ablation of the prostate: indications and outcome. Curr Opin Urol. 2009; 19(1):38–43.
7. Naspro R, et al. A review of the recent evidence (2006–2008) for 532-nm photoselective laser vaporisation and holmium laser enucleation of the prostate. Eur Urol. 2009;55(6):1345–57.
8. Son H, et al. Modified vaporization-resection for photoselective vaporization of the prostate using a GreenLight high-performance system 120-W Laser: the Seoul technique. Urology. 2011;77(2):427–32.
9. Te AE. The next generation in laser treatments and the role of the GreenLight high-performance system laser. Rev Urol. 2006;8 Suppl 3:S24–30.
10. Chughtai B, Te A. Photoselective vaporization of the prostate for treating benign prostatic hyperplasia. Expert Rev Med Devices. 2011;8(5):591–5.
11. Reich O. Greenlight: from potassium-titanyl-phosphate to lithium triborate or from good to better? Curr Opin Urol. 2011;21(1):27–30.
12. Mosli HA, et al. Photoselective vaporization of the prostate using GreenLight 120-W lithium triborate laser to treat symptomatic benign prostatic hyperplasia: a single-centre prospective study. Can Urol Assoc J. 2012;6(3):1–4.
13. Chung AS, et al. Photoselective vaporization of the prostate using the 180 W lithium triborate laser. ANZ J Surg. 2012;82(5):334–7.
14. Brunken C, et al. The 532-nm 180-W (GreenLight(R)) laser vaporization of the prostate for the treatment of lower urinary tract symptoms: how durable is the new side-fire fiber with integrated cooling system? Lasers Med Sci. 2013
15. Dusing MW, et al. Holmium laser enucleation of the prostate: efficiency gained by experience and operative technique. J Urol. 2010;184(2):635–40.
16. Brunken C, et al. Transurethral GreenLight laser enucleation of the prostate–a feasibility study. J Endourol. 2011;25(7):1199–201.

Holmium Ablation of Prostate

9

Lori B. Lerner, Joseph Shirk, and Tony Nimeh

Introduction

Lasers and BPH

The use of laser technology in surgical treatment of benign prostatic hyperplasia (BPH) is still relatively young with only 15 years in accumulated experience thus far. Despite this, it is already a complex field, partly due to rapidly developing technological innovations leading to multiple types of lasers each with its own varieties and settings and partly due to the various technical usage possibilities for each type of laser. The result is an intersecting matrix of different laser types (Nd:YAG, Ho:YAG, Tm:YAG, KTP, diode), methods of delivery (end-firing, side-firing, and interstitial), delivery systems and techniques, and different usages (ablation, visual ablation, contact ablation, interstitial coagulation, resection, enucleation, vaporization, vaporesection, vapoenucleation, enucleation, and photoselective vaporization). The multiplicity of possibilities has left clinicians with a seemingly endless number of possibilities, most of which have yet to be proven over a significant amount of time. Given all the different lasers that have hit the market – now, more than ever – it has become important that urologists learn about the various modalities available and appreciate the differences between them. As all lasers interact differently with tissue, a basic understanding of each energy source is vital.

From HoLAP to HoLRP to HoLEP and Back to HoLAP

The use of lasers for BPH dates back to 1992 when an Australian urologist, Dr. Anthony Costello, published the first series of patients post prostate laser ablation using the neodymium:yttrium-aluminum-garnet (Nd:YAG) laser [1]. However, due to significant side effects including prolonged catheter time, delayed clinical improvement, and irritative symptoms that were severe and persistent, Nd:YAG laser's use was abandoned rather quickly [2]. That said, the ease of use and decreased bleeding left many with a desire to explore other lasers and the era of laser prostate surgery was born.

Shortly after Dr. Costello's publication, Drs. Mark Fraundorfer and Peter Gilling elected to apply

L.B. Lerner, M.D. (✉)
Section of Urology, VA Boston Healthcare System, Boston University School of Medicine, 12 Water St, Hingham, MA 02043, USA

Department of Urology, Boston University School of Medicine, Boston, MA, USA
e-mail: Lerner_lori@hotmail.com

J. Shirk, M.D.
Department of Urology, David Geffen School of Medicine at University of California-Los Angeles, Los Angeles, CA, USA

T. Nimeh, M.D.
Department of Urology, VA Boston Healthcare System, 1400 VFW Parkway, West Roxbury, MA 02132, USA
e-mail: tony.nimeh@va.gov

B. Chughtai et al. (eds.), *Treatment of Benign Prostatic Hyperplasia: Modern Alternative to Transurethral Resection of the Prostate*, DOI 10.1007/978-1-4939-1587-3_9,

Table 9.1 Reimbursement and CPT code

CPT®	Work	Practice	Malpractice	Total	Work	Practice	Malpractice	Total
Code	RVU	RVU	RVU	RVUs	RVU	RVU	RVU	RVUs
52648	12.15	7.1	1.2	20.45	12.15	44.7	1.2	58.05
CPT® code	MD in office		MD in facility allowed amount[a]		Hospital outpatient allowed amount[a,b]		Ambulatory surgicenter[c]	
52648	$1,976		$696		$3,204		$1,847	

Department of Health and Human Services. Center for Medicare and Medicaid Services. https://www.cms.gov/PhysicianFeeSched/ 2012 National average Medicare physician payment rates calculated using a 2012 conversion factor $34.0376. [CMS-1524-CN]

[a]"Allowed amount" is the amount Medicare determines to be the maximum allowance for any Medicare-covered procedure. Actual payment will vary based on the maximum allowance less any applicable deductibles, coinsurance, etc

[b]The hospital outpatient payment rates are 2012 Medicare national averages. Source: January 4, 2012 Federal Register, CMS-1525-CN

[c]The ASC payments rates are 2012 Medicare national averages. ASC rates are from the 2012 Ambulatory Surgical Center Covered Procedures List – Addendum AA. Source: November 30, 2011 Federal Register, CMS-1525-FC

holmium:YAG (Ho:YAG) rather than Nd:YAG energy to prostate tissue hoping that the properties of holmium would be better suited than neodymium for transurethral surgery. Holmium laser technology had well-established applications in treating urinary calculi at that time, but this was its first application in treating the prostate [2]. They developed a combination approach using holmium to create a channel in the prostate and the Nd:YAG to coagulate (holmium laser ablation of the prostate or HoLAP) but discovered shortly thereafter that holmium could actually be used alone with fewer side effects. The laser used at the time was only 60 W (rather slow and tedious compared to the currently used 100 W lasers), and in an effort to become more efficient, they expanded on their HoLAP technique by resecting portions of the prostate and retrieving the pieces (holmium laser resection of the prostate – HoLRP). They quickly discovered that the properties of holmium allowed them to identify the prostatic capsule quite easily and led them to question if an endoscopic adenomectomy similar to an open procedure was possible. Once a proper tissue morcellator was developed that allowed for morcellation of large prostate pieces, they further developed the idea of the removal of the adenoma along the surgical capsule and the modern-day HoLEP was born (holmium laser enucleation of the prostate) [3].

HoLAP was temporarily abandoned with the advent of HoLEP. But with the emergence of other ablation lasers such as KTP (potassium titanyl phosphate) and the development of higher-power versions of the Ho:YAG (80 W then 100 and now a new 120 W unit), HoLAP reemerged [3]. Further improvement of the side-firing fiber allowed HoLAP to compete with other energy sources, and today, HoLAP has an established place in the armamentarium for BPH. In fact, both of the most recent guidelines for the treatment of BPH published by the American Urological Association and European Association of Urology include HoLAP [4, 5].

It is clear that ablation procedures are here to stay: they are now performed extensively in the urologic community worldwide. In the United States, there is a dedicated CPT code for prostate ablation: 52648 – "Laser vaporization of prostate including control of postoperative bleeding, complete vasectomy, meatotomy, cystourethroscopy, urethral calibration and/or dilation, internal urethrotomy, and transurethral resection of the prostate are included if performed" (Table 9.1). In this chapter, we will describe the holmium wavelength and its benefits in prostate surgery, indications for surgery, surgical technique of the modern HoLAP, and postoperative care and review published outcomes.

Physics

Mechanism of Action

Light amplification by stimulated emission (LASER) is a physical mechanism that can be used to deliver heat to a target tissue. Its effect on tissue (reflection, scattering, absorption, and extinction) varies depending on the wavelength, energy density, wattage, medium, tissue properties, and time of application. For example, at the same power wattage, a laser wavelength with a long extinction length may create deep necrosis, whereas a shorter extinction length will vaporize the tissue by bringing its temperature above boiling point. The most important phase of interaction between the laser and physiological tissue is absorption: the transformation of light energy to heat, causing the intended physiological changes. This is possible thanks to the presence of chromophores in human tissue. Chromophores are physiological chemical groups capable of absorbing light such as melanin, blood, and water. Depending on the absorption dynamics of specific types of lasers by a particular type of physiological tissue, the urologist might opt for a specific laser type and settings to achieve an intended effect such as coagulation, vaporization, resection, or enucleation via incision. Tissue coagulation is produced if the tissue is heated to temperatures between 70 °C and 100 °C, beyond which immediate vaporization occurs [6].

Ho:YAG Uses a Longer Pulsatile Wavelength

Both neodymium:yttrium-aluminum-garnet (Nd:YAG) lasers and holmium:yttrium-aluminum-garnet lasers (Ho:YAG) are solid-state lasers. They utilize a solid medium (crystals rather than liquid or gas) to derive optical gain. By comparison to the Ho:YAG, Nd:YAG has a shorter wavelength (1,064 vs. 2,140 nm) leading to absorption not only by water but also by hemoglobin: it can travel through a liquid environment resulting in deeper tissue penetration and more thermal injury with the ensuing side effects [3].

In contrast, Ho:YAG laser's wavelength is longer (2,140 nm, non-visible/infrared) and has a high absorption in water, which explains its favorable absorption coefficient in the prostate (high water density) and good tissue conductance of thermal energy [7]. The energy absorption by the prostate cell results in tissue heating to 100 °C, effectively causing vaporization/ablation with excellent hemostasis. The depth of penetration of holmium energy is quite shallow (0.4–0.5 mm). Furthermore, in urologic endoscopic surgery, there are no effects on the tissue if the laser is further than 0.5 mm from its target because urologists use a water medium, which completely dissipates holmium energy.

The Ho:YAG laser delivers its wavelength through rapid pulses rather than continuous. This is a distinguishing element that separates it from the continuous wavelength of the Nd:YAG and KTP lasers and explains Ho:YAG laser's lower hemostatic effects. On the other hand, pulse delivery leads to slower and shorter absorption as compared to continuous lasers. For these reasons, Ho:YAG has a more predictable tissue response and a lower side effect profile [2].

Ho:YAG laser's energy travels to water (its chromophore) and creates vapor bubbles, separating the tissue layers with a heating and shearing effect – called the "Moses Effect." During the pulse of laser energy, there is a microscopic air bubble on the tip of the fiber that allows the laser energy to travel further than through the fluid medium directly transmitting the laser energy into tissue. This "parting of the water" has been coined the "Moses Effect" in reference to the Biblical parting of the Red Sea by Moses [8]. The tissue effect is rapid and results in excellent hemostasis.

Ho:YAG Delivery

Holmium energy is delivered via small, flexible fibers and is controlled with precision by the operating surgeon. Energy is stored within the laser resonator and is released in a pulsed fashion controlled by a foot pedal. It travels along the laser fiber through internal reflections (also called "bounces"). Depending on how the fiber is used, ablation, coagulation, or cutting can be achieved. By lowering the *fluence*, either by decreasing the energy pulse or by increasing the distance between the fiber and the target, the tissue temperature is decreased and ablation is avoided; rather, the heat is absorbed into the tissue and results in coagulation [9].

Surgical Indications

In general, all patients with voiding symptoms secondary to bladder outlet obstruction are candidates for holmium surgery.

Prostate Size

While HoLAP is best done in glands under 60 cc [10, 11], newer studies show that the technique maintains its effectiveness in much larger glands. In fact, HoLAP has been performed in patients with prostates measuring up to 232 g [12]. Nevertheless, significant experience is required when approaching large glands, and beginners should limit themselves to small and moderate-sized glands (this recommendation stands not just for holmium laser, but for all lasers used for ablation) [13]. HoLAP has a relatively longer operative time as compared to resection techniques and other hemoglobin-based lasers on the market, particularly when treating men with a large prostate size [14]. That said, the differences in time between holmium and KTP published in the literature have been under 15 mins [13].

Patients with Comorbidities

Of special note is HoLAP's applicability to patients on anticoagulants. These patients can be treated very effectively even while at therapeutic levels of anticoagulation. In fact, the laser energy retains its hemostatic properties because it mainly depends on the cell's water content. Overall bleeding, regardless of coagulation status at the time of surgery, is much lower in all patients compared to TUR and open procedures [15].

In addition, normal saline can be utilized instead of water or glycine, which relieves the urologist from concerns related to TUR syndrome and time limitations related to absorption of hypotonic irrigants. The lower risks of operative and postoperative side effects may allow fragile, elderly patients' access to definitive BPH therapeutic options previously unavailable to them.

Radiated Patients

Water-based lasers, such as holmium, are the best energy sources for radiated patients regardless of the type of radiation used (external beam or brachytherapy). While these patients are at much greater risk for postoperative complications such as incontinence [16], poor healing, and stricture/bladder neck contractures, investigators have found only a minimal increase in risk when using holmium ablation and feel that holmium is the safest energy source available.

Furthermore, patients having undergone previous radiation therapy are best treated by holmium over all other energy modalities available because the penetration depth and risk for "overtreatment" is minimal. Holmium energy carries a lower risk of bleeding, fibrosis, urethral strictures, and irritative symptoms. Lastly, since normal saline is used during laser therapy, TUR syndrome risk is eliminated.

Surgical Equipment

Protective eyewear for the operating physician and those working with the fiber is recommended. Patients should have the eyes closed or blocked by a sheet. The machine is controlled by a key and relatively user-friendly. Regular maintenance is recommended to ensure proper functioning, and blast shield replacements should be kept in stock.

It is recommended to use a 26 F continuous flow resectoscope with a 30° lens. It is counter-recommended to use a cystoscope because the fiber would be too difficult to control. In addition, the lack of continuous irrigation makes visualization challenging, particularly at the beginning of the case when the channel is still obstructed. It is essential to use a laser bridge (see Fig. 9.1). This stabilizes the fiber and allows for efficient and predictable movement.

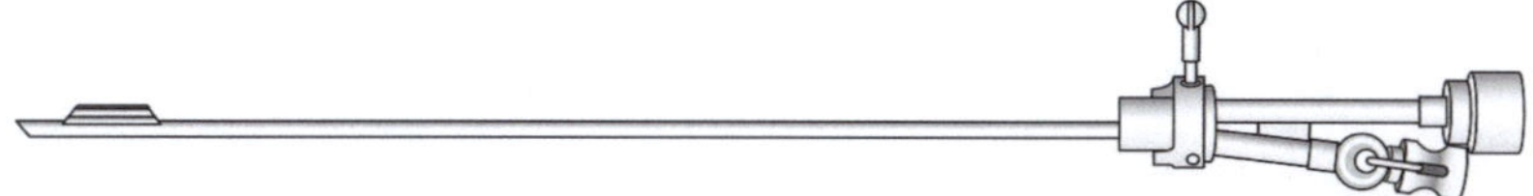

Fig. 9.1 Equipment: it is recommended to use a 26 F continuous flow resectoscope with a 30° lens

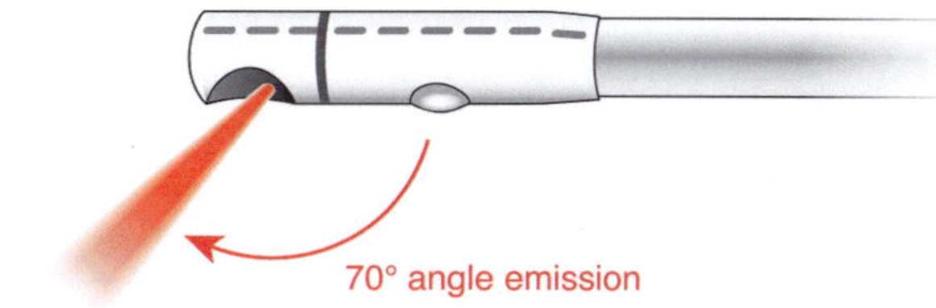

Fig. 9.2 The laser energy is directed at a 70° angle from the tip

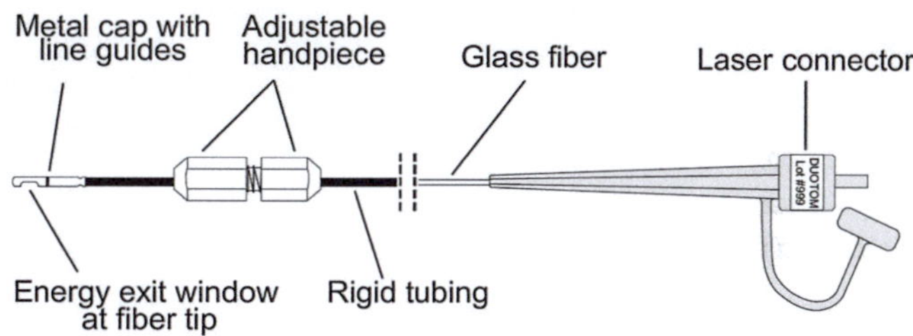

Fig. 9.3 Descriptive illustration of the laser device (DuoTome fiber image used with permission from Lumenis)

While other fibers are available and marketed, the authors prefer the DuoTome SideLite. This is a 550 μm fiber housed in a jacket made of biocompatible materials. The jacket contains an angled polished tip in a glass capillary (round glass "ball") that allows for the delivery of refractive side-fire energy. The total fiber diameter with the jacket is 7.2 F [17]. The laser energy is directed at a 70° angle from the tip (Fig. 9.2). An 80 W or 100 W holmium laser unit is utilized (preferably 100 W). Normal saline is used for irrigation, and a 20 F standard 2-way Foley catheter (sized based on surgeon preference) is used postoperatively.

Device Highlights

Please refer to Fig. 9.3 for a descriptive illustration of the device:
Line guide
Adjustable hand piece
Fiber cable
Laser connector
Side opening at fiber tip
Rigid tubing
Surgical technique – HoLAP

Settings

The laser is set to 2 J/50 Hz, which is the most frequently used setting with a 100 W laser; however, other settings have been described including 3.2 J and 25 Hz [18].

Preparation

The 550 micron side-fire fiber is advanced through the laser bridge until it exits from the end of the resectoscope, as confirmed by visualization of the solid line (Fig. 9.4). This line must always be visible throughout the ablation procedure to avoid thermal injury to the resectoscope and lens. The aiming beam is identified, which emerges at a 70° angle from the fiber.

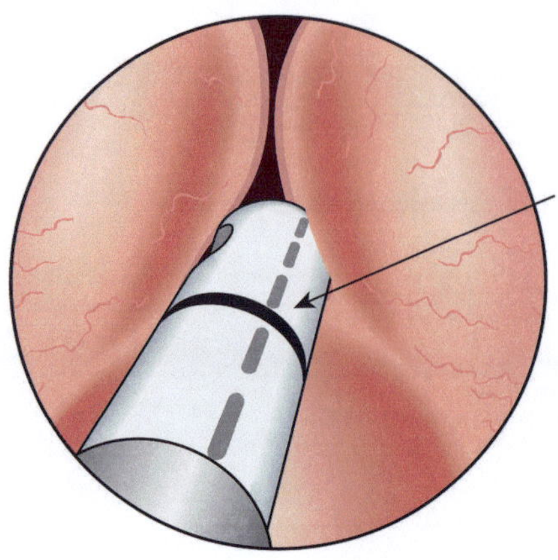

Fig. 9.4 The 550 micron side-fire fiber is advanced through the laser bridge until it exits from the end of the resectoscope, as confirmed by visualization of the *solid line*

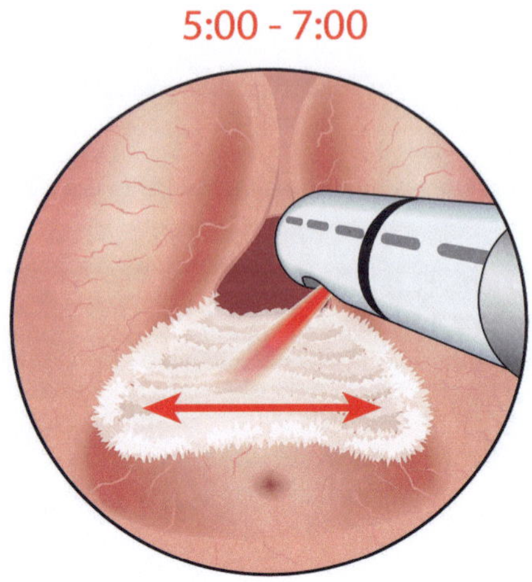

5:00 - 7:00

Fig. 9.5 Create troughs at 5 o'clock or 7 o'clock by using the side fire to cut the tissue posteriorly

Surgical Procedure

Surgeons tend to develop an approach that works well for them with the goal being to ablate all adenoma until prostatic capsule is visualized circumferentially from the bladder neck to the verumontanum. The fiber is designed to ablate tissue without charring or overheating. Since the holmium absorption depth is approximately 0.4 mm, tissue ablation is generally quickly achieved, which limits heat conduction to the surrounding tissue. If the fiber does not move, once the tissue within the zone has been ablated, the energy dissipates into the irrigant and there is no effect on the tissue. It is important not to "dig into" the tissue with the side-fire fiber. If tissue adheres to the housing material, it may reach very high temperatures when the laser is activated and can cause melting or breakdown of the housing material. In extreme cases, the glass "ball" may disconnect and need to be retrieved with graspers.

1. *Create troughs at 5 o'clock or 7 o'clock* (Fig. 9.5). This is achieved by using the side fire to cut the tissue posteriorly. The fiber is kept close to, but not touching, the prostate. The fiber is left in a fixed, slightly lateral position, and the camera end of the scope is lifted upwards, while pulling the entire scope back from the bladder neck to the veru. This is repeated until the fibers of the capsule are identified. Once the capsule is clearly visible, the scope and fiber are advanced to the bladder neck. The aiming beam is then directed laterally from the incision, at the level of the capsule, and the tissue is "pushed" towards the side. By leaving the aiming beam in the same position while moving laterally, absorption and heat generation are maximized, leading to more efficient ablation. Clearing tissue from 3:00 to 9:00 is essential; that is the most crucial area. If significant tissue remains anteriorly, this can be addressed at the end, time permitting. The fiber is utilized in each lateral direction, clearing the prostate off the capsule at the bladder neck from 5:00 to 7:00, widening the outlet. This maximizes flow and visualization.
2. *Lateral tissue ablation* (Fig. 9.6). The fiber is rotated slightly in a "cupping" fashion from 7:00 to 9:00 and 5:00 to 3:00. This is akin to an ice cream scooper, cupping the tissue in the open port of the fiber and "pushing" the tissue laterally then rotating upwards. It is important not to rotate too quickly; otherwise, the tissue temperature might not reach sufficient levels for efficient vaporization. This is a common mistake, particularly among urologists accustomed to laser energies which have a high absorption in hemoglobin, where rapid

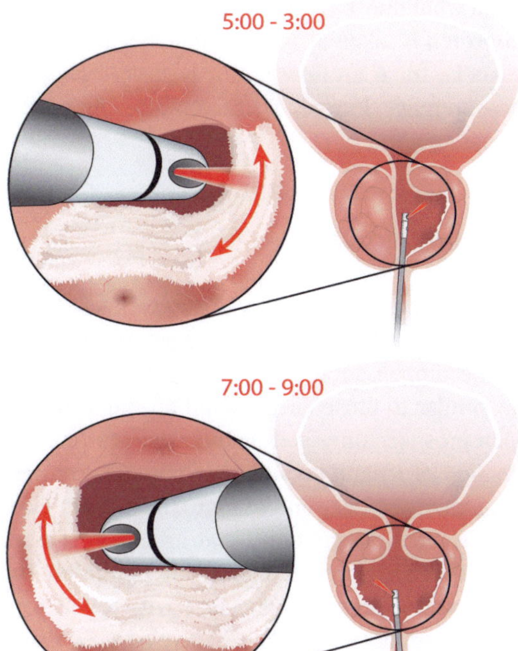

Fig. 9.6 Lateral tissue ablation: the fiber is rotated slightly in a "cupping" fashion from 7:00 to 9:00 and 5:00 to 3:00

rotations are important in order to prevent too deep of a defect. With water-based lasers, the surgeon must allow sufficient time for the energy to be absorbed, and rapid rotations will lead to merely heating the irrigant rather than ablating the tissue.

3. *Proximal to distal tissue ablation*. The resectoscope is gradually withdrawn from the bladder neck, ablating lateral tissue along the way. This is done using the same technique, moving towards the veru, with the surgeon clearing the prostate from the capsule upwards towards 3:00 or 9:00. As the tissue disappears, the prostate may "fall" into the operating field, and bands of tissue might become apparent. It is essential to ablate these as they appear, always working from the capsule up/anteriorly and from the bladder neck to the veru. If desired, the resectoscope can be turned upside down so the fiber is exiting at 12:00, and anterior tissue can be ablated (Fig. 9.7).

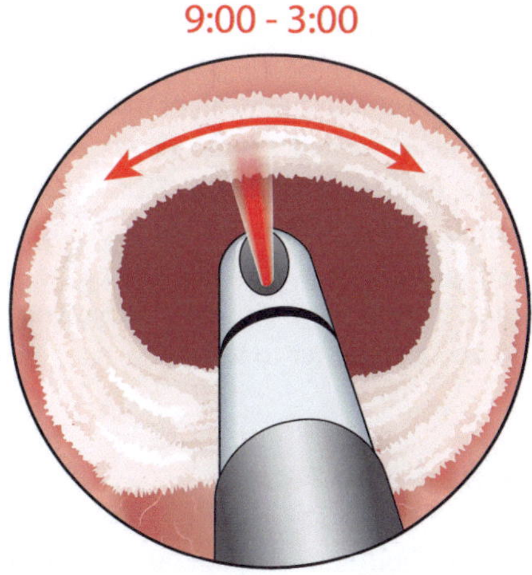

Fig. 9.7 Proximal to distal tissue ablation: the resectoscope is gradually withdrawn from the bladder neck, ablating lateral tissue along the way moving towards the veru, with the surgeon clearing prostate from capsule upwards towards 3:00 or 9:00

Postoperative Irrigation

It is recommended to give all patients 10 mg of furosemide at the end of the case to assist with short-term "natural irrigation," as 3-way Foley catheters are usually not used. Patients tend to be very comfortable after HoLAP, but should there be symptoms of bladder overactivity, they are given a belladonna and opium suppository in the recovery room and discharged on antimuscarinic therapy. Narcotic pain medication is very rarely necessary.

Special Considerations

Approach

While there may be a temptation to start at the veru, this approach is inefficient because the obstructed prostate tissue will impede flow and make visualization more difficult. Occasionally, if the tissue is "falling," making visualization difficult when ablating on the capsule, the surface mucosa can be cleared from top to bottom to open a channel large enough for flow. But once this is achieved, it is best to return to the capsule posteriorly and proceed as previously described.

Anterior Prostate

To address the anterior portion of the prostate, the resectoscope is turned upside down so that the laser fiber is exiting at 12:00. Rotate the fiber, sweeping the laser beam over the prostate tissue. Positioning the fiber directly over the scope brings the laser energy closer to the anterior tissue and makes it easier to ablate.

In the Irradiated Patient

When using holmium in patients having undergone radiation therapy, it is best to consider a bladder neck incision or transurethral incision of the prostate and keep ablation to a strict minimum. The goal is to simply open the outlet, not remove all the tissue. Regrowth is minimal after radiation, and symptoms in a postradiated patient are more likely to be caused by a high bladder neck, elevated middle lobe, or "tight" coaptation of the lateral lobes rather than by a large prostate.

Postoperative Care

Basic Management

Postoperatively, the patients are managed with a standard 2-way 20 F Foley catheter for 1–2 days.

Stretching of the bladder during the procedure often renders patients transiently hypotonic, and placing an overnight Foley catheter preemptively manages the risk of urinary retention, which could result in a return visit to the emergency department. If a patient was self-catheterizing or in urinary retention before the procedure, it is recommended for the catheter to be left for 3–5 days to be removed at home by the patient or in clinic after a voiding trial.

The vast majority of patients are discharged the same day as the procedure, with a smaller percentage staying overnight for observation. Therapeutically, anticoagulated patients may be kept overnight, but 3-way irrigation is rarely required.

Patients are discharged with antimuscarinic medication to be taken on an as-needed basis. They either stop alpha blockers and 5-ARI's or finish what they have at home. Acetaminophen or ibuprofen is taken as needed. Patients are seen at 4 weeks for a uroflow and a post-void residual measurement. Further follow-up after that point is case specific.

Bladder Recovery

Bladder recovery is a process that varies between patients according to the level of preexisting bladder decompensation prior to surgery. Symptoms are similar to those encountered after a TURP or open prostatectomy and include short-term exacerbation of irritative voiding symptoms, transient incontinence (stress and/or urge), retrograde ejaculation, urethral strictures, and urinary retention. True dysuria is uncommon with holmium, but some patients might have overactivity felt as pain at the tip of the penis. With ablative surgical therapies, stress incontinence is unusual. Antimuscarinic medication should be used in patients with persistent urge symptoms and continued until resolution is achieved. It is important to clearly communicate to the patient prior to surgery that the duration of recovery varies from patient to patient.

Radiated Patients

Most patients do not experience dysuria postoperatively; however, radiated patients are the one exception to this rule. As their prostatic tissue and urethra have already been "burned" by radiation, these patients may be more susceptible to dysuria after any transurethral procedure. Pyridium may have some effect, but in general, time is the best healer and pain medication may be necessary in the short term.

Published Outcomes

Surgical Outcomes

Since the mid-1990s, a number of HoLAP studies were conducted to evaluate the efficacy of HoLAP, including Drs. Fraundorfer and Gilling's paper. Holmium surgical treatments are attractive

Table 9.2 Long-term holmium laser ablation of the prostate results

Study	Participants (*n*)	Time to follow-up (year)	Prostate volume (cc) (range)	IPSS Pre (range)	IPSS Post (range)	Q_{max} (mL/s) Pre (range)	Q_{max} (mL/s) Post (range)	PVR (mL) Pre (range)	PVR (mL) Post (range)	Reoperation rate (%)
Kumar et al. [12]	15	0.25	121.82 (80–203)	20.41**	5.7**	6.92	15.06	_	_	5
Herrick et al. [23]	37	1	34.1	21.2	11.5	_	_	169.3	64	10.8
Tan et al. [24]	34	7	40.5 (14–133)	18.8 (8–34)**	10.0 (0–26)**	9.2 (4–16)	16.8 (5–35)	_	_	15
Barski et al. [25]	42	3	40 (10–130)	18.1 (4–35)	7.7 (1–21)	10.6 (1.7–29)	17.8 (3–36.9)*	80 (0–1,600)	0 (0–270)*	17.4
Elmansy et al. [26]	57	3	33.1 (10–60)	20 (8–35)	5.9 (0–20)	6.7 (3.1–15)	17.7 (5.4–42.8)	205 (10–900)	38.8 (0–340)	7
Mottet et al. [15]	8	1	36.7	21.7	6.5	8.8	19.9	_	_	5.8

*Longest follow-up was 12 months
**AUA score instead of IPSS

Table 9.3 Long-term complications of holmium laser ablation of the prostate

Study	Participants (*n*)	Time to follow-up (year)	Prostate volume (cc) (range)	Urge incontinence (%)	Urethral stricture (%)	Bladder neck contracture (%)	Prostate CA (%)	Reoperation rate (%)
Kumar et al. [12]	15	0.25	121.82 (80–203)	0	0	5		5
Herrick et al. [23]	37	1	34.1	_	_	_	_	10.8
Tan et al. [24]	34	7	40.5 (14–133)	_	_	_	_	15
Barski et al. [25]	42	3	40 (10–130)	2.2	3	0.7	_	17.4
Elmansy et al. [26]	57	3	33.1 (10–60)	1.8	3.5	5.3	1.8	7
Mottet et al. [15]	8	1	36.7	4.3	_	_	_	5.8

*Longest follow-up was 12 months
**AUA score instead of IPSS

because they produce minimal bleeding and tissue edema, virtually no delayed tissue sloughing, and are safe to use in therapeutically anticoagulated patients [13, 19–21]. HoLAP improves early functional outcomes with same-day discharge, early return to normal activity, and minimal impact on erectile function [10]. Results of the major studies conducted using HoLAP are displayed in Tables 9.2 and 9.3. In a study evaluating sexual function after HoLAP, Elshal et al. found no difference between the pre- and postop International Index of Erectile Function 15-item questionnaire scores when evaluating the group as a whole. Specifically, the IIEF was unchanged in 24.4 %, improved in 29.4 %, and declined in 41.2 % [22]. Outcomes from various published studies are depicted in Tables 9.1 and 9.2 [12, 15, 23–26].

Operative Time

In a study by Elzayat [13] comparing HoLAP to photoselective vaporization (PVP), the most commonly used comparative laser technique, HoLAP was shown to require more time (approximately 14 min longer than PVP). This is probably due to the thermomechanical effect of holmium being more suited to the cutting of tissue as opposed to ablation [11]. That said, due to its high absorption by water, prostate glands with high water content will ablate more quickly, such as with prostate edema from an indwelling catheter and/or BPH that has not been treated with finasteride. Despite the slower ablation time, all other operative and postoperative results have been shown to be similar with significant improvements in flow rate, post-void residual, and International Prostate Symptom (IPSS) and bother scores. In addition, outcomes have been durable with up to 3 years of follow-up [26].

User-Friendliness and Convenience

In addition to the benefits provided by early and long-lasting symptom relief, HoLAP is urologist-friendly because it offers a relatively short learning curve. Unlike other surgical techniques for BPH, the learning curve for HoLAP is relatively flat as the steps are relatively simple [27]. Yap et al. evaluated the difference in operative time and outcomes between an experienced HoLAP practitioner and residents in their third year of training, under the supervision of the experienced surgeon. There was a difference of 11 min in procedure time favoring the experienced practitioner over the learner. However, the outcomes and complications were no different suggesting that HoLAP, even in the hands of a learner, is safe and yields excellent outcomes [23].

In addition, holmium lasers are more polyvalent than other laser energy sources because they can also be used simultaneously for other endourological applications (e.g., bladder stones or urethral strictures).

Summary

While TURP has long held the throne of "gold standard" for endoscopic surgical treatment of BPH, there is no doubt that newer technologies have challenged the crown. Holmium laser energy exhibits a number of favorable characteristics that make it an ideal energy source for BPH treatment. The superficial absorption in a fluid environment makes it arguably one of the safest energies available. The ability of the surgeon to use either an end-fire or side-fire fiber allows for surgeons of all abilities to treat most prostates. While slightly slower than some of the other energy sources available for ablation, the time difference is actually rather minimal, and efficiency does increase as the surgeon gains more experience. Prostate enucleation requires a greater skill set and takes longer to learn than ablation, making HoLAP an attractive technique to many surgeons. HoLAP outcomes are excellent with durable results and minimal complications. Holmium energy has stood the test of time for over a decade and continues to be a valuable tool for use in patients requiring transurethral surgery of the prostate.

References

1. Costello AJ, Bowsher WG, Bolton DM, Braslis KG, Burt J. Laser ablation of the prostate in patients with benign prostatic hypertrophy. Br J Urol. 1992; 69(6):603–8.
2. Gilling PJ, Cass CB, Malcolm AR, Fraundorfer MR. Combination holmium and Nd:YAG laser ablation of the prostate: initial clinical experience. J Endourol. 1995;9(2):151–3.
3. Gilling PJ, Kennett K, Das AK, Thompson D, Fraundorfer MR. Holmium laser enucleation of the prostate (HoLEP) combined with transurethral tissue morcellation: an update on the early clinical experience. J Endourol. 1998;12(5):457–9.

4. AUA. AUA guidelines on the management of benign prostatic hyperplasia: diagnosis and treatment recommendations. American Urological Association Education and Research, Inc.
5. Oelke M, Bachmann A, Descazeaud A, Emberton M, Gravas S, Michel MC, et al. EAU guidelines on the treatment and follow-up of non-neurogenic male lower urinary tract symptoms including benign prostatic obstruction. Eur Urol. 2013;64(1):118–40.
6. Tanagho EA, McAninch J. Smith's general urology. 15th ed. New York: Lange Medical Books/McGraw Hill; 2000. p. 451–63.
7. Te AE. The development of laser prostatectomy. BJU Int. 2004;93(3):262–5.
8. Teichmann HO, Herrmann TR, Bach T. Technical aspects of lasers in urology. World J Urol. 2007; 25(3):221–5.
9. Jansen ED, van Leeuwen TG, Motamedi M, Borst C, Welch AJ. Temperature dependence of the absorption coefficient of water for midinfrared laser radiation. Lasers Surg Med. 1994;14(3):258–68.
10. Lerner LB, Tyson MD. Holmium laser applications of the prostate. Urol Clin North Am. 2009;36(4):485–95, vi.
11. Te AE, Lee R. Holmium laser enucleation of the prostate: an evolving prostatectomy technique. J Urol. 2010;184(2):641–2.
12. Kumar SM. Rapid communication: holmium laser ablation of large prostate glands: an endourologic alternative to open prostatectomy. J Endourol. 2007;21(6):659–62.
13. Elzayat EA, Al-Mandil MS, Khalaf I, Elhilali MM. Holmium laser ablation of the prostate versus photoselective vaporization of prostate 60 cc or less: short-term results of a prospective randomized trial. J Urol. 2009;182(1):133–8.
14. Tan AH, Gilling PJ. Holmium laser prostatectomy: current techniques. Urology. 2002;60(1):152–6.
15. Mottet N, Anidjar M, Bourdon O, Louis JF, Teillac P, Costa P, et al. Randomized comparison of transurethral electroresection and holmium: YAG laser vaporization for symptomatic benign prostatic hyperplasia. J Endourol. 1999;13(2):127–30.
16. Kollmeier MA, Stock RG, Cesaretti J, Stone NN. Urinary morbidity and incontinence following transurethral resection of the prostate after brachytherapy. J Urol. 2005;173(3):808–12.
17. Lumenis. Lumenis laser fibers for the VersaPulse® PowerSuite™ Family. The Lumenis Group of Companies; 2009 [5/26/2013]; Available from: http://www.lumenis.com/urologyekit/media/PDF/3PB-006360_rC_fibers_br_lores.pdf.
18. Goldfischer EKS, Kuo RL, David R, Hurley L. HoLAP technique and tips. San Antonio: Lumenis; 2005 [cited 5/26/2013]; Available from: http://www.surgical.lumenis.com/pdf/AUABooth Abstracts.pdf.
19. Aho TF, Gilling PJ, Kennett KM, Westenberg AM, Fraundorfer MR, Frampton CM. Holmium laser bladder neck incision versus holmium enucleation of the prostate as outpatient procedures for prostates less than 40 grams: a randomized trial. J Urol. 2005; 174(1):210–4.
20. Gilling PJ, Aho TF, Frampton CM, King CJ, Fraundorfer MR. Holmium laser enucleation of the prostate: results at 6 years. Eur Urol. 2008;53(4): 744–9.
21. Kuntz RM, Lehrich K, Ahyai SA. Holmium laser enucleation of the prostate versus open prostatectomy for prostates greater than 100 grams: 5-year follow-up results of a randomised clinical trial. Eur Urol. 2008;53(1):160–6.
22. Elshal AM, Elmansy HM, Elkoushy MA, Elhilali MM. Male sexual function outcome after three laser prostate surgical techniques: a single center perspective. Urology. 2012;80(5):1098–104.
23. Herrick BW, Yap RL. It is safe to teach residents laser prostate surgery in the private practice setting. Urology. 2013;81(3):629–32.
24. Tan AH, Gilling PJ, Kennett KM, Fletcher H, Fraundorfer MR. Long-term results of high-power holmium laser vaporization (ablation) of the prostate. BJU Int. 2003;92(7):707–9.
25. Barski D, Richter M, Winter C, Arsov C, de Geeter P, Rabenalt R, et al. Holmium laser ablation of the prostate (HoLAP): intermediate-term results of 144 patients. World J Urol. 2012.
26. Elmansy HM, Elzayat E, Elhilali MM. Holmium laser ablation versus photoselective vaporization of prostate less than 60 cc: long-term results of a randomized trial. J Urol. 2010;184(5):2023–8.
27. Seki N, Naito S. Holmium laser for benign prostatic hyperplasia. Curr Opin Urol. 2008;18(1):41–5.

Holmium Enucleation of Prostate

10

Arman Adam Kahokehr and Peter J. Gilling

Introduction

Surgical techniques for the endoscopic management of patients with bladder outlet obstruction (BOO) resulting from BPH can be divided into three groups. These are vaporisation (removal of tissue by ablation), resection of tissue (excision of small chips and subsequent irrigation from bladder) and enucleation (removal of the adenoma from the surgical capsule and subsequent morcellation). Coagulation, a fourth group, is rarely employed currently. Enucleation is the endoscopic equivalent to open prostatectomy (OP) and a sophisticated form of laser prostatectomy involving dissection in anatomical planes with the energy source being a secondary consideration to the technique itself.

Laser use has evolved for a range of diseases faced by urologists. Many centres around the globe now rely on the advantages offered by lasers compared to other technologies both for endoscopic stone surgery and for endoscopic surgery for symptomatic benign prostate hyperplasia (BPH).

A.A. Kahokehr, M.B.Ch.B., Ph.D.
Department of Urology, Tauranga Hospital, Bay of Plenty District Health Board, Tauranga, New Zealand

P.J. Gilling, M.D. (Otago), FRACS (✉)
Department of Urology, Tauranga Hospital, Suite 6, 850 Cameron Road, 3112 Tauranga, New Zealand
e-mail: peter@urobop.co.nz

Laser Properties: Holmium: Yttrium-Aluminium-Garnet (Ho:YAG)

Absorption is the most important component in the light–tissue interaction, and laser energy is mostly absorbed by components of the treated tissue resulting in thermal effects and tissue penetrance. Molecular excitation leads to temperature increases which results in coagulation, vaporisation or carbonisation. The wavelength of laser light and type of tissue (based on the tissue chromophores present which absorb the radiation) define the effect of the laser on tissue.

The Ho:YAG laser operates at 2,120 nm with tissue water as the chromophore. High energy concentration in a pulsed manner results in steam bubbles with resultant disruption of prostate tissue. The laser heats water which absorbs energy at this wavelength. The vaporisation bubble is produced at the tip of the quartz or silica fibre (that is used to deliver the laser beam), and rapid expansion of the vapour bubble occurs. Molecules in contact with this bubble are destabilised. The tissue penetration of this laser is only 0.4 mm in prostate tissue. Coagulation is achieved simultaneously via dissipating heat, with minimal but sufficient coagulative necrosis and minimal charring. The physical properties of this laser make it suitable for use in different tissues, including stones, due to the fact that water makes up a significant component of most calculi. During soft

B. Chughtai et al. (eds.), *Treatment of Benign Prostatic Hyperplasia: Modern Alternative to Transurethral Resection of the Prostate*, DOI 10.1007/978-1-4939-1587-3_10,

tissue use in the prostate, the plane of enucleation is easy to develop due to the superior visibility offered by the pulsed holmium laser compared to alternative continuous mode energy sources. Good haemostasis is possible.

The simplest BPH procedure to learn and perform using the Ho:YAG laser is a bladder neck incision. This can be performed bilaterally or with a single incision using the high-powered (>50-W) holmium laser. Ablation (HoLAP), resection (HoLRP) and enucleation (HoLEP) are all possible, and dealing with bladder calculi at the same setting makes this a very versatile laser.

HoLEP Technique Evolution

The holmium laser for treatment of BPH was first reported in 1995. This technology for BPH evolved initially from HoLAP to HoLRP and subsequently into the HoLEP. Holmium prostatectomy was first reported by Gilling et al. [1]. By initially combining the neodymium:YAG laser for circumferential coagulation and then the Ho:YAG laser for ablation (later utilising the Ho:YAG beam only), all parameters measured were significantly improved. HoLAP has been compared with TURP in only one RCT that showed a similar improvement in International Prostate Symptom Score (IPSS) and Qmax between the two groups at 12 months follow-up [2]. With the development of holmium resection and enucleation techniques, there has been less interest in HoLAP, but with the introduction of the high-powered 100-W Ho-laser, ablation has become more efficient and remains a viable technique.

HoLRP was next developed as a way to overcome the inefficiencies of laser ablation while using the precise incisional qualities of the holmium wavelength [3]. The procedure involves complete resection of the prostatic adenoma, using a piecemeal incisional technique, down to the surgical capsule, with the creation of a transurethral resection of the prostate (TURP-like) cavity.

HoLRP has been studied in three RCTs and six reports [3–8]. Based on meta-analysis of these RCTs, HoLRP is as effective as TURP in terms of improvement of Qmax, improved symptoms, quality of life scores and durability [9]. HoLRP appeared to be superior to TURP in terms of transfusion rates, duration of catheterisation and hospitalisation and was more cost-effective than TURP [9–11]. The main disadvantage of HoLRP was the longer operative time, which can be up to 20–30 % longer than for standard TURP. This is primarily because of the time it takes to incise the lateral lobes into fragments small enough to be safely extracted by way of the urethra. With the evolution from HoLRP to HoLEP, the former technique has been performed less often; however, HoLRP remains a useful tool in those needing 'channel' prostatectomy in malignancy or repeat procedures for regrowth of benign adenoma.

With the development of a transurethral tissue morcellator and the evolution of the enucleation technique, HoLEP has become the main holmium-based technique. This most recent step in the evolution of the holmium laser prostatectomy has involved the development of a technique involving enucleation of the entire prostatic lobes using existing surgical tissue planes. Thus, the holmium laser fibre acts much like the index finger of the surgeon during an open prostatectomy in shelling out the adenoma. The lobes are then morcellated in the bladder using a customised tissue morcellator.

HoLEP results in an anatomically complete removal of adenoma from the surgical capsule and is the endoscopic equivalent to OP. The completeness of adenomatous tissue removal results in an average postoperative decrease in both PSA and prostate volume in the range of 70–90 % of the preoperative value in comparison to 30–45 % for ablation techniques. In terms of the surgical approach, laser enucleation in particular has proven to be a size-independent procedure, challenging the role of open prostatectomy as well as TURP, with equal efficiency and significantly reduced morbidity.

A tissue morcellator is utilised in this technique once the enucleated lobes are placed in the bladder. This allows histological assessment of retrieved tissue [8]. This anatomically complete technique has also resulted in a shift from resection to surgical enucleation for the proponents of plasmakinetic (bipolar) technology [12].

Fraundorfer and Gilling published the first HoLEP experience with the use of a morcellator in 1998 [13]. Fourteen patients with a mean gland volume of 98.6 ml were treated with a mean operating time of 98 min. Twelve patients were discharged catheter-free the following day. At 4 weeks, the mean Qmax was 25.2 ml/s and the mean IPSS score was 7.2. A later update of 64 patients, also in 1998, in the controlled clinical trial was published by Gilling et al. [14]. This confirmed the safety profile and the advantages of treating larger prostates with HoLEP.

The completeness of adenoma removal can be assessed indirectly by the change in serum PSA. Tinmouth et al. investigated 509 HoLEP patients at two leading institutions with preoperative transrectal ultrasonographic (TRUS) volume measurements: postoperative pathology and TRUS volume [15]. The mean weight of adenoma resected was 49.8 g (range 5–300 g) in the first group and 90.4 g (range 7.9–312 g) in the second group. The mean decrease in PSA was an impressive 81.7 % (range 6.0–1.1 ng/ml; $P<0.0001$) and 86.0 % (range 8.6–1.2 ng/ml; $P<0.0001$). TRUS volume decreased significantly from 111.9 cc to 26.5 cc. PSA correlated well with the weight of adenoma resected. Hence, PSA was shown to be a useful tool for the objective assessment of adenoma removal, as the reduction in PSA corresponds well to the weight of removed adenoma.

Randomised Trials

HoLEP has the highest number of RCTs comparing it to TURP and OP compared to any other laser technology available [16–28]. Based on meta-analysis of randomised trials, catheter time and hospital stay appear to be shortened consistently in patients undergoing HoLEP, and it is also superior to TURP with regard to postoperative complications [29].

The risk of clinically relevant bleeding and the need for blood transfusion are also minimal (none of the RCT reports suggest the need for blood transfusion). Perioperative and late adverse events are similar to TURP, including AUR secondary to blood clot formation, UTI, and bladder neck stricture disease or urethral stricture formation. Postoperative urgency occurs in 5.6 % and 2.2 % of cases after HoLEP and TURP, respectively. When compared to TURP, HoLEP results in a greater improvement in Qmax (weighted mean difference 1.48 ml/s, 95 % CI: 0.58–2.40; $p=0.002$), superior urodynamics and a greater IPSS reduction [30, 31] making HoLEP the only endoscopic procedure to date with superior functional efficacy compared to TURP.

HoLEP has been compared to OP in two RCTs in four published reports [18, 22, 32, 33] with reduced catheterisation, hospital stay and blood loss seen in the HoLEP arms and equivalence in durability and low reoperation rates with up to 5 years follow-up. This evidence makes HoLEP an alternative to OP and questions the role of OP in the laser era.

In a study looking at patients with urinary retention, the mean preoperative catheter time was 7 months, and a mean 56 g of tissue was enucleated [34]. The initial trial without catheter was successful in 81 % of patients in Group 1. All those who failed initially had a successful removal 1–2 weeks later. Hence, these data confirm that HoLEP can be safely performed in patients with urinary retention and is not associated with any increased morbidity when compared to HoLEP performed for lower urinary tract symptoms. HoLEP is effective in treating urinary retention.

Durability

Long-term RCT data with a mean follow-up of 7–10 years show that HoLEP results are durable, and most patients remain satisfied with less need for re-intervention than TURP patients with a mean IPSS score of 3.6 and mean Qmax of 26.9 cc/s described [28, 35]. Reoperation due to residual, or regrowth, of BPH occurred in 0.7 % of patients [35]. In prostates >100 ml, HoLEP proved to be as effective as OP, regarding improvement in micturition with equally low reoperation rates at 5-year follow-up [33] with

AUA symptom score of 3.0, and the mean Qmax was 24.4 cc per second in the HoLEP arm. Late complications comprised of urethral strictures and bladder neck contractures in 5 % of patients. No patient developed a recurrence of their bladder outlet obstruction.

Morcellation

The first morcellator employed by Gilling and Fraundorfer was a modified arthroscopic shaver introduced suprapubically. The technology and idea evolved into the first commercially available morcellator, the Versacut (Coherent, Inc.) (Fig. 10.1). Several other commercially available morcellators are now available including the Piranha (Richard Wolf UK Ltd) (Fig. 10.2), a Karl Storz prototype and the Morcelmed (Elmed). Mechanical morcellation was confirmed to be safe in 2002 by an Italian group in 114 patients soon after its release [36]. Bladder mucosal damage has been reported in some early case reports. This complication can generally be avoided by following the safety principles of morcellation:

- Distension of the bladder achieved by utilising two inflow irrigation channels
- Good visualisation of the morcellator blades at all times with excellent haemostasis
- Morcellating with the blades at the 6-o'clock position at the bladder neck and above the trigone

The maximum morcellation rates of the various morcellators have been recorded in an ex vivo study using cooked bovine heart to be Piranha 20 (19.3–21.4) g/min, Versacut 10.8 (8.2–13.1) g/min, Karl Storz prototype 9.8 (7.9–10.76) g/min and Richard Wolf prototype 38.6 (35.3–42.9) g/min [37]. These findings need to be assessed in clinical trials and in in vivo studies. Another recent objective evaluation of the commercially available morcellators by Cornu et al. reveals that the Wolf and Lumenis morcellators have similar aspiration power parameters (20.4 and 22.2 mL/s), and the morcellating power was 2.5 and 6 g of tissue per minute, respectively [38]. The cutting part of the Wolf morcellator was under visual control, whereas the distal part of the cutting device was out of view with the Lumenis device. Evaluation of the nephroscopes showed that the field of vision was larger with the Storz compared to the Wolf, and irrigation flow was 0.35 and 0.52 l/min, respectively.

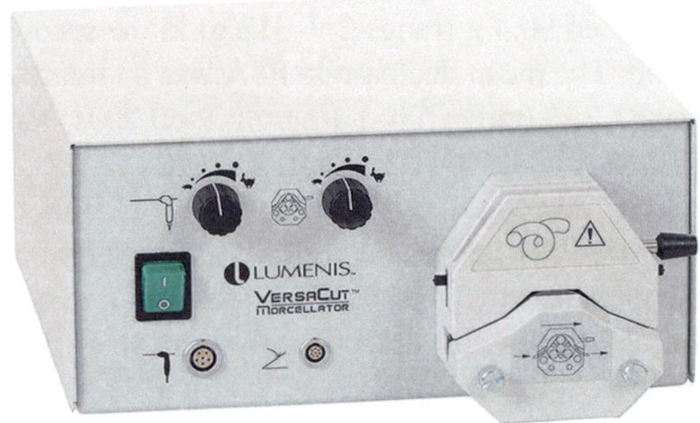

Fig. 10.1 Versacut morcellator (Lumenis Ltd.) (Used with permission)

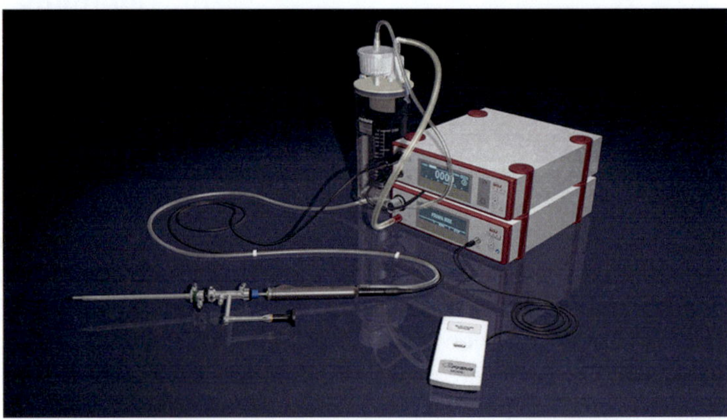

Fig. 10.2 Richard Wolf Piranha morcellator (Used with permission)

As suggested by the authors, these objective data could be the basis for a prospective trial comparing the two devices.

Cost

Holmium prostatectomy is a cost-effective approach (25 % cheaper than TURP) with reduced nursing to manage bladder irrigation and clot retention due to the reduced risk of bleeding following this procedure [11]. The cost advantage of both reusable laser fibres and morcellator blades utilised during HoLEP eliminates the costly disposals incurred by other techniques. In a prospective study, the cost of HoLEP was almost 10 % (about $600) less than that of OP [39] with the majority of savings in the length of hospital stay and in favour of HoLEP. Long-term follow-up of HoLEP shows the durability of the excellent postoperative results. These findings, plus the fact that the HoLEP procedure is prostate size independent, make a strong case for it being the new reference standard for transurethral surgery of symptomatic BPH.

Histology

The advantage of HoLEP over other ablative laser technologies, such as photovaporisation of the prostate (PVP), is that tissue is retrieved for histology. Histological findings between tissue specimens after standard TURP and HoLEP have been compared in a prospective study by Naspro et al. [40] in 80 patients. Prostatic architecture was maintained in the HoLEP group, especially in the central areas of the enucleated tissue. A percentage of prostatic tissue obtained from HoLEP is lost by vaporisation and coagulation. These differences did not alter the pathologist's ability in detecting malignancy.

Sexual Function

Randomised data shows no significant differences in postoperative erectile and orgasmic function assessed by the international index of erectile function (IIEF), a validated questionnaire, between patients undergoing either TURP or HoLEP [20]. Both TURP and HoLEP seem to cause an alteration of the IIEF orgasmic function domain due to retrograde ejaculation. This is an issue that needs to be discussed preoperatively with patients undergoing any transurethral surgery for BPH involving tissue removal.

Other Aspects of Safety

Intraoperative concerns regarding noise level of the laser machine have been raised. Using a handheld decibel metre to measure sound levels at six different areas within the operating theatre during three different phases of laser activity, it has been shown that laser machine noise levels (VersaPulse, Lumenis) during HoLEP are well within the limits described by the European Physical Agents Directive on Noise, which have been devised to protect against noise-induced hearing loss [41].

Technique

Equipment Required

We currently utilise a VersaPulse holmium laser (Lumenis, Santa Clara, California) with a 550-μm end firing fibre. The setting is 2.0 J at 50 Hz (100 W). The laser fibre is placed through a protective 6-F *ureteral catheter* and secured with a Luer-Lock injection port. HoLEP is performed using a 27-F continuous flow resectoscope (Karl Storz, Germany). The inner sheath is modified by incorporating a *laser fibre channel* and bridge as a single instrument. A standard 30° telescope is used. The irrigating solution is 0.9 % saline. The morcellator telescope (Storz long nephroscope) has an offset lens and a 5-mm working channel. The Versacut morcellator (Lumenis) (Fig. 10.1) comprises a handpiece with reciprocating blades, controller box with high-powered suction pump, and foot pedal. There are other commercially available morcellators, and we also utilised the Piranha morcellator (Wolf) (Fig. 10.2).

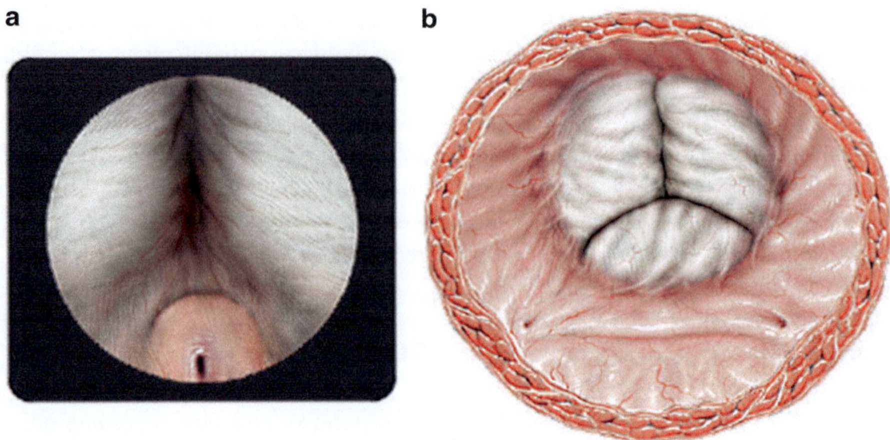

Fig. 10.3 (**a**) Endoscopic and (**b**) intravesicle view of the obstructing prostate (From Gilling P. Holmium Laser Enucleation of the Prostate (HoLEP). BJU Int 2007;101:131–142. Reprinted with permission from John Wiley and Sons)

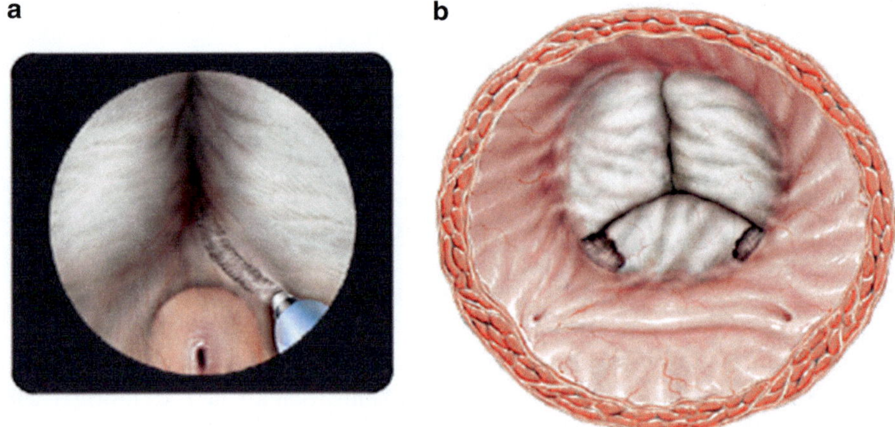

Fig. 10.4 (**a**) Endoscopic and (**b**) intravesicle view of the bladder neck incisions made at the 5- and 7-o'clock positions (From Gilling P. Holmium Laser Enucleation of the Prostate (HoLEP). BJU Int 2007;101:131–142. Reprinted with permission from John Wiley and Sons)

Step 1: Bladder Neck Incisions

After insertion of the resectoscope and general cystoscopy to assess for secondary pathology and the location of the ureteric orifices (Fig. 10.3), bladder neck incisions are made, either a single one at the 5-o'clock position or at both the 5- and 7-o'clock positions. The depth is increased until all circular fibres have been divided (Fig. 10.4). This aids in identifying the surgical capsule of the prostate. The landmark for the depth of dissection for the rest of the procedure is thus set. The incisions are lengthened down just adjacent to the verumontanum. The laser fibre is *kept close* to the beak of the resectoscope so that the resectoscope beak can be used to separate tissue during the dissection. The incision(s) is widened slightly laterally by undermining the lateral lobes. This aids to define the plane of dissection for the enucleation of the lateral lobes, which comes later, and also allows irrigant to flow more easily along these incisions to improve vision. If the bladder neck is particularly high, with a

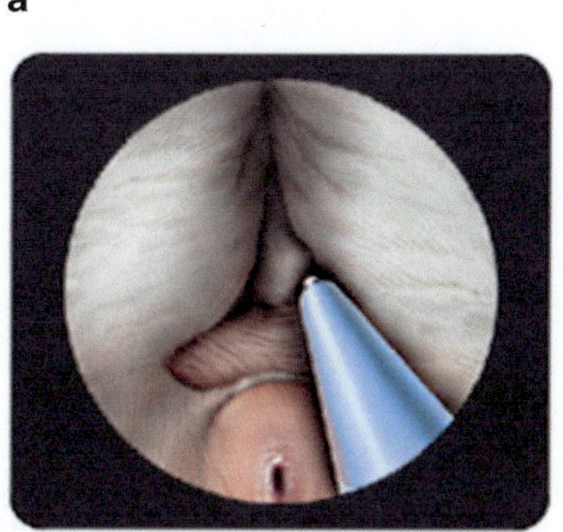

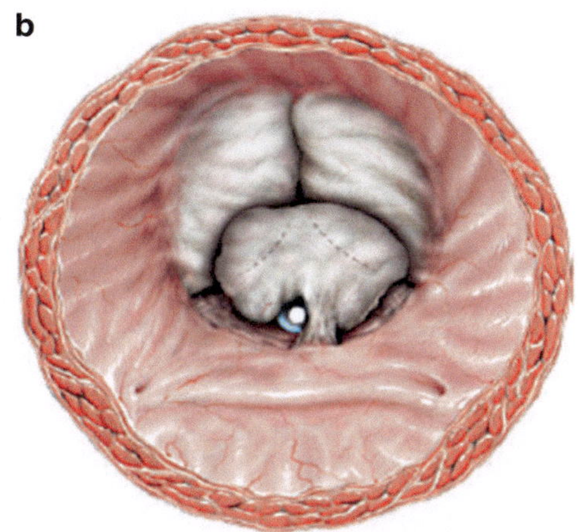

Fig. 10.5 (**a**) Endoscopic and (**b**) intravesicle view of median lobe enucleation (From Gilling P. Holmium Laser Enucleation of the Prostate (HoLEP). BJU Int 2007;101:131–142. Reprinted with permission from John Wiley and Sons)

large median lobe, it is often easier to find the correct plane just proximal to the verumontanum on either side of it, and then later connect this transverse incision with one made at the bladder neck at the 5- or 7-o'clock position. Bothersome superficial mucosal bleeding can occur at the apex on either side of the verumontanum, and defocusing the beam by pulling the fibre back slightly can coagulate these vessels effectively.

Step 2: Median Lobe Enucleation

The distal ends of the bladder neck incisions are then joined just proximal to the verumontanum with a transverse incision, and the median lobe is dissected on the capsule in a retrograde fashion toward the bladder neck. The beak of the resectoscope is important during this step, as it manipulates the median lobe up into the bladder allowing the laser to dissect the adenoma off the capsule (Fig. 10.5). Care must be taken not to go too deeply and undermine the bladder neck. After some experience, this step can usually be performed in a continuous manner with a side to side cradle type of movement moving proximally. Often a smaller median lobe is taken with the right lateral lobe as a single fragment.

Step 3: Enucleation of the Lateral Lobes

The lateral lobes are then undermined on each side by extending the initial bladder neck incision laterally and circumferentially at the apex (in a *hockey stick* curved-type incision initially) (Fig. 10.6), working toward the 2- and 10-o'clock positions in turn and keeping the landmark position of the verumontanum in mind. The depth of the initial bladder neck incisions is used as a guide to the surgical capsule and the plane of dissection. Once found, the plane is clearly visible, and the lobes strip away easily as the lobe is enucleated (Fig. 10.7). The plane is developed from the apex toward the bladder neck (Fig. 10.8).

Once the limit of the *hockey stick* incision is reached, a bladder neck incision is then also made at the 12-o'clock position down to the capsule. Occasionally, the enucleation can be done circumferentially, and the entire adenomatous mass can be enucleated in a single piece. A sweeping motion is used to continue the incision circumferentially laterally, as well as distally (in a reverse *hockey stick* incision), until the resectoscope can be partially withdrawn, and the upper and lower resection planes can be visualised and connected (Fig. 10.8). *This is probably the most challenging part of the procedure as the lobes get larger*. In large prostates, it is occasionally difficult to judge how far back to carry the upper incision before sweeping down. Coming down too early leads to creating a new plane of dissection inside the proper plane, and continuing

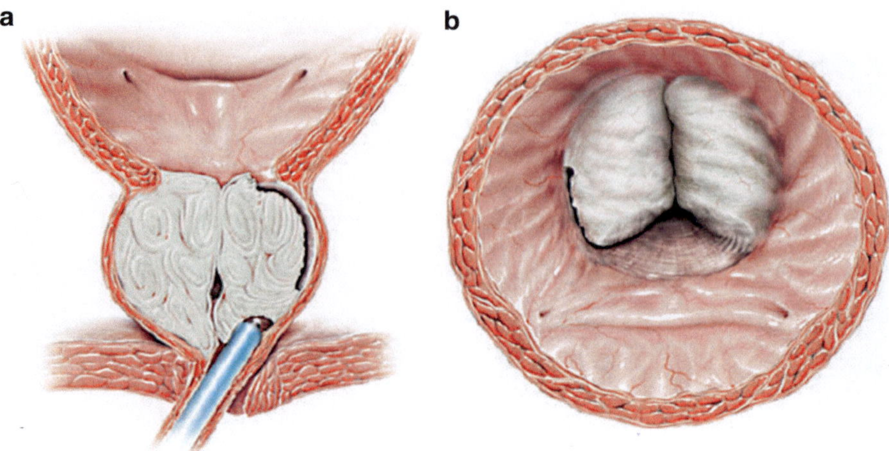

Fig. 10.6 (**a**) Frontal and (**b**) intravesicle view of right lateral lobe enucleation (From Gilling P. Holmium Laser Enucleation of the Prostate (HoLEP). BJU Int 2007;101:131–142. Reprinted with permission from John Wiley and Sons)

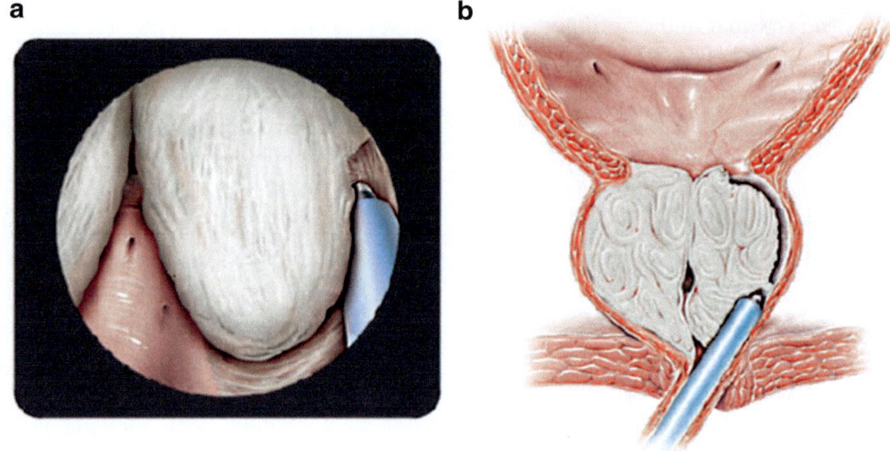

Fig. 10.7 (**a**) Endoscopic and (**b**) frontal view of right lateral lobe enucleation (From Gilling P. Holmium Laser Enucleation of the Prostate (HoLEP). BJU Int 2007;101:131–142. Reprinted with permission from John Wiley and Sons)

the upper incision too far runs the risk of injuring the external sphincter by going beyond the dissection limit.

Once each of the lateral lobes has been released from the bladder neck in turn (Fig. 10.9), haemostasis should be attended to with the defocused laser beam (Fig. 10.10). *This is important to achieve optimal visibility* for the next part of the operation, the morcellation of the enucleated prostate lobes.

Step 4: Morcellation of the Enucleated Prostate

Morcellation is via a dedicated nephroscope with a 5-mm working channel and offset telescope lens. The morcellator has two blades with a hollow inner lumen. One blade fits inside the other. These blades are 5 mm in outer diameter and are designed to pass down a working channel of similar size. A vacuum pump is connected to the morcellator handle to provide suction through the blades, and

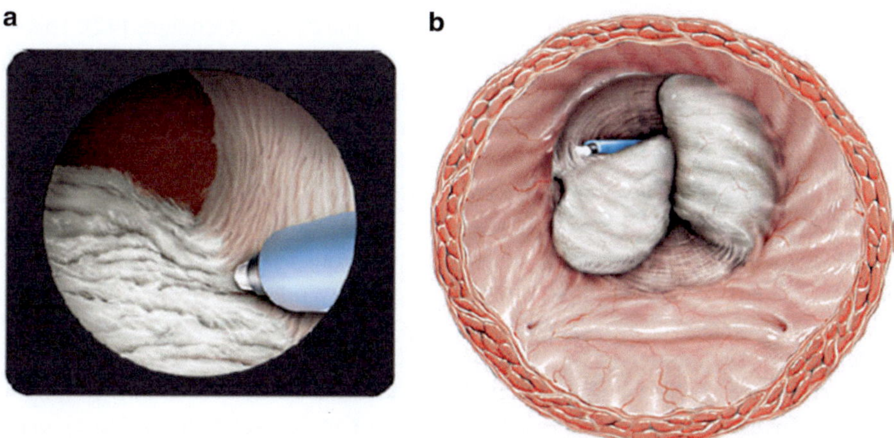

Fig. 10.8 (**a**) Endoscopic and (**b**) intravesicle view of completing right lateral lobe enucleation (From Gilling P. Holmium Laser Enucleation of the Prostate (HoLEP). BJU Int 2007;101:131–142. Reprinted with permission from John Wiley and Sons)

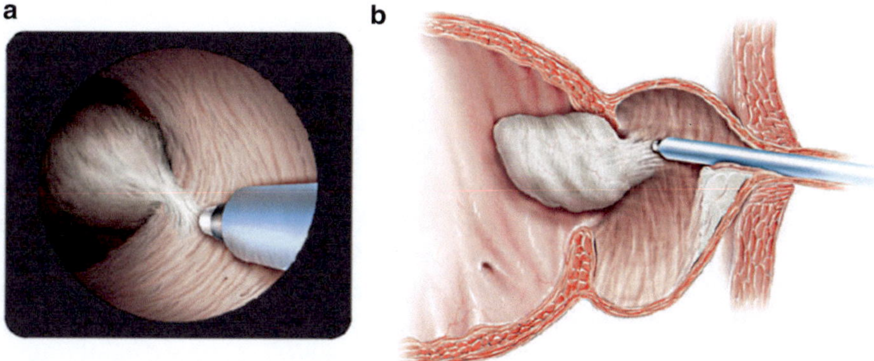

Fig. 10.9 (**a**) Endoscopic and (**b**) lateral view of completing right lateral lobe enucleation (From Gilling P. Holmium Laser Enucleation of the Prostate (HoLEP). BJU Int 2007;101:131–142. Reprinted with permission from John Wiley and Sons)

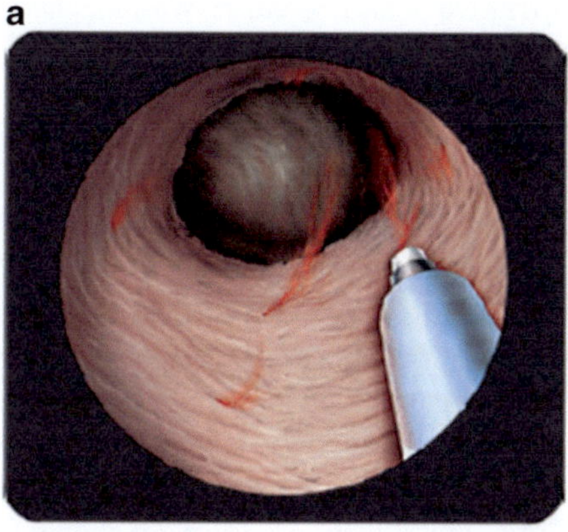

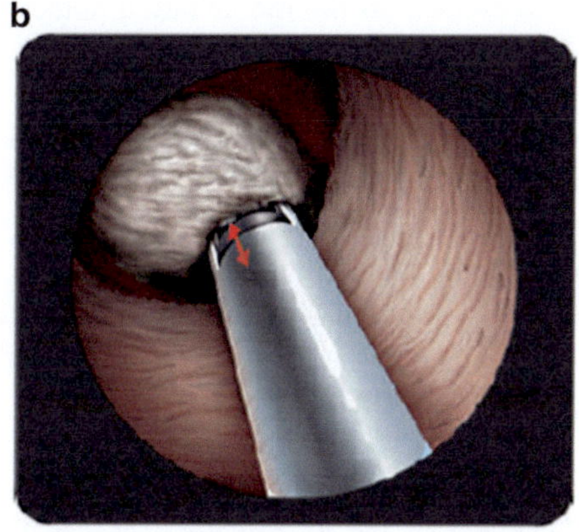

Fig. 10.10 (**a**) and (**b**) Endoscopic views of the prostate cavity at the end of enucleation, and subsequent morcellation (From Gilling P. Holmium Laser Enucleation of the Prostate (HoLEP). BJU Int 2007;101:131–142. Reprinted with permission from John Wiley and Sons)

device activation is controlled through a foot pedal. Saline should *be connected to both inflow ports* (outer resectoscope sheath and nephroscope) to ensure that the bladder remains distended during the morcellation process. This is crucial as the collapse of the bladder can lead to a morcellation injury to the bladder wall. The bladder is distended to full capacity. Perfect haemostasis is essential. The high-powered suction tubing is used to engage the prostate fragments (which are at this stage floating free in the bladder). The operator controls the variable suction using a graduated foot pedal (Versacut morcellator, Lumenis) to attract and then engage the fragments (Fig. 10.10). The foot pedal also controls the speed of the morcellator blades. The action of the blades slices off fragments of tissue that then pass through the hollow inner sheath and the suction tubing. This tissue is collected in netting fitted over the end of the tubing.

The operator must be careful not to engage the bladder mucosa. If this happens, the foot should be taken off the pedal immediately, and the pump suction released by opening the hinged gate on the roller pump. The injury to the bladder mucosa is generally minor and should not interfere with continuing the procedure. Large, full-thickness injuries can rarely lead to extravasation of irrigant or excessive bleeding, which will hamper visibility.

Prostatic tissue can be removed at a rate of up to and exceeding 10 g/min, but if the prostatic tissue is particularly fibrous, morcellation tends to proceed more slowly as these balls of dense fibrous tissue tend to bounce off the morcellation blades. Any smaller fragments ('beach balls') that are remaining can be evacuated with a Toomey syringe by way of the resectoscope sheath or by extraction with a tissue-grabbing loop. A 20-F 3-way urethral Foley catheter is then introduced into the bladder and removed the following morning.

Modified Tissue Removal

Initially, electrocautery was employed to resect the attached lobes before the morcellator was developed to facilitate tissue removal. Investigators subsequently described this modified tissue retrieval as the 'mushroom' technique [42]. This is when the enucleated prostate lobes are initially left attached at the bladder neck by a small pedicle of tissue. An electrocautery loop is then utilised to resect the lobe into small pieces retrievable with an evacuator such as a Toomey syringe or Ellik evacuator. While this may reduce the need for a mechanical morcellator overall, the morcellator is an efficient method of tissue removal following adequate enucleation. By employing the safety measures described, morcellation is safe and accepted.

Summary videos outlining the steps described above can be watched on-line at the following Web sites:

http://www.youtube.com/watch?v=mVW6uIagOgI
http://www.youtube.com/watch?v=A8Q_BkFKfTA

Power

Recently, there has been interest in utilising a moderate-powered holmium:YAG laser for performing HoLEP. One study evaluating a 50W device found similar safety profiles [43]. Utilisation of 70W and 80W holmium lasers seems to be also effective [44, 45]. At our institution, there is a randomised trial currently recruiting patients to compare the effects of the pulsed 50-W low-power laser and the 100-W laser.

Learning Curve

Operative learning curve was reached after 25 cases in another series from Korea [46] and about 15 cases in moderate-sized prostates in a series from China [47] and 20 patients from a series from Canada [48]. In a dedicated training centre, the efficiency of enucleation and morcellation during the learning curve peaked around 50 cases. The use of postoperative irrigation, catheter time and duration of hospitalisation was decreased as the medical and nursing staff also changed practice to take advantage of the excellent haemostatic properties of the holmium:YAG laser. With mentoring, complication rates were shown to be low, and outcome measures of success were consistent throughout the course of the 'learning curve' [41].

Summary

Various lasers and techniques are now available. The decision regarding which laser is most appropriate for a given patient should depend on the patient's comorbidities, the surgeon's expertise with different procedures and the availability of different laser resources. The selection of energy source in the future is likely to be a matter of personal choice [49]. However, to answer the question of 'which laser is best for BPH surgery', HoLEP has the greatest level 1 evidence with the longest follow-up to date, is cost-effective and is the only technique which can reliably replace open prostatectomy.

References

1. Gilling PJ, Cass CB, Malcolm AR, Fraundorfer MR. Combination holmium and Nd:YAG laser ablation of the prostate: initial clinical experience. J Endourol. 1995;9(2):151–3.
2. Mottet N, Anidjar M, Bourdon O, Louis JF, Teillac P, Costa P, et al. Randomized comparison of transurethral electroresection and holmium: YAG laser vaporization for symptomatic benign prostatic hyperplasia. J Endourol. 1999;13(2):127–30.
3. Gilling PJ, Kennett KM, Fraundorfer MR. Holmium laser resection versus transurethral resection of the prostate: results of a randomized trial with 2 years of follow-up. J Endourol. 2000;14(9):757–60.
4. Westenberg A, Gilling P, Kennett K, Frampton C, Fraundorfer M. Holmium laser resection of the prostate versus transurethral resection of the prostate: results of a randomized trial with 4-year minimum long-term followup. J Urol. 2004;172(2):616–9.
5. Kitagawa M, Furuse H, Fukuta K, Aso Y. A randomized study comparing holmium laser resection of the prostate to transurethral resection of the prostate. Br J Urol. 1997;Suppl 80:209.
6. Gilling PJ, Mackey M, Cresswell M, Kennett K, Kabalin JN, Fraundorfer MR. Holmium laser versus transurethral resection of the prostate: a randomized prospective trial with 1-year followup. J Urol. 1999;162(5):1640–4.
7. Hammad FT, Mark SD, Davidson PJ, Gowland SP, Gordon B, English SF. Holmium:YAG laser resection versus transurethral resection of the prostate: a randomized prospective trial with 1-year follow-up. ANZ J Surg. 2002;72:A138.
8. Das A, Kennett KM, Sutton T, Fraundorfer MR, Gilling PJ. Histologic effects of holmium:YAG laser resection versus transurethral resection of the prostate. J Endourol. 2000;14(5):459–62.
9. Tooher R, Sutherland P, Costello A, Gilling P, Rees G, Maddern G. A systematic review of holmium laser prostatectomy for benign prostatic hyperplasia. J Urol. 2004;171(5):1773–81.
10. Das A, Kennett K, Fraundorfer M, Gilling P. Holmium laser resection of the prostate (HoLRP): 2-year follow-up data. Tech Urol. 2001;7(4):252–5.
11. Fraundorfer MR, Gilling PJ, Kennett KM, Dunton NG. Holmium laser resection of the prostate is more cost effective than transurethral resection of the prostate: results of a randomized prospective study. Urology. 2001;57(3):454–8. Clinical Trial Comparative Study Randomized Controlled Trial Research Support, Non-U.S. Gov't.
12. Zhao Z, Zeng G, Zhong W, Mai Z, Zeng S, Tao X. A prospective, randomised trial comparing plasmakinetic enucleation to standard transurethral resection of the prostate for symptomatic benign prostatic hyperplasia: three-year follow-up results. Eur Urol. 2010;58(5):752–8.
13. Fraundorfer MR, Gilling PJ. Holmium:YAG laser enucleation of the prostate combined with mechanical morcellation: preliminary results. Eur Urol. 1998; 33(1):69–72.
14. Gilling PJ, Kennett K, Das AK, Thompson D, Fraundorfer MR. Holmium laser enucleation of the prostate (HoLEP) combined with transurethral tissue morcellation: an update on the early clinical experience. J Endourol. 1998;12(5):457–9.
15. Tinmouth WW, Habib E, Kim SC, Kuo RL, Paterson RF, Terry CL, et al. Change in serum prostate specific antigen concentration after holmium laser enucleation of the prostate: a marker for completeness of adenoma resection? J Endourol. 2005;19(5):550–4.
16. Tan AH, Gilling PJ, Kennett KM, Frampton C, Westenberg AM, Fraundorfer MR. A randomized trial comparing holmium laser enucleation of the prostate with transurethral resection of the prostate for the treatment of bladder outlet obstruction secondary to benign prostatic hyperplasia in large glands (40 to 200 grams). J Urol. 2003;170(4 Pt 1):1270–4.
17. Kuntz RM, Ahyai S, Lehrich K, Fayad A. Transurethral holmium laser enucleation of the prostate versus transurethral electrocautery resection of the prostate: a randomized prospective trial in 200 patients. J Urol. 2004;172(3):1012–6.
18. Kuntz RM, Lehrich K, Ahyai S. Transurethral holmium laser enucleation of the prostate compared with transvesical open prostatectomy: 18-month follow-up of a randomized trial. J Endourol. 2004;18(2): 189–91.
19. Montorsi F, Naspro R, Salonia A, Suardi N, Briganti A, Zanoni M, et al. Holmium laser enucleation versus transurethral resection of the prostate: results from a 2-center, prospective, randomized trial in patients with obstructive benign prostatic hyperplasia. J Urol. 2004;172(5 Pt 1):1926–9.
20. Briganti A, Naspro R, Gallina A, Salonia A, Vavassori I, Hurle R, et al. Impact on sexual function of holmium laser enucleation versus transurethral resection

of the prostate: results of a prospective, 2-center, randomized trial. J Urol. 2006;175(5):1817–21.
21. Gupta N, Sivaramakrishna, Kumar R, Dogra PN, Seth A. Comparison of standard transurethral resection, transurethral vapour resection and holmium laser enucleation of the prostate for managing benign prostatic hyperplasia of >40 g. BJU Int. 2006;97(1):85–9.
22. Naspro R, Suardi N, Salonia A, Scattoni V, Guazzoni G, Colombo R, et al. Holmium laser enucleation of the prostate versus open prostatectomy for prostates >70 g: 24-month follow-up. Eur Urol. 2006;50(3):563–8.
23. Neill MG, Gilling PJ, Kennett KM, Frampton CM, Westenberg AM, Fraundorfer MR, et al. Randomized trial comparing holmium laser enucleation of prostate with plasmakinetic enucleation of prostate for treatment of benign prostatic hyperplasia. Urology. 2006;68(5):1020–4.
24. Wilson LC, Gilling PJ, Williams A, Kennett KM, Frampton CM, Westenberg AM, et al. A randomised trial comparing holmium laser enucleation versus transurethral resection in the treatment of prostates larger than 40 grams: results at 2 years. Eur Urol. 2006;50(3):569–73.
25. Ahyai SA, Lehrich K, Kuntz RM. Holmium laser enucleation versus transurethral resection of the prostate: 3-year follow-up results of a randomized clinical trial. Eur Urol. 2007;52(5):1456–63.
26. Gilling PJ, Aho TF, Frampton CM, King CJ, Fraundorfer MR. Holmium laser enucleation of the prostate: results at 6 years. Eur Urol. 2008;53(4):744–9.
27. Montorsi F, Naspro R, Salonia A, Suardi N, Briganti A, Zanoni M, et al. Holmium laser enucleation versus transurethral resection of the prostate: results from a 2-center prospective randomized trial in patients with obstructive benign prostatic hyperplasia. J Urol. 2008;179(5 Suppl):S87–90.
28. Gilling PJ, Wilson LC, King CJ, Westenberg AM, Frampton CM, Fraundorfer MR. Long-term results of a randomized trial comparing holmium laser enucleation of the prostate and transurethral resection of the prostate: results at 7 years. BJU Int. 2012;109(3):408–11.
29. Tan A, Liao C, Mo Z, Cao Y. Meta-analysis of holmium laser enucleation versus transurethral resection of the prostate for symptomatic prostatic obstruction. Br J Surg. 2007;94(10):1201–8.
30. Ahyai SA, Gilling P, Kaplan SA, Kuntz RM, Madersbacher S, Montorsi F, et al. Meta-analysis of functional outcomes and complications following transurethral procedures for lower urinary tract symptoms resulting from benign prostatic enlargement. Eur Urol. 2010;58(3):384–97.
31. Lourenco T, Pickard R, Vale L, Grant A, Fraser C, MacLennan G, et al. Alternative approaches to endoscopic ablation for benign enlargement of the prostate: systematic review of randomised controlled trials. BMJ. 2008;337:a449.
32. Kuntz RM, Lehrich K. Transurethral holmium laser enucleation versus transvesical open enucleation for prostate adenoma greater than 100 gm.: a randomized prospective trial of 120 patients. J Urol. 2002; 168(4 Pt 1):1465–9.
33. Kuntz RM, Lehrich K, Ahyai SA. Holmium laser enucleation of the prostate versus open prostatectomy for prostates greater than 100 grams: 5-year follow-up results of a randomised clinical trial. Eur Urol. 2008;53(1):160–6.
34. Aho T, Fernando H, Suraparaju L. Safety and efficacy of holmium laser enucleation of the prostate for urinary retention. Eur Urol. 2006;Suppl 5(2):272.
35. Elmansy HM, Kotb A, Elhilali MM. Holmium laser enucleation of the prostate: long-term durability of clinical outcomes and complication rates during 10 years of followup. J Urol. 2010;186(5):1972–6.
36. Ivano V, Rodolfo H, Alberto M, Aleasundro P, Valenti S, Alberto V. Holmium laser enucleation of the prostate combined with mechanical morcellation: Initial Italian experience in 114 patients. Eur Urol. 2002;Suppl 1:169.
37. Ritter M, Krombach P, Bolenz C, Martinschek A, Bach T, Haecker A. Standardized comparison of prostate morcellators using a new ex-vivo model. J Endourol. 2012;26(6):697–700.
38. Cornu JN, Terrasa JB, Lukacs B. Ex-Vivo comparison of available morcellation devices during holmium laser enucleation of the prostate through objective parameters. J Endourol. 2012.
39. Salonia A, Suardi N, Naspro R, Mazzoccoli B, Zanni G, Gallina A, et al. Holmium laser enucleation versus open prostatectomy for benign prostatic hyperplasia: an inpatient cost analysis. Urology. 2006; 68(2):302–6.
40. Naspro R, Freschi M, Salonia A, Guazzoni G, Girolamo V, Colombo R, et al. Holmium laser enucleation versus transurethral resection of the prostate. Are histological findings comparable? J Urol. 2004; 171(3):1203–6.
41. Aho T, Maan Z, Pillai R. Noise levels during holmium laser enucleation of the prostate (HOLEP). Eur Urol. 2006;Suppl 5(2):272.
42. Hochreiter WW, Thalmann GN, Burkhard FC, Studer UE. Holmium laser enucleation of the prostate combined with electrocautery resection: the mushroom technique. J Urol. 2002;168(4 Pt 1):1470–4.
43. Rassweiler J, Roder M, Schulze M, Muschter R. Transurethral enucleation of the prostate with the holmium: YAG laser system: how much power is necessary? Urologe A. 2008;47(4):441–8.
44. Hurle R, Vavassori I, Piccinelli A, Manzetti A, Valenti S, Vismara A. Holmium laser enucleation of the prostate combined with mechanical morcellation in 155 patients with benign prostatic hyperplasia. Urology. 2002;60(3):449–53.
45. Vavassori I, Hurle R, Vismara A, Manzetti A, Valenti S. Holmium laser enucleation of the prostate combined with mechanical morcellation: two years of experience with 196 patients. J Endourol. 2004;18(1):109–12.
46. Jeong CW, Oh JK, Cho MC, Bae JB, Oh SJ. Enucleation ratio efficacy might be a better predictor

to assess learning curve of holmium laser enucleation of the prostate. Int Braz J Urol. 2012;38:362–71. Discussions 72.
47. Du C, Jin X, Bai F, Qiu Y. Holmium laser enucleation of the prostate: the safety, efficacy, and learning experience in China. J Endourol. 2008;22:1031–6.
48. El-Hakim A, Elhilali MM. Holmium laser enucleation of the prostate can be taught: the first learning experience. BJU Int. 2002;90:863–9.
49. Gilling PJ. Laser enucleation is increasingly becoming the standard of care for treatment of benign prostatic hyperplasia of all sizes. Eur Urol. 2013.

11 Thulium Resection of Prostate

Joseph J. Pariser and Doreen E. Chung

Introduction

The high-power thulium laser was introduced in 2005 for the treatment of BPH [1]. Its peak absorption, 2 μm, is very close to the peak absorption of water in tissue. This theoretically translates to high vaporization efficiency without deep thermal damage. An ex vivo study using porcine kidneys by Wendt-Nordahl et al. demonstrated a lower bleeding rate with the 70 W thulium laser and the 80 W KTP laser as compared to electrocautery transurethral resection of the prostate (TURP) [2]. In comparison to the 80 W KTP laser, the 70 W laser had a higher tissue ablation rate.

So far most published studies using the thulium laser for BPH have employed enucleation, vapoenucleation, or laser resection techniques (see Chap. 12), which this laser is ideal for. Studies using the 70–120 W thulium laser systems demonstrate good efficacy of these procedures with low morbidity and few complications in mostly small- and medium-sized prostates [3]. Safety and efficacy have also been demonstrated in patients taking oral anticoagulation [4]. Comparative studies have been published comparing thulium laser prostatectomy to monopolar TURP, bipolar TURP, and HoLEP. Compared to all these techniques, thulium laser prostatectomy had a longer operative time and demonstrated superior blood loss compared to TURP techniques.

However, the thulium laser is also a very safe and effective tool for laser vaporization of the prostate with very few studies describing the outcomes of this technique [5–7]. In this chapter, we will discuss our preferred technique for thulium laser vaporization of the prostate and associated data.

Technique

Our technique for thulium laser vaporization of the prostate (ThuVP) is simple and systematic. It is easily learned by the general urologist and is similar to a traditional TURP (see Fig. 11.1).

Equipment needed includes a continuous flow laser cystoscope, with a minimum caliber of 23 French. The irrigation is hung at approximately 70 cm above the patient. We begin at a low setting of 80 W for demarcating the borders of vaporization. Vaporization itself can be done at the maximum power setting of the laser.

J.J. Pariser, M.D.
Section of Urology, Department of Surgery, University of Chicago Medical Center, Chicago, IL, USA
e-mail: joseph.pariser@uchospitals.edu

D.E. Chung, M.D., FRCSC (✉)
Section of Urology, Department of Surgery, University of Chicago Medical Center and Mount Sinai Hospital, Chicago, IL, USA
e-mail: doreenechung@gmail.com

B. Chughtai et al. (eds.), *Treatment of Benign Prostatic Hyperplasia: Modern Alternative to Transurethral Resection of the Prostate*, DOI 10.1007/978-1-4939-1587-3_11,

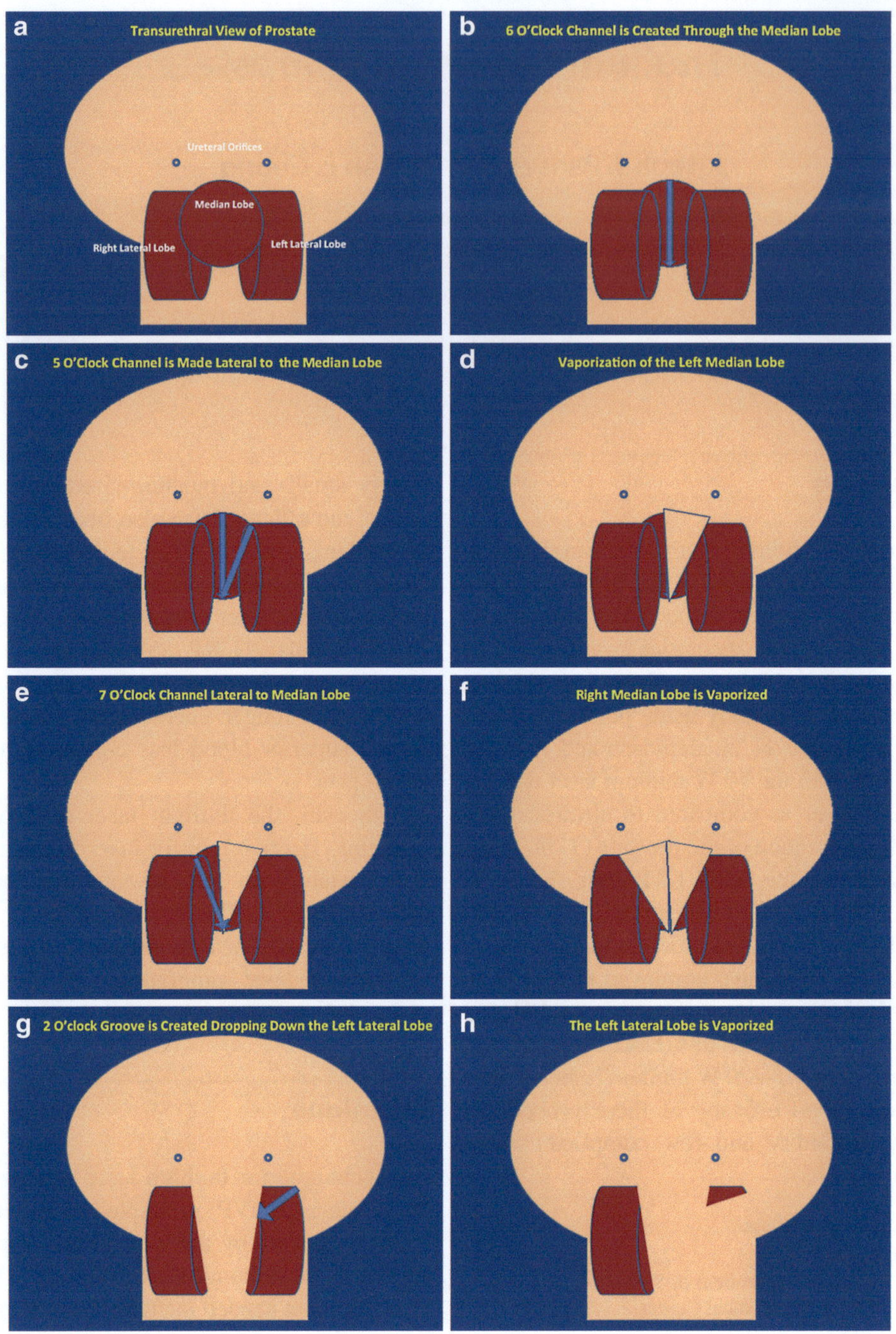

Fig. 11.1 (**a**) This is a transurethral view of the prostate with trilobar hypertrophy. (**b**) A groove is created at the 6 o'clock position facilitating the flow of irrigation and visualization of the ureteral orifices. (**c**) Next a channel is made at the 5 o'clock position lateral to the median lobe, separating the median and lateral lobes. (**d**) Vaporization of the left median lobe between these two channels is performed. (**e**) A channel is made at the 7 o'clock position separating the right median and lateral lobes. (**f**) The right median lobe is vaporized. (**g**) Next a groove is created at the 2 o'clock position, dropping down the left lateral lobe. (**h**) The left lateral lobe is vaporized. (**i**) A groove is made at the 10 o'clock position dropping down the right lateral lobe. (**j**) The right lateral lobe is vaporized. (**k**) The anterior tissue between 10 o'clock and 2 o'clock is vaporized. Any remaining apical tissue is vaporized as well

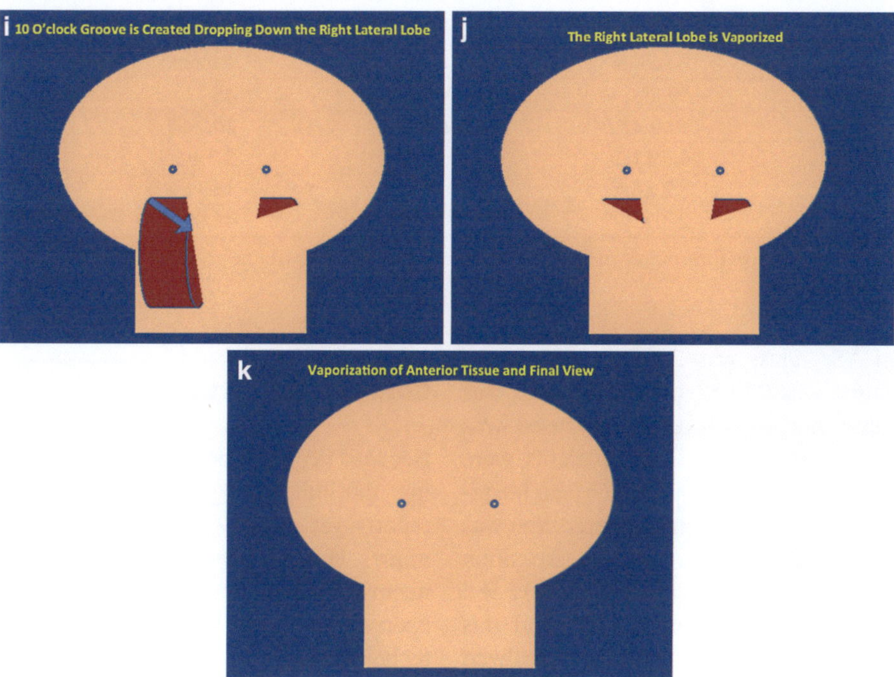

Fig. 11.1 (continued)

A channel is made at the 6 o'clock position to facilitate the flow of saline and to optimize visualization. It is very important at this point in the procedure to ensure that both ureteral orifices are visualized with certainty. Next a groove is made at the 5 o'clock position separating the left median from lateral lobe. The intervening tissue is vaporized. The same steps are performed to vaporize the right median lobe. To drop down the left lateral lobe, a channel is made at the 2 o'clock position. The lateral left lateral lobe is then vaporized. The right lateral lobe is dropped down by making a channel at the 10 o'clock position and then is vaporized. The anterior tissue between 10 and 2 o'clock is then vaporized. Finally, any remaining apical tissue is vaporized. In order to attempt to preserve antegrade ejaculation, some apical tissue near the verumontanum may be left intact.

At the end of the procedure, a 20Fr 2-way Foley catheter with a 30 cc balloon is inserted and connected to straight drainage. It is kept in place for 1–2 nights. Most patients are discharged the same day as surgery.

Data

Thus far, few studies have described outcomes of thulium laser vaporization of the prostate. We have been performing a simple methodical anatomically based technique for thulium laser vaporization of the prostate since 2010. Following institutional review board approval, we retrospectively reviewed medical records from December 2010 to October 2013, including 68 men who underwent ThuVP by a single surgeon [5].

Nine patients with known prostate cancer who underwent ThuVP were excluded. At baseline, mean age was 66 ± 10 years. Mean IPSS and QoL were 19.8 ± 8.0 and 4.5 ± 1.1. Mean Qmax, PVR, and prostate volume were 5.3 ± 4.5 mL/s, 220 ± 397 mL, and 57 ± 30 mL. Twenty-eight (47 %) patients were anticoagulated preoperatively. The most common indication for surgery was refractory LUTS (71 %) with urinary retention as the next most common reason (25 %). Other indications included recurrent hematuria, recurrent UTI, and bladder calculi.

Table 11.1 Efficacy parameters during follow-up

Parameter	Baseline	1 week	1 month	3 months
No. of patients (*n*)	59	52	45	43
IPSS	19.9±8.0	n/a	10.7±7.3	8.7±6.5
QoL	4.5±1.1	n/a	2.3±1.3	2.1±1.4
Qmax (mL/s)	5.2±4.5	15.3±6.6	16.1±8.0	14.6±6.8
PVR (mL)	220±397	28.4±54.3	48.0±86.9	45.1±62.8

$p<0.05$ for all postoperative time points in all measurements compared to baseline

Median ASA class was 2 (IQR 2–3). Mean operative time was 97±52 min, laser time was 34.6±18 min, and total laser energy used was 234±139 kJ. Forty-seven (78 %) patients were discharged the same day as surgery. Mean hospital stay was 0.4±1.0 days, and catheter time was 2.9±2.6 days. Continuous bladder irrigation (CBI) was administered in seven patients (12 %). Initially all patients were given CBI, and this practice was discontinued when it was realized that this was unnecessary. No blood transfusions were required. No significant change in serum sodium was seen (0.0±2.8 mEq/L, $p=0.78$).

Significant improvements were seen in all voiding parameters at each measured time interval, depicted in Table 11.1. Statistically significant improvements from baseline Qmax and PVR were noted at all time intervals (Fig. 11.1). Significant improvements were also seen in subjective measurements including IPSS and QoL. All 15 patients who presented in retention were voiding spontaneously at the time of their last follow-up. There were no major (≥Clavien class III) complications. Within 30 days of surgery, 6 (10 %) patients were treated for symptomatic UTI, and three patients (5 %) experienced clot retention requiring catheterization.

Between 30 and 60 days, 2 (3 %) patients developed postoperative urethral strictures requiring endoscopic treatment within 90 days of surgery. One patient with detrusor underactivity required repeat ThuVP 26 months following initial surgery for symptomatic regrowth of tissue. Overall these short-term results demonstrate that the ThuVP is a safe and effective procedure for the treatment of BPH. Studies with longer follow-up are needed to assess the durability of this procedure.

Comparative Studies

Because very few published studies exist regarding thulium laser vaporization, there are no reports yet directly comparing it to other techniques. However, thulium laser prostatectomy by means of vapoenucleation and vaporesection has been compared to TURP and to a HoLEP-type technique.

Several studies have been published comparing thulium laser prostatectomy with standard monopolar TURP [8]. Using a 50 W continuous wave thulium laser (LISA laser products OHG, Germany), Xia et al. performed thulium laser resection of the prostate-tangerine technique (TmLRP) and compared outcomes up to 12 months to standard TURP [8]. Fifty-two patients were randomized to TmLRP and 48 to TURP. There was a smaller decrease in hemoglobin in the TmLRP group versus TURP (0.92±0.82 vs. 1.46±0.65 g/dL, $p=0.0004$). At 1, 6, and 12 months, no significant differences were seen between groups in IPSS, QoL, Qmax, or PVR. No significant changes in IIEF-5 scores were seen compared to pre-op in either group. Overall this study suggested that subjective and objective improvements of this technique are similar to TURP but with lower morbidity.

More recently, a study was performed to compare the short-term efficacy and safety of TmLRP with a 50 W thulium laser to bipolar transurethral plasmakinetic prostatectomy (BiTURP) [9]. One hundred patients were randomized to TmLRP or BiTURP. Operative time was significantly longer in the TmLRP group (61±24 vs. 30±6 min, $p<0.05$), while catheterization time

(1.8 ± 0.4 vs. 3.2 ± 0.6 days, $p < 0.05$) and hospital stay (3.3 ± 0.8 vs. 4.1 ± 1.3 days, $p < 0.05$) were significantly shorter. No transfusions were required in either group. Significant improvements were seen in both groups at 1 and 3 months post-op. Compared to BiTURP, TmLRP was superior in safety, blood loss, and urethral stricture rate with similar improvements in IPSS, Qmax, and PVR.

Yang et al. published a comparative study of 158 patients randomized to TmLRP with a 100 W thulium laser and BiTURP, with all patients returning for 18-month follow-up [10]. TmLRP required a longer operation time (65 vs. 47 min, $p = 0.22$) than BiTURP but resulted in shorter hospital stay (2.5 vs. 4.6 days, $p = 0.026$), shorter catheterization time (2.1 cs. 3.5 days, $p = 0.026$), and lower drop in hemoglobin (−0.15 vs. −0.30 g/dL, $p = 0.045$). Similar improvements were seen in IPSS, QoL, Qmax, and PVR.

Conclusions

In summary, thulium laser vaporization of the prostate is a safe and effective procedure for the surgical treatment of BPH. Short-term data demonstrate significant improvements in objective and subjective voiding with few complications, but additional comparative studies are needed.

References

1. Fried N, Murray K. High-power thulium fiber laser ablation of urinary tissues at 1.94. J Endourol. 2005;19:25.
2. Wendt-Nordahl G, Huckele S, Honeck P, et al. Systemic evaluation of a recently introduced 2-μm continuous-wave thulium laser for vaporesection of the prostate. J Endourol. 2008;22:1041.
3. Gross A, Netsch C, Knipper S, et al. Complications and early postoperative outcome in 1080 patients after thulium vapoenucleation of the prostate: results at a single institution. Eur Urol. 2012;63:859.
4. Macchione L, Mucciardi G, Gali A, et al. Efficacy and safety of prostate vaporesection using a 120-W 2-μm continuous-wave Tm:YAG (RevoLix 2) in patients on continuous oral anticoagulant or antiplatelet therapy. Int Urol Nephrol. 2013;45:1545–51.
5. Pariser JJ, Famakinwa OJ, Pearce SM, et al. High-power thulium laser vaporization of the prostate: Short-term outcomes of safety and effectiveness. J Endourol. 2014.
6. Mattioli S, Munoz R, Recasens R, et al. Treatment of benign prostatic hyperplasia with the Revolix laser. Arch Esp Urol 2008;61:1037–43.
7. Vargas C, Garcia-Larrosa A, Capdevila S, et al. Vaporization of the prostate with 150-W thulium laser: complications with 6-month follow-up. J Endourol 2014;28:841–45.
8. Xia S, Zhuo J, Sun X, et al. Thulium laser versus standard transurethral resection of the prostate: a randomized prospective trial. Eur Urol. 2008;53:383.
9. Peng B, Wang G, Zheng J, et al. A comparative study of thulium laser resection of the prostate and bipolar transurethral plasmakinetic prostatectomy for treating benign prostatic hyperplasia. BJU Int. 2013;111:633.
10. Yang Z, Wang X, Liu T. Thulium laser enucleation versus plasmakinetic resection of the prostate: a randomized prospective trial with 18-month follow-up. Urology. 2013;81:396.

12 Thulium Enucleation of Prostate

Doreen E. Chung

Introduction

The thulium laser has several properties that make it an effective and versatile tool for use in urology. Its wavelength is adjustable between 1.75 and 2.22 μm to match the peak absorption of water in tissue, which is 1.94 μm. Higher absorption of laser radiation in the water in tissues theoretically translates to more efficient vaporization [1]. The fiber is diode pumped which gives it the capability of operating in either a pulsed mode or continuous wave mode. The pulsed mode is better suited for treating stones, whereas the continuous wave mode is more suitable for hemostasis and coagulation of tissue.

This laser has potential applications in the kidney, ureter, bladder, and prostate [2–5]. For minimally invasive prostate procedures, the thulium laser is ideal, with properties that make it comparable to both the holmium and GreenLight® laser.

D.E. Chung, M.D., FRCSC (✉)
Section of Urology, Department of Surgery, University of Chicago Medical Center and Mount Sinai Hospital, Chicago, IL, USA
e-mail: doreenechung@gmail.com

Laser Properties

The thulium laser has been previously evaluated for medical applications. However, power output was limited to <5 W, which was inadequate for the majority of urology applications. A new thulium laser system was introduced in 2005 with power output up to 150 W, making it a competitive for urologic applications [1].

Because the peak absorption of the thulium laser is closer to the peak absorption of water in tissue (see Fig. 12.1), there is a smaller zone of thermal damage created by this laser as compared to the holmium laser by a factor of 4 [6]. Decreasing thermal damage may help to decreased postoperative dysuria following minimally invasive prostate procedures, an adverse effect that is commonly associated with the GreenLight® laser.

The thulium laser system produces a single-mode perfect Gaussian spatial beam profile with a diameter of approximately 18 μm. Like the holmium laser beam, this beam can be confined to a standard silica optical fiber in a variety of diameters. In general silica fibers are flexible, robust, and reusable, decreasing the production cost and increasing the duration of usage of the fibers.

B. Chughtai et al. (eds.), *Treatment of Benign Prostatic Hyperplasia: Modern Alternative to Transurethral Resection of the Prostate*, DOI 10.1007/978-1-4939-1587-3_12,

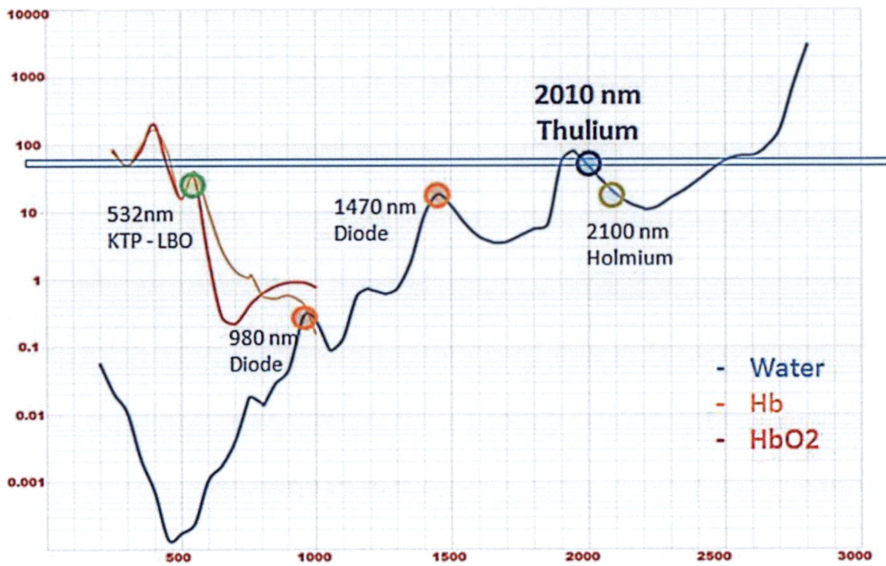

Fig 12.1 Peak absorption spectra

Ex Vivo Studies

Fried et al. studied the effect of a 40-W thulium laser (Model TLR-40-1940; IPG Photonics, Oxford, MA) on ex vivo animal tissues including canine prostate, canine bladder, and porcine ureter [1]. The animal models were used to represent the application of the laser for the following procedures: minimally invasive prostate surgery, incision of bladder neck contracture, and laser direct visual internal urethrotomy.

Eight canine prostates with a mean mass of 16.4±7.2 g were vaporized with the thulium laser with an ablation rate of 0.21±g/min. The efficacy rate was 7.6±kJ/g. The area of thermal coagulation was measured on H&E staining for all the tissues. This zone measured 500–2,000 μm in the canine prostate and 400–500 μm in the bladder. The extent of thermal damage in the ureter was to a radius of 600 μm.

These animal studies demonstrated that the thulium laser did indeed show promise as an effective tool for vaporization of the prostate as well as incision of bladder neck contractures. The ablation rate was relatively low in this study compared to the high-power holmium laser and the 80 and 100-W GreenLight® lasers, which have published ablation rates of 1–2 g/min [7, 8], but the power of the system used in the study was 40 W, far lower than the commercially available thulium systems available at that time, with maximum power up to 150 W of power.

In this study, the thermal coagulation zone was more extensive than predicted by the authors who hypothesized that the pulse of 10 ms used in this study was too long. Higher-power thulium lasers with up to 150 W should allow for the laser to provide sufficient energy for soft tissue ablation at shorter pulse widths.

An ex vivo study was done in isolated blood-perfused porcine kidneys to evaluate the effect of the continuous wave thulium laser on the prostate compared to electrocautery transurethral resection of the prostate (TURP) and the 80-W potassium-titanyl-phosphate (KTP) laser [9]. At the thulium laser power setting of 70 W, the thulium demonstrated a higher tissue ablation rate compared to the 80-W KTP laser (6.6±0.7 g after 10 min for the thulium vs. 4±0.5 g for the KTP laser). With TURP the ablation rate was much higher than for either of the lasers. Only 30 s were required to resect tissue with the same surface area, 8.3±0.4 g. It is notable, however, that the contemporary GreenLight XPS® was not used in this study.

Hemostasis and coagulation zones were also compared. The thulium laser and KTP lasers demonstrated similar hemostasis with a bleeding rate of 0.16±0.07 g/min and the KTP 0.21±0.07 g/min. This was significantly less than with TURP, which had a bleeding rate of 20.14±2.03 g/min ($p<0.05$). Coagulation zone depth was significantly deeper with the KTP laser (265±41 μm for the thulium vs. 667±64 μm for the KTP, $p<0.05$) and comparable to TURP (287±28 μm). Overall the 70-W continuous wave thulium laser demonstrated higher tissue ablation rate, similar hemostatic properties, and shallower coagulation zone depth than the 80-W KTP laser. Compared to TURP both tissue ablation and bleeding rate were reduced.

In Vivo Studies

The first human studies were performed with the 70-W RevoLix™ laser system in small prostates [10, 11] with a wavelength of 2,013 nm. Findings of thulium vapoenucleation and laser resection studies are summarized in Table 12.1. Bach et al. reported on a single surgeon series of 54 men with a mean prostate volume 30.3 (range 12–38) cc who underwent vaporesection of the prostate [11]. The vaporesection technique was performed with a 550 μm optical core diameter fiber.

The steps of this technique are similar to a holmium laser enucleation of the prostate. It is done with a 26 French continuous flow laser resectoscope with a trocar cystostomy and continuous suction. The distal resection margin is marked first. Due to the vaporizing properties of the laser, the thulium laser is capable of simultaneous vaporization and resection. Next the median lobe is vaporesected. The lateral lobes are resected and finally the apical tissue is vaporized. The authors did not use a morcellator and advised maintenance of tissue chip size small enough to allow for easy evacuation through the resectoscope sheath.

The goal of this study was to determine feasibility of the procedure. Exclusion criteria included prostate volume above 40 ml, maximum flow rate (Qmax) greater than 15 ml/s, or International Prostate Symptom Score (IPSS) less than 7. Outcome measures were improvements in Qmax, post-void residual volume (PVR), and IPSS at discharge and 1 year after the procedure.

Table 12.1 Thulium vapoenucleation and laser resection studies

Study	No. subjects	Mean/median prostate size (cc)	OR time (min)	Laser time (min)	Follow-up (months)	Complications
Bach et al. [11]	54	30 (12–38)		52 (28–72)	12	11 % UTI
Bach et al. [12]	88	61±24	72±27	32±10	n/a	17 % overall
						2 % transfusion
						7 % UTI
						2 % reoperation
Bach et al. [13]	208	46±22 and 43±24	72±29 and 68±29	36±12 and 34±12	n/a	1 % transfusion
						8 % UTI
						3 % reoperation
Gross et al. [14]	1,080	51 (IQR 36–78)	56 (IQR 40–80)	33 (IQR 33–71)	n/a	2 % UTI
						2 % transfusion
						5 % reoperation
Macchione et al. [16]	76	65±15	47±8	Not reported	6	7 % UTI
						1 % transfusion
						0 % reoperation
Xia et al. [10]	52	59±17	46±16	Not reported	12	4 % UTI
						0 % transfusion
Peng et al. [18]	50	58±12	61±24	Not reported	3	0 % transfusion
Zhang et al. [20]	71	76±10	72±19		18	0 % transfusion

Other outcomes assessed were operating time, decrease in hemoglobin, transfusion rate, and catheter time.

Mean patient age was 61 (56–82) years. Despite the small prostate size of the population in this study, 14 (26 %) patients had acute urinary retention prior to surgery. Mean resection time was 52 (28–72) minutes and the calculated tissue removal rate after "crossing the learning curve" was 1.5 g/min. The mean catheter time was 1.7 (1–3) days with an average hospital stay of 3.5 (2–6) days. No patients required transfusion or re-hospitalization. Six (11 %) patients developed a symptomatic urinary tract infection requiring antibiotic therapy. The criteria for diagnosis of this complication were not specified. Improvements were seen in mean IPSS (19.8–6.9), Qmax (4.1–20.1 ml/s), and PVR (86–12 ml).

After this feasibility study, this same group of authors investigated the feasibility and efficacy of thulium:YAG (Tm:YAG) laser vapoenucleation of the prostate in larger prostates [12]. In this short-term study, with follow-up to discharge, 88 patients with prostate volume 61.3 ± 24.0 cc underwent vapoenucleation of the prostate with the 70-W RevoLix® Tm:YAG laser. In contrast to the previous study in smaller prostates, morcellation was performed in all patients following enucleation.

Inclusion criteria for the study were Qmax <15 cc/s and IPSS >7. The technique was the same as in the abovementioned study except that morcellation was carried out after enucleation. Continuous bladder irrigation was applied overnight for all patients with a 22 or 24-French 3-way Foley catheter. Outcomes assessed were Qmax, PVR, intraoperative parameters, postoperative course, and complications.

Mean age was 71 ± 8 years and mean prostate volume was 61 ± 24 cc (range 30–160). 31 % of patients were in retention prior to surgery and the rest of the subjects had surgery due to refractory lower urinary tract symptoms. Mean preoperative IPSS was 18 ± 7. The mean operative time was 72 ± 27 min and mean laser time was 32 ± 10 min. Mean applied laser energy was 124 ± 40 kJ and an average of 32 ± 18 g of tissue was retrieved. The amount of tissue retrieved is not comparable to tissue retrieved from a holmium laser enucleation of the prostate (HoLEP) due to the fact that much tissue is also vaporized in this procedure. Foley catheter time was mean 2.1 days, and those with a suprapubic tube had it removed on average on postoperative day 3. Patients were discharged the day after catheter removal. Four (5 %) patients were found to have incidental prostate adenocarcinoma. No significant changes were seen in serum sodium.

Complication rate was 16.6 % with 12 patients having complications. Two (2.2 %) patients required blood transfusions for postoperative bleeding. Six (6.8 %) patients developed symptomatic UTIs, three (3.4 %) patients experienced intra- or postoperative bleeding, and two (2.2 %) underwent a second-look procedure during the same hospital stay due to inability to void. Significant improvements were seen at discharge in Qmax (3.5 ± 4.7 to 19.8 ± 11.6 ml/s) and PVR (121 ± 340 to 22 ± 33 ml).

Bach et al. next compared outcomes of Tm:YAG vapoenucleation (ThuVEP) of the prostate in patient with and without an indwelling catheter secondary to recurrent urinary retention arising from BPH [13]. Outcomes of the procedure in 65 patients with recurrent retention before surgery were compared to outcomes in 143 men without. In this study, three surgeons performed the procedures.

Patients with and without a catheter prior to surgery had similar prostate volumes with mean sizes 46 ± 22 and 43 ± 24 ml. Follow-up for this study was only until the day of discharge with mean hospital stay unrecorded. Transfusion rate was very low with only one patient in each group requiring transfusion (1 % overall). Not surprisingly ten patients in the retention group developed a UTI in the perioperative period versus six in the nonretention group. Overall Tm:YAG vapoenucleation was safe and effective in the short term even for patients in retention.

This same group published a paper describing complications and early postoperative outcomes of ThuVEP performed by 11 surgeons at a single institution in a very large series of 1,080 patients [14]. This was a short-term analysis examining preoperative status, surgical details, and immediate outcomes.

Median age at surgery was 71 years; prostate size was 52 ml (IQR 36–79) with a median operation time of 56 min. Twenty-two percent of patients were in retention prior to surgery. Median enucleation time was 33 min (IQR 22–50), and median resected tissue weight was 30 g (IQR 36–78). Significant changes were seen after surgery in median maximum flow rate (8.9 vs. 18.4 ml/s, $p<0.001$) and post-void residual volume (120 vs. 20 ml, $p<0.001$) compared to before surgery. Median catheterization time was 2 days (IQR 2–2), and median hospital stay was 4 days (IQR 3–5). Incidental prostate cancer was discovered in 59 (5.5 %) patients.

Overall immediate morbidity rate was 16.9 %. Minor complications (Clavien class 1 and 2) occurred in 262 (24.6 %) patients. Within 4 weeks 71 (6.6 %), patients required intervention (Clavien 3a: 0.6 %; Clavien 3b: 6 %). One patient had a Clavien 4a complication and had an acute myocardial infarction. No mortalities were seen.

The most frequently reported complications were urinary retention after catheter removal (9 %), UTI without bacteremia (6.9 %), clot retention without surgical revision (3.5 %), residual prostate tissue requiring reoperation (2.7 %), capsular perforation (2.1 %), hemorrhage requiring reoperation (2 %), bleeding requiring blood transfusion (1.7 %), UTI with signs of bacteremia (1.5 %), extraperitoneal fluid collection (1.5 %), superficial bladder injury due to morcellation (1.4 %), ureteral orifice injury (0.7 %), and hydronephrosis due to ureteric orifice injury (0.6 %). The overall reoperation rate was 4.7 % and the readmission rate was 4.1 %.

A subanalysis was done and patients were stratified by prostate size. Group A had prostate size <40 ml (28 %), group B had prostate size 40–79 ml (47 %), and group C had prostate size ≥80 ml (25 %). No differences were seen in complications rates between the groups.

Complication rate using the Clavien Classification System (CCS) were then compared to those in published series of holmium laser enucleation of the prostate (HoLEP), photoselective vaporization of the prostate (PVP), TURP, and open prostatectomy. Overall in this large series, immediate outcomes and complication rates for ThuVEP were similar to those in large series of HoLEP and PVP and lower than in TURP and open prostatectomy. This large series confirmed that ThuVEP is a safe and effective procedure for the treatment of symptomatic BPH with low perioperative morbidity.

With the introduction of the 120-W thulium laser, Netsch et al. evaluated the ablative and hemostatic properties of the 120-W Tm:YAG laser with those of the 70-W Tm:YAG laser and concluded that the 120-W Tm:YAG laser ablation offers significantly higher ablation with a comparable rate of bleeding and tissue penetration depth [15]. Further studies have been done with the higher-power 120-W laser.

Macchione et al. investigated the safety and efficacy of ThVEP using the 120-W Tm:YAG laser (Revolix Duo) in 76 patients who were taking oral antiplatelet or anticoagulation [16]. In 41 patients (group A), the procedure was performed while patients continued oral anticoagulation, and in 35 patients (group B), oral anticoagulation was discontinued 10 days prior to surgery and patients were bridged with low molecular weight heparin (LMWH) for 2 weeks, with 3 (8 %) patients from this group taking warfarin.

In group A, 5 (12 %) patients were taking warfarin, 20 (48 %) acetylsalicylic acid (ASA), 12 (29 %) ticlopidine, and 4 (10 %) ASA and clopidogrel. In group B, 3 (8 %) patients were taking warfarin, 15 (42 %) ASA, 11 (31 %) ticlopidine, and 6 (17 %) ASA and clopidogrel. All procedures were performed by a single surgeon. Decision for discontinuing oral anticoagulation was made by the consultant cardiologist. In both groups, mean age was similar (69 ± 7 for both) as well as mean prostate size (65 ml for both). Median ASA for both groups was 3.

Operative times (48 ± 8, 47 ± 5 min), catheterization time (1.5 ± 6, 1.6 ± 6 days), hospital stay (2.3 ± 0.9 and 2.4 ± 9 days), mean drop in sodium (0.52 ± 2.0 and 1.34 ± 1.1 g/l), and mean hemoglobin drop (0.35 ± 0.2 and 0.85 ± 0.2 g/l) were similar between groups A and B. Only one patient in group A required a transfusion. Three (4 %) patients overall required continuous bladder irrigation for postoperative hematuria. Significant improvements were seen compared to baseline in Qmax, IPSS, PVR, and QoL at 3 and 6 months postop.

Overall, this study demonstrated that ThuVEP is a safe and effective treatment for patients with BPH who require oral anticoagulation therapy with few perioperative complications.

Learning Curve

The learning curve of ThuVEP was first examined in Gross et al.'s large series of 1,080 patients undergoing the procedure [14]. The 1,080 cases were divided into five consecutive subgroups of 216 patients each. Overall complication rates decreased significantly over time (see Fig. 12.2). The complication rate was 41.7 % within the first 216 cases and 19.4 % within the last 216 cases ($p<0.001$). Transfusion rates also improved (3.2 % vs. 0 %, $p<0.007$). Significant differences were seen between the first and last 216 patients in terms of Clavien 3b complications (11.1 % vs. 3.3 %, $p=0.0012$). No changes in the rate of UTI were seen between the first and last 216 cases. Few institutions would be able to have the case volume to reach the lower complication rate on this learning curve.

These authors next decided to prospectively evaluate the learning curve of ThuVEP [17]. Implementing a mentor-based system, 3 surgeons of different backgrounds were assigned 32 patients each to perform ThuVEP on. Surgeon A was a resident without any experience in transurethral prostate surgery. Surgeon B was experienced in transurethral prostate surgery such as TURP, but not ThuVEP. Surgeon C acted as the mentor and was an experienced surgeon in ThuVEP. After studying videos extensively, surgeons A and B assisted in ten procedures and then were assigned cases independently. In cases of difficulty, the mentor was always available for help. Significant differences were seen in laser energy used, enucleation time, and operative time. However, improvements were seen in Qmax, PVR, and IPSS in all groups to 12 months. There were few differences in complications. For surgeons A and B, transient stress urinary incontinence was seen in 5 (16 %) patients each and persisted in 1 (3 %) patient each for surgeons A and B. Overall the authors concluded that ThuVEP was performed by surgeons A and B with reasonable enucleation, morcellation, and overall operation efficiency after 8–16 procedures.

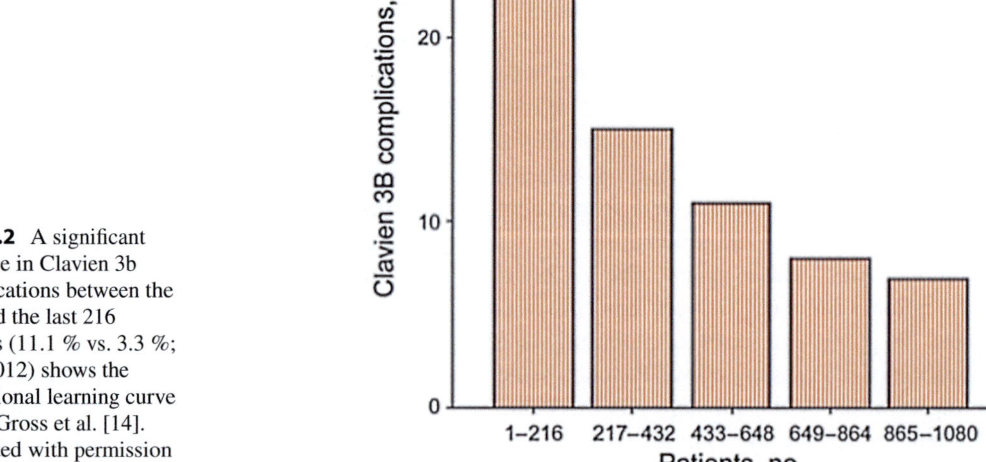

Fig. 12.2 A significant decrease in Clavien 3b complications between the first and the last 216 patients (11.1 % vs. 3.3 %; $p\leq 0.0012$) shows the institutional learning curve (From Gross et al. [14]. Reprinted with permission from Elsevier Limited)

The differences in learning curve between the retrospective and prospective studies done at the same institution may be due to the evolving institutional learning curve. The prospective study is also limited by the highly specialized environment that would be difficult to mimic elsewhere and could not be applied to a more litigious environment such as practice in North America.

Comparative Studies

Several studies have been published comparing thulium laser prostatectomy with standard monopolar TURP [10]. Using a 50-W continuous wave thulium laser (LISA laser products OHG, Germany), Xia et al. performed thulium laser resection of the prostate-tangerine technique (TmLRP) and compared outcomes up to 12 months to standard TURP [10]. Inclusion criteria included urodynamic bladder outlet obstruction and prostate volume less than 100 g. Patients with an indwelling Foley catheter were excluded. Fifty-two patients were randomized to TmLRP and 48 to TURP.

The tangerine technique is similar to ThuVEP. However, instead of using a morcellator, long narrow strips of tissue are carved out, pushed into the bladder, and then evacuated. It may still be considered a vapoenucleation procedure.

Baseline characteristics between the groups were similar, with mean age in both groups of 69. Mean TRUS volume was 59 ± 17 ml for the TmLRP group and 55 ± 16 ml for the TURP group. Baseline IPSS (22 ± 7, 21 ± 6), Qmax (8 ± 3 and 8 ± 3 ml/s), and PVR (93 ± 32 and 85 ± 37 ml) were similar in both groups prior to procedure.

Operative for both procedures were also similar for TmLRP and TURP (46 ± 16 and 50 ± 20 min, $p = 0.28$). As expected, resected weight was less in the TmLRP group (21 ± 10 vs. 19 ± 14, $p = 0.0001$). There was a smaller decrease in hemoglobin in the TmLRP group versus TURP (0.92 ± 0.82 vs. 1.46 ± 0.65 g/dl, $p = 0.0004$). Hospital stay (115 ± 24 vs. 161 ± 34 h, $p < 0.0001$) and catheterization time (46 ± 26 and 87 ± 34 h, $p < 0.0001$) were also shorter in the TmLRP group compared to TURP. At 1, 6, and 12 months, no significant differences were seen between groups in IPSS, QoL, Qmax, or PVR. No significant changes in IIEF-5 scores were seen compared to preop in either group.

Regarding adverse effects, there were 2 (4 %) transfusions required in the TURP group, but none required in the TmLRP. No significant differences were found with regard to rate of transfusion, TUR syndrome, or UTI. No differences were seen either in the rate of de novo stress urinary incontinence or urethral strictures seen. However, this may be due to the relatively small number of subjects in this study. Overall this study suggested that subjective and objective improvements of this technique are similar to TURP but with lower morbidity.

More recently, a study was performed to compare the short-term efficacy and safety of TmLRP with a 50-W thulium laser to bipolar transurethral plasmakinetic prostatectomy (BiTURP) [18]. One hundred patients were randomized to TmLRP or BiTURP. Baseline characteristics of the TmLRP and BiTURP patients were similar with regard to mean prostate volume (58 ± 12 and 58 ± 15 ml), IPSS (20 ± 8 and 19 ± 8), QoL score (5 ± 3 and 5 ± 1), Qmax (8 ± 4 ml/s for both groups), and PVR 97 ± 35 and 88 ± 38 ml). Operative time was significantly longer in the TmLRP group (61 ± 24 vs. 30 ± 6 min, $p < 0.05$), while catheterization time (1.8 ± 0.4 vs. 3.2 ± 0.6 days, $p < 0.05$) and hospital stay (3.3 ± 0.8 vs. 4.1 ± 1.3 days, $p < 0.05$) were significantly shorter.

Following the procedures, no significant differences were seen between groups in serum sodium and hemoglobin. No transfusions were required in either group. Significant improvements were seen in both groups at 1 and 3 months postop. Compared to BiTURP, TmLRP was superior in safety, blood loss, and urethral stricture rate with similar improvements in IPSS, Qmax, and PVR.

Yang et al. published a comparative study of 158 patients randomized to TmLRP with a 100-W thulium laser and BiTURP, with all patients returning for 18-month follow-up [19]. Baseline parameters were similar in both groups. Mean prostate volume was 62 ± 7 in the TmLRP group and 69 ± 23 ml in the BiTURP group. Mean baseline IPSS in both groups was 23. Patients were relatively young for both groups, 62±7 years and 61±7 years. TmLRP required a longer operation time (65 vs. 47 min, $p=0.22$) than BiTURP but resulted in shorter hospital stay (2.5 vs. 4.6 days, $p=0.026$), shorter catheterization time (2.1 cs. 3.5 days, $p=0.026$), and lower drop in hemoglobin (−0.15 vs. −0.30 g/dl, $p=0.045$). Similar improvements were seen in IPSS, QoL, Qmax, and PVR up to 18 months.

In terms of complications, no transfusions were required in either group. Clot retention was observed in 3 (4 %) BiTURP patients and in 1 (1 %) TmLRP patient. No other perioperative complications were mentioned, and no reoperations were reported in either group.

Thulium laser enucleation of the prostate with the "mushroom technique" (ThuLEP-M) has also been compared to holmium laser enucleation of the prostate with the "mushroom technique" (HoLEP –M). Zhang et al. randomized 133 consecutive patients with BPH to ThuLEP-M with a 70-W (Revolix®, Katlenburg, Germany) thulium laser system ($n=71$) or HoLEP-M with a 100-W holmium (VersaPulse®, Lumenis, Santa Clara, CA) laser system ($n=62$) [20]. This technique is very similar to ThuVEP and HoLEP where median and lateral lobes are demarcated and lifted off the capsule. However, instead of being pushed into the bladder, the lobes are left attached to the bladder neck. Next, using a monopolar electrocautery loop, the lobes are mechanically fragmented into pieces small enough to be evacuated through the resectoscope sheath. Mannitol solution was used for the entire procedure.

For the ThuLEP-M and HoLEP-M groups mean patient age at baseline was similar (76±10 and 74±10 years). Mean prostate volume was also similar and overall relatively small (47±25 and 44±23). Operative time was comparatively longer for ThuLEP-M versus HoLEP-M (72±19 vs. 62±20 min), but no significant differences were seen in the weight of resected tissue (38±12 vs. 40±10 g, $p=0.072$), decrease in hemoglobin (0.5±0.1 vs. 0.5±0.1 g/dl, $p=0.107$), or catheterization time (2.4±10 vs. 2.5±1.0 days). Improvements in IPSS, QoL, Qmax, PVR, and PSA reduction were similar in both groups at 1, 6, 12, and 18 months.

With regard to complications, one patient from each group experienced intraoperative capsular perforation necessitating suprapubic tube insertion. No transfusions were required in either group. No short- or long-term reoperations were mentioned.

This study demonstrated that enucleation of the prostate with the thulium and holmium lasers is comparably safe and effective with good and similar clinical outcomes to 18 months.

Conclusions

The thulium laser has several properties that confer some theoretical advantages over other lasers used for treating BPH. Thulium laser resection, vapoenucleation, and enucleation techniques appear safe and effective with low morbidity. Further comparative and long-term studies are needed for this promising technology, particularly in larger prostates.

References

1. Fried N, Murray K. High-power thulium fiber laser ablation of urinary tissues at 1.94. J Endourol. 2005; 19:25.
2. Pierce MC, Jackson SD, Dickinson MR, et al. Laser–tissue interaction with a high-power 2-μm fiber laser: preliminary studies with soft tissue. Lasers Surg Med. 1999;25:407.
3. Sumiyoshi T, Sekita H, Arai T, et al. High-power continuous-wave 3- and 2μm cascade Ho3+:ZBLAN fiber laser and its medical applications. EEE J Sel Top Quant Electr. 1999;5:936.
4. Pierce M, Jackson S, Dickinson M, et al. Laser–tissue interaction with a continuous wave 3-μm fibre laser: preliminary studies with soft tissue. Lasers Surg Med. 2000;26:491.
5. El-Sherif A, King T. Soft and hard tissue ablation with short- pulse high peak power and continuous thulium-silica fibre lasers. Lasers Med Sci. 2003;18:139.
6. Schomacker K, Domankevitz Y, Flotte T, et al. Co:MgF2 laser ablation of tissue: effect of wavelength on ablation threshold and thermal damage. Lasers Surg Med. 1991;11:141.
7. Hai M, Malek R. Photoselective vaporization of the prostate: initial experience with a new 80 W KTP

laser for the treatment of benign prostatic hyperplasia. J Endourol. 2003;17:93.
8. Tan A, Gilling P, Kennett K, et al. A randomized trial comparing holmium laser enucleation of the prostate with transurethral resection of the prostate for the treatment of bladder outlet obstruction secondary to benign prostatic hyperplasia in large glands (40 to 200 grams). J Urol. 2003;170:1270.
9. Wendt-Nordahl G, Huckele S, Honeck P, et al. Systemic evaluation of a recently introduced 2-μm continuous-wave thulium laser for vaporesection of the prostate. J Endourol. 2008;22:1041.
10. Xia S, Zhuo J, Sun X, et al. Thulium laser versus standard transurethral resection of the prostate: a randomized prospective trial. Eur Urol. 2008;53:383.
11. Bach T, Hermann T, Ganzer R, et al. Revolix vaporesection of the prostate: initial results of 54 patients with 1-year follow-up. World J Urol. 2007;25:257.
12. Bach T, Wendt-Nordahl G, Michel M, et al. Feasibility and efficacy of thulium:YAG laser enucleation (VapoEnucleation) of the prostate. World J Urol. 2009;27:541.
13. Bach T, Hermann T, Hacker A, et al. Thulium:yttrium-aluminum-garnet laser prostatectomy in men with refractory urinary retention. BJU Int. 2009;104:361.
14. Gross A, Netsch C, Knipper S, et al. Complications and early postoperative outcome in 1080 patients after thulium vapoenucleation of the prostate: results at a single institution. Eur Urol. 2012;63:859.
15. Netsch C, Bach T, Hermann T, et al. Thulium:YAG VapoEnucleation of the prostate in large glands: a prospective comparison using 10- and 120-W 2-μm lasers. Asian J Androl. 2012;14:325.
16. Macchione L, Mucciardi G, Gali A, et al. Efficacy and safety of prostate vaporesection using a 120-W 2-μm continuous-wave Tm:YAG (RevoLix 2) in patients on continuous oral anticoagulant or antiplatelet therapy. Int Urol Nephrol. 2013;45:1545–51.
17. Netsch C, Bach T, Hermann T, et al. Evaluation of the learning curve for Thulium VapoEnucleation of the prostate (ThuVEP) using a mentor-based approach. World J Urol. 2013;31:1231.
18. Peng B, Wang G, Zheng J, et al. A comparative study of thulium laser resection of the prostate and bipolar transurethral plasmakinetic prostatectomy for treating benign prostatic hyperplasia. BJU Int. 2013;111:633.
19. Yang Z, Wang X, Liu T. Thulium laser enucleation versus plasmakinetic resection of the prostate: a randomized prospective trial with 18-month follow-up. Urology. 2013;81:396.
20. Zhang F, Shao Q, Hermann T, et al. Thulium laser versus holmium laser transurethral enucleation of the prostate: 18-month follow-up data of a single center. Urology. 2012;79:869.

13 Diode Laser Treatment of Prostate

Malte Rieken and Alexander Bachmann

Technical Background

Diodes are semiconductors with the ability to generate and emit monochromatic light. The wavelength depends on the semiconductor used. The emitted light is passed through a crystal, which defines the final wavelength. The production of relatively cheap semiconductors in the 1990s leads to a widespread use of 1,064 nm-based Nd:YAG laser systems. These early lasers were characterized by deep optical penetration depth, which led to a coagulative necrosis of the tissue causing sloughing and severe storage symptoms.

Current diode laser systems aim to overcome these disadvantages by modulating frequency, pulsation, maximum power, or fiber design. The main advantage of diode lasers in comparison to Nd:YAG lasers is a much smaller laser generator size. Diode lasers consume less energy and can be operated from a standard power outlet. It is important to notice that diode lasers come in various forms that have to be differentiated from each other. Currently, laser types with wavelengths of 940, 980, 1,318, and 1,470 nm are available for application in prostate surgery [1] (Table 13.1). Regarding fiber design, front-fire and side-fire fibers are available. Wavelength, power output, pulse mode, and fiber design influence laser-tissue interaction. Optical penetration depth varies strongly between different wavelengths and even between different models of the same wavelength. Tissue necrosis induced by diode laser application ranges from around 1 to 5 mm in ex vivo models. In canine experiments, a necrotic zone of up to 6 mm has been described [2].

Equipment and Surgical Technique

The equipment consists of the laser generator and the laser fiber, which is introduced in a specific laser cystoscope. Models from different manufacturers are available (Table 13.1).

Various surgical techniques exist for the application of diode laser in the treatment of BPO:

- Diode laser vaporization of the prostate (DiVAP) with side-firing fibers in noncontact mode
- Diode laser vaporization of the prostate (DiVAP) with quartz head in contact mode
- Diode laser enucleation of the prostate (DiLEP) with front-firing fiber in contact mode

The surgical technique of DiVAP resembles that of PVP, whereas DiLEP is comparable to other enucleating techniques like HoLEP.

M. Rieken, M.D. (✉) • A. Bachmann, M.D.
Department of Urology, University Hospital Basel, Spitalstrasse 21, 4031 Basel, Switzerland
e-mail: malte.rieken@usb.ch; alexander.bachmann@usb.ch

B. Chughtai et al. (eds.), *Treatment of Benign Prostatic Hyperplasia: Modern Alternative to Transurethral Resection of the Prostate*, DOI 10.1007/978-1-4939-1587-3_13,

Table 13.1 Overview of diode laser types and manufacturers

Laser name	Manufacturer	Wavelength (nm)	Surgical technique	References
Ceralas™[a]	Biolitec, Jena, Germany	980 nm, 1,470 nm	DiVAP, noncontact	[5, 8, 6]
			DiVAP, contact	[9, 14]
			DiLEP	[12, 13]
Diolas™	Limmer Laser, Berlin, Germany	980 nm	DiVAP	[3, 4, 15]
Eraser™	Rolle + Rolle, Salzburg, Austria	1,318 nm	DiLEP	[10, 16]
K2 diode laser system™	Huentek, Seoul, Korea	980 nm	DiVAP	[7]
Medilas D UroBeam™	Dornier MedTech, Wessling, Germany	940 nm	DiLEP	[11]

[a]The laser systems and fibers changed within recent years

Diode Laser Vaporization of the Prostate

Outcomes

Various studies show that DiVAP leads to a rapid and significant improvement of voiding parameters and micturition symptoms (Tables 13.2 and 13.3). A major drawback is the lack of any randomized trial comparing DiVAP with other surgical techniques. Furthermore, maximum follow-up is limited to 1 year. Two prospective trials including 139 and 117 patients compared PVP with the 120-W GreenLight Laser and DiVAP with a 200-W 980 nm diode laser [3, 4] (Table 13.2). In both studies, lasing time, operation time, and hospitalization time were comparable. In contrast, the amount of applied energy was significantly higher in patients operated with the 200-W 980 nm diode laser [3, 4]. Within 6- and 12-month follow-up, both laser types achieved comparable functional results [3, 4]. Other cohort studies report comparable functional results within a maximum follow-up of 6–12 months after treatment with 100-W, 120-W, or 132-W 980 nm diode lasers [5–7] (Table 13.3). In a pilot study with a 50-W 1,470 nm diode laser, micturition symptoms (IPSS, QoL) and voiding parameters (Q max, PVR volume) were significantly improved at 12-month follow-up [8]. However, the study was limited by the low number of included patients ($n = 10$).

A recent modification of diode laser prostatectomy is the covering of the laser tip with quartz. This concentrates the laser energy at the tip of the fiber, which does not emit a free beam. The laser fiber works in contact mode, which resembles TURP. The surgical properties of this novel fiber were compared to a standard side-firing fiber used with a 980 nm diode laser. 120 patients were randomized into two groups; at a follow-up of 6 months, both groups showed a significant improvement in micturition symptoms and voiding parameters which were more pronounced in patients operated with the quartz head fiber [9] (Table 13.2).

Safety and Complications

DiVAP is characterized by excellent hemostatic properties and high intraoperative safety. Impaired visibility due to intraoperative bleeding is significantly less with the 200-W 980 nm diode lasers than with 120-W PVP [4]. Furthermore, no perioperative blood transfusions are reported. The use of the TURP loop to control bleeding is significantly less frequent than with the 120-W PVP (0–4 % vs. 8–12 %) [3, 4] (Table 13.2). Comparative studies have reported a significantly higher rate of dysuria and reoperations with the

Table 13.2 Overview of diode laser, randomized and comparative trials

Author	Year	Study type	Follow-up (months)	Laser type, technique	Compared to	Number of patients	Complications; type/number	Surgical reintervention, reoperation	Functional outcome
Lusuardi et al. [10]	2011	RCT	6	1,318 nm 120-W	Bipolar TURP	DiLEP: 30	Transient incontinence	None	Comparable
							DiLEP: 1 (3.3)		
				DiLEP		Bipolar TURP: 30	Bipolar TURP: (6.7)		
							Symptomatic UTI		
							DiLEP: 1 (3.3)		
Xu et al. [11]	2013	RCT	12	940 nm 250-W	Bipolar enucleation of the prostate (BEP)	DiLEP: 40	Transient incontinence	None	Comparable
				DiLEP		BEP: 40	DiLEP: 3 (7.5)		
							BEP: 4 (10)		
							Storage symptoms		
							DiLEP: 5 (8)		
							BEP: 14 (35)		
Yang et al. [12]	2013	Comparative study	12	980 nm 80-W	TURP	DiLEP: 74	Blood transfusion	None	Comparable
				DiLEP		TURP: 52	DiLEP: 2 (2.7)		
							TURP: 3 (5.8)		
							Bladder mucosal injury		
							DiLEP: 7 (9.5)		
							TURP: 0		
Chiang et al. [3]	2010	Comparative study	12	980 nm 200-W	532 nm 120-W PVP	DiVAP: 55	Transient incontinence	Re-TURP	Comparable
				DiVAP		PVP: 84	DiVAP: 8 (14.5)	DiVAP: 5 (9.1)	
							PVP: 2 (2.4)	PVP: 3 (3.6)	
							Dysuria with tissue sloughing	Urethral stricture	
							DiVAP: 10 (18.2)	DiVAP: 3 (5.5)	
							PVP: 0	PVP: 2 (2.4)	
								Bladder neck contracture	
								DiVAP: 5 (9.1)	
								PVP: 2 (2.4)	

(continued)

Table 13.2 (continued)

Author	Year	Study type	Follow-up (months)	Laser type, technique	Compared to	Number of patients	Complications; type/number	Surgical reintervention, reoperation	Functional outcome
Ruszat et al. [4]	2009	Comparative study	6	980 nm 200-W	532 nm 120-W PVP	DiVAP: 55	Blood transfusion	Re-TURP	Comparable
				DiVAP		PVP: 62	DiVAP: 0	DiVAP: 10 (18.2)	
							PVP: 1 (1.6)	PVP: 1 (1.6)	
							Transient incontinence	Bladder neck contracture	
							DiVAP: 4 (7.3)	DiVAP: 8 (14.5)	
							PVP: 0	PVP: 1 (1.6)	
							Dysuria		
							DiVAP: 13 (23.6)		
							PVP: 11 (17.7)		
Shaker et al. [9]	2012	RCT	6	980 nm DiVAP	980 nm DiVAP	Contact mode: 56	Hematuria	Urethral stricture	Comparable
				Contact mode fiber	Noncontact mode fiber	Noncontact mode: 57	Contact mode: 2 (3.5)	Contact mode : 2 (3.6)	
							Noncontact mode: 6 (10.5)	Noncontact mode: 3 (5.3)	
							Prolonged dysuria > 1 month:	Bladder neck contracture	
							Contact mode: 10 (17.2)	Contact mode: 2 (3.6)	
							Noncontact mode: 24 (42.1)	Noncontact mode: 3 (5.3)	
							Passage of tissue remnants		
							Contact mode: 9 (16.1)		
							Noncontact mode: 30 (52)		

Table 13.3 Overview of diode laser case series

Author	Year	Maximum follow-up (months)	Laser type	Surgical technique	Number of patients	Mean prostate volume	Perioperative complications	Surgical reintervention, reoperation	Functional outcome
Seitz et al. [8]	2007	12	1,470 nm 50- W	DiVAP	10	48	Transient dysuria: 2 (20)	Re-TURP: 2 (20)	Significantly improved
Yang et al. [7]	2011	6	980 nm 120-W	DiVAP	96	45	Transient dysuria: 16 (16.7)	None	Significantly improved
Erol et al. [5]	2009	6	980 nm 132-W	DiVAP	47	51	Transient dysuria: 11 (23.4)	Catheterization due to late bleeding: 1 (2.1)	Significantly improved
							Transient incontinence: 2 (4.2)		
							Late bleeding: 1 (2.1)		
Leonardi et al. [6]	2009	12	980 nm 100-W	DiVAP	52	45	Late bleeding: 1 (1.9)	Catheterization due to late bleeding: 1 (1.9)	Significantly improved
Yang et al. [13]	2013	6	980 nm 80-W	DiLEP	120	63	Bladder mucosal injury: 8 (6.7)	Bladder neck contracture: 1 (0.8)	Significantly improved
							Blood transfusion: 2 (1.7)	Urethral stricture: 2 (1.7)	
							Febrile UTI: 3 (2.5)	Bladder clot tamponade: 2 (1.7)	
Hruby et al. [16]	2013	6	1,318 nm 120- W	DiLEP	43	60	Transient incontinence: 1 (2.3)	Needle aspiration of periprostatic abscess: 1 (2.3)	Significantly improved
							Symptomatic UTI: 1 (2.3)		

200-W 980 nm diode lasers in comparison to 120-W PVP [3, 4].

These high reoperation rates were not observed in case series of lower-powered diode lasers. In series with 120-W and 132-W 980 nm diode lasers, no reoperation occurred during a follow-up of 6 months [5, 7]. After treatment with a 50-W 1,470 nm diode laser, two of ten patients required re-TURP within 2 months [8] (Table 13.3). In the prospective randomized comparison of side-firing fiber and quartz head fiber, patients operated in contact mode with the quartz head fiber showed significantly less postoperative passage of tissue remnants and dysuria [9].

Diode Laser Enucleation of the Prostate

Outcomes

In recent years, an increasing number of studies report on diode laser enucleation of the prostate (DiLEP). Prospective randomized studies compared DiLEP with bipolar TURP [10] and bipolar enucleation of the prostate [11]. In one study, 60 patients were assigned to treatment with a 1,318 nm 120-W diode laser or bipolar TURP. Operating time was on average 9 min longer with DiLEP to retrieve a comparable amount of tissue [10]. Another prospective study randomized 80 patients to DiLEP with a 940 nm 250-W diode laser or bipolar enucleation of the prostate [11]. In this study, operating time with DiLEP was on average 16 min shorter, while the amount of resected tissue was comparable. In both studies, catheterization time and hospitalization time were significantly shorter after DiLEP. Improvements in micturition symptoms (IPSS, QoL) and voiding parameters (Qmax, PVR volume) were comparable at 6- and 12-month follow-up [10, 11] (Table 13.2). Similar results were observed in a prospective non-randomized comparison between a 980 nm 80-W diode laser and TURP [12]. A case series including 120 men confirmed the efficacy of DiLEP in patients with a prostate volume of 60 ml and larger [13] (Table 13.3).

Safety and Complications

Similar to DiVAP, DiLEP is characterized by high intraoperative safety. In the two randomized trials, no blood transfusion was necessary in patients operated with DiLEP [10, 11]. Estimated blood loss was significantly lower after DiLEP. Transient incontinence occurred in one of 30 [10] and three of 40 patients after DiLEP [11] (Table 13.2). No reoperations due to adenoma, urethral strictures, or bladder neck contractures have been reported during follow-up of 6 and 12 months. Among patients operated with DiLEP by a 980 nm 80-W diode laser, blood transfusions were necessary in 2 of 74 patients. Furthermore, bladder mucosal injury during morcellation was recorded in 10 % of the patients, which may be attributed to the learning curve [12].

Summary

- Various laser types and techniques are available for diode laser prostatectomy.
- Diode laser prostatectomy is characterized by high intraoperative safety.
- DiVAP has been associated with a high reoperation rate in some studies.
- DiLEP appears to have superior physical properties leading to an improved safety profile.
- Intermediate- and long-term data on functional outcomes and complications are not available.

References

1. Bach T, et al. Laser treatment of benign prostatic obstruction: basics and physical differences. Eur Urol. 2012;61(2):317–25.
2. Rieken M, et al. Laser vaporization of the prostate in vivo: experience with the 150-W 980-nm diode laser in living canines. Lasers Surg Med. 2010;42(8):736–42.
3. Chiang PH, et al. GreenLight HPS laser 120-W versus diode laser 200-W vaporization of the prostate: comparative clinical experience. Lasers Surg Med. 2010; 42(7):624–9.
4. Ruszat R, et al. Prospective single-centre comparison of 120-W diode-pumped solid-state high-intensity system laser vaporization of the prostate and 200-W

high-intensive diode-laser ablation of the prostate for treating benign prostatic hyperplasia. BJU Int. 2009; 104(6):820–5.

5. Erol A, et al. High power diode laser vaporization of the prostate: preliminary results for benign prostatic hyperplasia. J Urol. 2009;182(3):1078–82.
6. Leonardi R. Preliminary results on selective light vaporization with the side-firing 980 nm diode laser in benign prostatic hyperplasia: an ejaculation sparing technique. Prostate Cancer Prostatic Dis. 2009;12(3):277–80.
7. Yang KS, et al. Initial experiences with a 980 nm diode laser for photoselective vaporization of the prostate for the treatment of benign prostatic hyperplasia. Korean J Urol. 2011;52(11):752–6.
8. Seitz M, et al. The diode laser: a novel side-firing approach for laser vaporisation of the human prostate–immediate efficacy and 1-year follow-up. Eur Urol. 2007;52(6):1717–22.
9. Shaker HS, et al. Quartz head contact laser fiber: a novel fiber for laser ablation of the prostate using the 980 nm high power diode laser. J Urol. 2012;187(2):575–9.
10. Lusuardi L, et al. Safety and efficacy of eraser laser enucleation of the prostate: preliminary report. J Urol. 2011;186(5):1967–71.
11. Xu A, et al. A randomized trial comparing diode laser enucleation of the prostate with plasmakinetic enucleation and resection of the prostate for the treatment of benign prostatic hyperplasia. J Endourol. 2013;27(10): 1254–60.
12. Yang SS, et al. Diode laser (980 nm) enucleation of the prostate: a promising alternative to transurethral resection of the prostate. Lasers Med Sci. 2013;28(2): 353–60.
13. Yang SS, et al. Prostate volume did not affect voiding function improvements in diode laser enucleation of the prostate. J Urol. 2013;189(3):993–8.
14. Shaker H, Alokda A, Mahmoud H. The Twister laser fiber degradation and tissue ablation capability during 980-nm high-power diode laser ablation of the prostate. A randomized study versus the standard side-firing fiber. Lasers Med Sci. 2012;27(5): 959–63.
15. Chen CH, et al. Preliminary results of prostate vaporization in the treatment of benign prostatic hyperplasia by using a 200-W high-intensity diode laser. Urology. 2010;75(3):658–63.
16. Hruby S, et al. Eraser laser enucleation of the prostate: technique and results. Eur Urol. 2013;63(2):341–6.

14 Modern Open Prostatectomy

Saman Shafaat Talab and Shahin Tabatabaei

History of Open Prostatectomy

Benign prostatic hyperplasia (BPH) is a common histologic condition that in many cases may lead to bladder outlet obstruction and lower urinary tract symptoms. Before the twentieth century, surgeons, who were familiar with transperineal bladder stone removal, chose the same approach for prostate adenoma enucleation. The approach however had a long learning curve and high risk of complications, especially urinary incontinence. Since 1894, when Eugene Fuller performed the first suprapubic prostatectomy and further popularized with Peter Freyer, who reported his experience with 1,000 cases in 1912, the operation became one of the most common urological procedures in the twentieth century [1]. The next evolution in benign prostate surgery happened in 1945, when the retropubic simple prostatectomy was described by Terence Millin [2]. Through the retropubic approach, there was no need to open the bladder. Prostate capsulotomy would be performed, followed by prostate adenoma enucleation. The exposure was better and hence bleeding control was thought to be more thorough. Furthermore, there was usually no need for suprapubic cystotomy.

Parallel to the improvements in open prostatectomy techniques, the second gradual (but revolutionary) change occurred in the early 1930s, when the Stern-McCarthy instrument was introduced. This allowed transurethral prostate tissue resection using a wire loop under direct vision [3]. This innovation paved the way for the subsequent advances in endoscopic prostate surgery, and finally, transurethral techniques have almost replaced the open approach in the surgical management of most BPH cases [4–6]. Less need for open incision, shorter hospitalization and postoperative recovery, and lower risk of perioperative hemorrhage were quoted as some of the appeals for transurethral approach. Still, when selecting the appropriate surgical approach in an individual with symptomatic BPH, prostate gland size is an important consideration. Although the prostate volume threshold between transurethral surgery and open prostatectomy remains an issue for debate, both AUA and EAU guidelines on the management of male lower urinary tract symptoms still recommend open prostatectomy as treatment of choice for large prostate glands (>80–100 mL) [7, 8]. More recently, the size limit for transurethral approach has been challenged in several studies, especially with the advent of more powerful laser energy sources.

Before the introduction of medical treatments for BPH, surgical therapies (open/endoscopic) and watchful waiting were the only available

S.S. Talab, M.D. • S. Tabatabaei, M.D. (✉)
Department of Urology, Harvard Medical School, Massachusetts General Hospital, 55 Fruit Street, GRB-1102, Boston, MA 02114, USA
e-mail: sshafaattalab@mgh.harvard.edu; stabatabaei@partners.org

B. Chughtai et al. (eds.), *Treatment of Benign Prostatic Hyperplasia: Modern Alternative to Transurethral Resection of the Prostate*, DOI 10.1007/978-1-4939-1587-3_14,

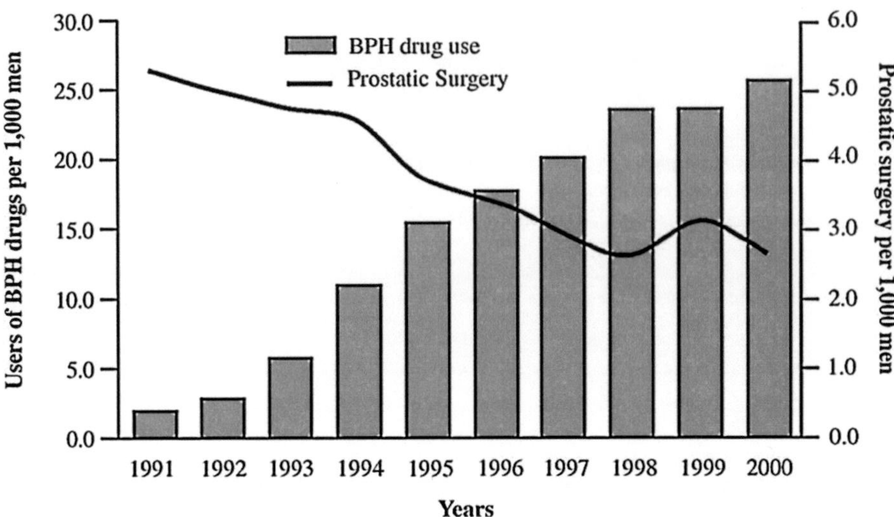

Fig. 14.1 BPH drug use and prostatic surgery in the PHARMO area 1991–2000 (Source: PHARMO Institute for Drug Outcomes Research. From Souverein et al. [9]. Reprinted with permission from Elsevier)

options for BPH patients. However, following promising results of BPH medical therapy, it became the first line of therapy for the majority of BPH patients. Surgical intervention was pushed to the second-line therapy and was offered to patients only when they failed medical therapy.

This change is reflected by a time-trend graph of the prevalence of BPH drug use and prostate surgery, among men aged 50 years and older, between 1991 and 2000 (Fig. 14.1) [9]. The increased use of BPH medical therapy corresponds to a proportional decline in BPH surgery in the same period.

It seems that the use of BPH medical therapy with its acceptable long-term symptom control has led to increased incidence of larger symptomatic prostate adenomas. Prostate grows in size, while early symptoms are controlled by medications. Therefore, patients who used to be traditionally operated by transurethral resection of prostate (TURP) – when the prostate was smaller – now need to undergo open adenomectomy because of larger prostate size. A report by Vela-Navarrete et al. has shown that the rate of open prostatectomy has risen from 18.8 % in 1992 to 28.6 % in 2002, and the mean adenoma weight has increased from 73 to 79 g [10].

Despite the increasing popularity of bipolar TURP, photoselective vaporization of the prostate (PVP), and holmium laser enucleation of the prostate (HoLEP), which are considered by some experts as the best treatment option for BPH regardless of prostate size [11, 12], open simple prostatectomy remains the procedure of choice for glands too large for safe endoscopic resection [7, 8]. Meanwhile, advancements in laparoscopic technology and the drive to apply the minimally invasive approach to most surgical procedures have led to the recent introduction of a variety of laparoscopic and robot-assisted simple prostatectomy techniques. In the current review, we will mainly focus on the available data regarding surgical outcomes and possible perioperative complications of the minimally invasive transabdominal simple prostatectomy techniques.

Laparoscopic Simple Prostatectomy (LSP)

In recent years, increasing amount of data has shown feasibility and encouraging initial outcomes of laparoscopic simple prostatectomy in patients with lower urinary tract symptoms (LUTS) due to large prostate adenomas.

Overall LSP can be categorized into conventional multi-port or single-port laparoscopic approach.

Conventional Multi-Port Laparoscopic Simple Prostatectomy

In this technique with the patient in Trendelenburg position, four or five ports including one 10–20 mm sub-umbilical camera port are placed. Most surgeons have explained the extraperitoneal approach toward Retzius space using finger or balloon dissection of the preperitoneal space [13–17]. In contrast, others prefer the transperitoneal approach to the prostate capsule and bladder neck [18, 19]. Regardless of the transperitoneal and extraperitoneal access to Retzius space, LSP is accomplished mainly through two different techniques of transcapsular (Millin) or transvesical prostate adenomectomy. The procedure is comprised of several steps, which vary, based on the type of approach and surgeon's preference. In general, they share similar steps that include cystotomy or prostate capsulotomy (depending on transvesical or transcapsular technique), development of the subcapsular plane to separate the prostate adenoma from the capsule, prostate adenomectomy, prostatic fossa reconstruction (trigonization), and hemostasis, followed by closure of cystotomy or capsulotomy.

The first laparoscopic prostatectomy for BPH was described by Mariano et al. in 2002 [20]. In that case report, anterior prostate capsulotomy was performed to extract a 120 g prostate adenoma. The estimated blood loss was 800 cc and the operative time was 3.8 h. Later on in 2006, the same group reported their 6-year experience on 60 patients who underwent laparoscopic prostatectomy [18]. At the final follow-up, significant improvement of both international prostate symptom score (IPSS) and Qmax was reported. The mean calculated prostate weight was 144.50 g (range, 80–422 g), and the mean resected prostate tissue weight was 131 g (range, 68–398 g). The average operation time was 138 min (range: 95–242 min). The technique also included hemostatic control of dorsal vein complex and lateral pedicles of the prostate before an anterior prostatic capsule incision that helped to reduce intraoperative blood loss. The mean estimated blood loss was 330 cc. More recently, Porpiglia et al. reported their extraperitoneoscopic transcapsular adenomectomy in 78 consecutive patients with large prostate glands [21]. The mean operative time was 103 ± 31 min with the average estimated blood loss of 333 ± 321 cc. The average volume of the excised prostate adenoma was 77 cc, which was about 80 % of the prostate volume of 96 cc. The functional results also demonstrated significant improvement in Qmax, IPSS, and quality of life 1 year after the surgery.

In Table 14.1, a summary of data from published studies has been depicted. Overall, the current body of literature shows a convincing functional outcome of LSP in patients with large prostate and the results that are comparable with open simple prostatectomy [22, 14]. However, one may point on three key issues of intraoperative hemostasis, operative time, and operative cost for laparoscopic approach compared to the standard open surgery, which may warrant further scrutiny.

Review of published data shows the evolution of LSP technique since its first inception. Surgeons have attempted various technical modifications to minimize intraoperative hemorrhage, and at the same time, they gained more experience with this technique, which helped them to overcome some technical challenges. In one study by Sotelo et al., it was shown that performing capsulotomy directly over the anterior surface of the prostate gland may violate the subcapsular venous plexus, contributing to increased blood loss. After their initial transcapsular adenomectomy technique led to significant blood loss in the first 5 cases, they decided to incise the bladder neck just proximal to the prostatovesical junction to gain entry to the bladder in the next 12 cases. As a result of this modification, average blood loss decreased about 75 % from 660 cc in the first 5 cases to 165 cc in the subsequent patients [19]. Another study in 16 patients using the similar transvesical approach reported average intraoperative blood loss of 134 cc (range: 50–300 cc) [17]. Overall, in a few published studies comparing laparoscopic versus open simple prostatectomy, significantly less intraoperative blood loss is reported with the laparoscopic technique [14, 22, 23]. In terms of

Table 14.1 Laparoscopic simple prostatectomy: data from published series

			Mean (range)						
Reference	Year	Pts	Operative duration (min)	Estimated blood loss (cc)	Prostate volume (cc)	Resected tissue weight (g)	Hospitalization (days)	Catheterization (days)	Transfusion (%)
Van Velthoven et al. [16]	2004	18	145	192	95.1	47.6	5.9	3[a]	0
Sotelo et al. [19]	2005	17	156 (85–380)	516 (100–2,500)	93	72 (32–120)	2 (0.6–4.6)	6.3 (3–7)	5 (29)
Mariano et al. [18]	2006	60	138.5 (95–242)	330.98 (85–850)	144.5 (80–422)	131 (68–98)	3.46 (2–7)	4.6 (3–7)	0
Baumert et al. [22][b]	2006	30	115	367	121.8	77.2	5.1	4	1 (3.3)[c]
Zhou et al. [13]	2009	45	105.4 (81–210)	360.1 (110–1,500)	85.4 (62–110)	78.2 (65–115)	6.3	4.6	3 (6.6)
McCullough et al. [23]	2009	96	95.1	350 (300–575)	111.3	–	6.3	5.2	15 (15.8)
Yun et al. [15]	2010	11	191.9 (132–276)	390.9 (200–800)	109.3 (75.9–190)	72.4 (58–103)	6.5 (5–9)	5.6 (4–8)	2 (18.2)
Chlosta et al. [40]	2011	66	55 (45–85)	200 (100–250)	85 (70–120)	85.5 (65–98)	5.2 (5–10)	7.3 (6–9)	0
Porpiglia et al. [21]	2011	78	103	333	96	77	5.4	3.5	2 (2.5)
Oktay et al. [17]	2011	16	133 (75–210)	134 (50–300)	147 (80–200)	–	3.9 (2–7)	6.3 (6–7)	1 (6.2)
García-Segui et al. [24]	2012	17	135	250	–	–	3.7	5.5	0

[a]In four patients (22.2 %), the catheter needed to be replaced
[b]In the first 17 cases, a Millin-type procedure and, in the following 13 cases, transvesical approach were used
[c]One patient who had previously undergone inguinal hernia repair using bilateral mesh had an abdominal wall hematoma which was managed conservatively

operative time, some reports demonstrated shorter operative time with open surgery [22–24], while others showed no significant difference between the two techniques [14]. With more experience, one may expect shortening of the operative time. Regarding the postoperative parameters, most of the recent studies report shorter duration of catheterization and hospital stay in patients, who underwent laparoscopic adenomectomy, compared to those treated with open technique [22–24]. Other studies, however, showed no significant difference between the two groups in terms of postoperative morbidity [25].

Overall, the available data suggests that when surgeons pass their learning curve, along with advances in surgical instruments and laparoscopic techniques, satisfactory functional outcomes as well as improvements in operative time, intraoperative hemostasis, and other postoperative parameters should be expected.

To our knowledge, there is no published data comparing the operation cost of open versus laparoscopic simple prostatectomy. The overall cost is the product of operating time, equipment cost, hospital stay, and perioperative complications. The experience of the surgical team has a significant impact on these variables. Therefore, one should expect the data to vary depending on the mentioned parameters.

Single-Port Laparoscopic Simple Prostatectomy

In standard laparoscopic surgery, three to five laparoscopic ports are used, which requires multiple skin incisions. There are continuous attempts aimed at minimizing morbidity and improving cosmetic outcomes of laparoscopy. The introduction of more sophisticated articulating and/or curved instruments and the presence of more experienced laparoscopic surgeons have led to the development of techniques, such as multichannel single-access ports with the use of novel bent/articulating instruments, which could allow the laparoscopic procedure to be performed through a single skin incision [26–29]. In this case, laparo-endoscopic single-site surgery (LESS) is a variant of the laparoscopic surgery that uses a single small incision through which a single multichannel access port is placed. The incision is usually at umbilicus and allows virtually scar-free surgery.

Sotelo et al. reported the first case of simple prostatectomy with LESS surgery (Fig. 14.2) [30]. They used an R-port channel that allows simultaneous passage of three laparoscopic instruments (two 5 mm and one 12 mm) through a single umbilical incision. Then following induction of pneumoperitoneum, adenoma was dissected through a transverse cystotomy at the bladder neck. The surgery was successful with no intraoperative or postoperative complications. However, authors reported that this procedure was technically more difficult than the standard laparoscopic approach and expected a long learning curve.

At the same time, Desai et al. reported the initial results of a modified single-site surgery technique, called single-port transvesical enucleation of the prostate (STEP), in three patients with large prostates [31]. In this technique, following an initial cystoscopy, the bladder was filled with normal saline, and the proposed suprapubic site of the skin incision was marked such that it overlaid the highest portion of the bladder with the aid of a needle inserted percutaneously and cystoscopic monitoring. Then the bladder wall was entered sharply, and the inner ring of the R-port was inserted into the bladder. In the next step, the inner and outer rings were approximated, thus assuring the abdominal and bladder wall between the rings of the R-port in an airtight seal. Then the bladder insufflated with carbon dioxide to create the pneumovesicum (Fig. 14.3). Later on, the same group published the results of 34 consecutive cases, who underwent STEP surgery [32]. The average patients' BMI was 26 with the range of 21–41 with the average prostate volume of 102.5 cc (range: 50–247 cc). The mean operative duration was 116 min (range, 45–360 min) with mean estimated blood loss of 460 cc (range, 50–2,500 cc), a transfusion rate of 15 %, and mean hospital stay of 3 days.

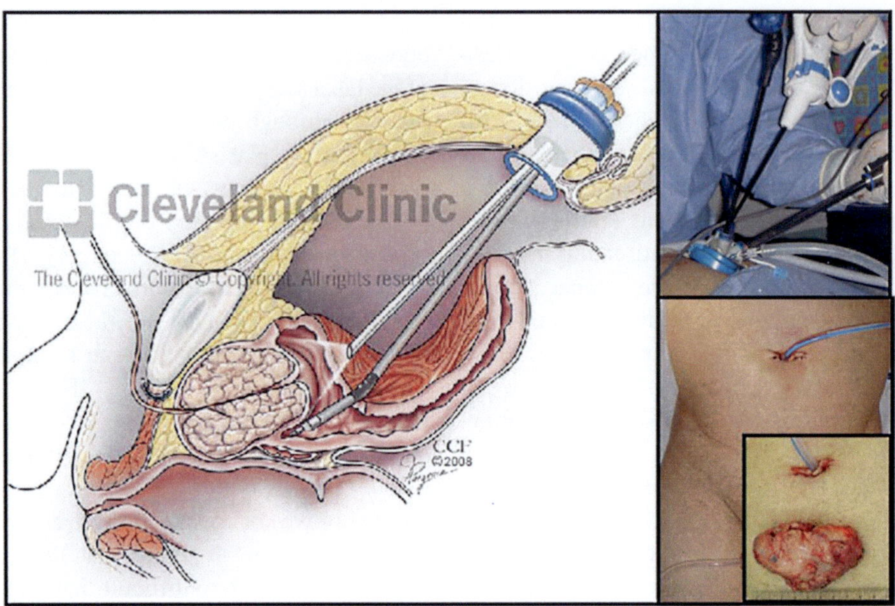

Fig. 14.2 Schematic diagram and pictures of LESS simple prostatectomy and postoperative appearance. The instruments dissect the adenoma through a cystotomy at the bladder neck (*left*). Photograph shows the R-port in place at the umbilicus (*up*). Completely, intraumbilical incision, urethral Foley catheter, and externalized closed suction drain. Inset shows the extracted adenoma (*down*) (Reprinted with permission, Cleveland Clinic Center for Medical Art & Photography © 2009. All Rights Reserved. From Sotelo et al. [30]. Reprinted with permission from Elsevier)

STEP complication rate however was significant. They reported one death of a Jehovah's Witness, who developed postoperative bleeding. In four cases, they had to convert to open surgery, either for complete enucleation of the adenoma or for management of the complications.

More recently, Oh and Park reported their surgical outcome in 32 patients who were treated with finger-assisted STEP (F-STEP) and compared the results with TURP outcome [33]. They showed better functional outcome in the F-STEP group compared to TURP patients, particularly in those with a medium- to large-size prostate and intravesical protruding adenomas.

The duration of the hospital stay (3.02±4.56 days vs. 1.90±3.82 days) and estimated blood loss (176.54±14.11 cc vs. 126.54±14.60 cc) were comparable in both groups. However, operative time (109.42±44.48 min vs. 68.03±25.02 min) and duration of catheterization (5.31±0.76 days vs. 2.09±1.74 days) were more favorable in TURP patients.

The main advantage of STEP is that the transvesical approach provides direct access to the large prostatic adenoma with no need for peritoneal violation or tissue dissection, thereby further reducing the access trauma. Furthermore, pneumovesicum may help control the intraoperative bleeding by providing tamponade-like effect on venous channels. Using this technique was successful in achieving complete enucleation of the prostate especially in those with prominent intravesical gland. In prostates with large apical portion, digital assistance was required for complete adenomectomy.

Despite multiple iterations regarding feasibility and satisfying functional outcome of STEP (Table 14.2), the approach has not been widely used. Several factors seem to be involved in this context. According to Autorino et al., laparoendoscopic single-site surgery including STEP was determined to be a very difficult and complex procedure with long learning curve that requires advanced laparoscopic training [32].

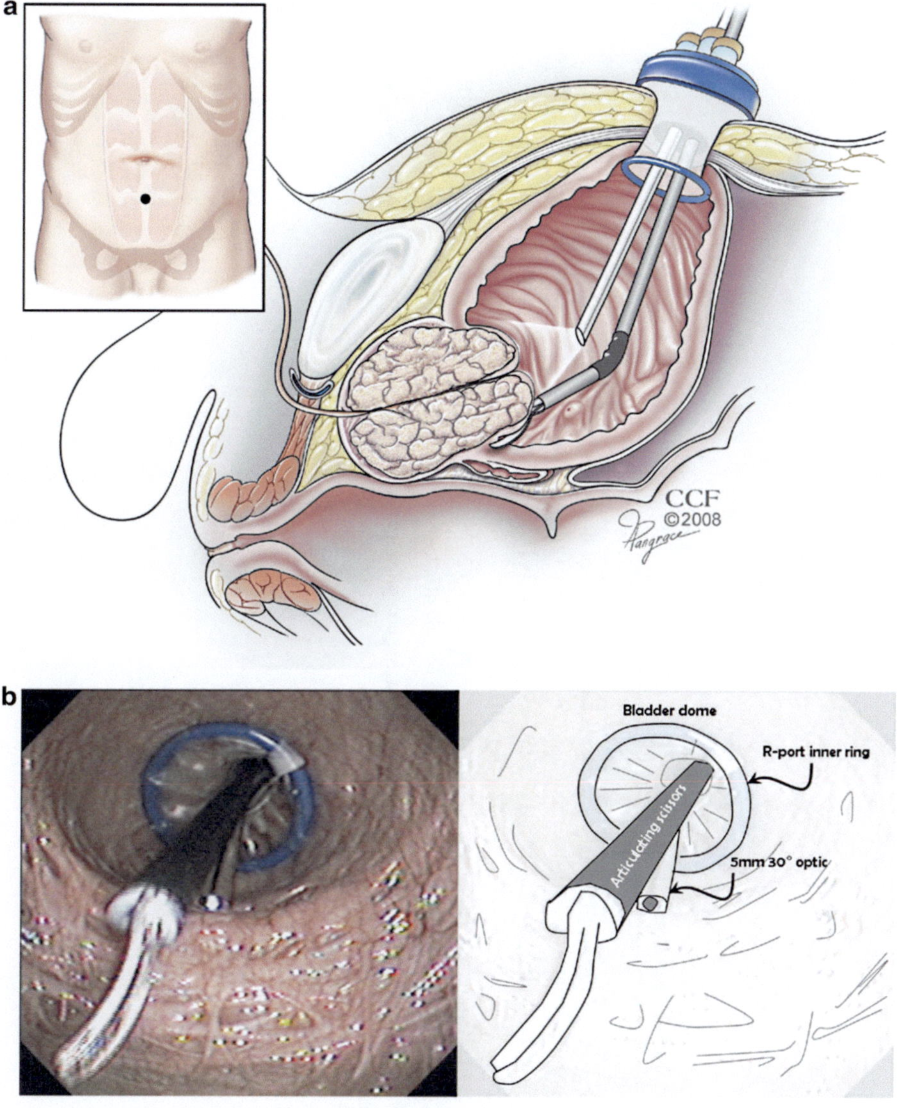

Fig. 14.3 (**a**) Diagrammatic representation of principles of STEP. R-port inserted through infraumbilical midline incision directly into bladder (Reprinted with the permission of The Cleveland Clinic Center for Medical Art & Photography © 2008. All Rights Reserved). (**b**) Cystoscopic view showing internal ring of R-port snuggly cinched inside bladder (From Desai et al. [31]. Reprinted with permission from Elsevier)

The complication rate in the most indicated group, who are patients with prostates larger than 100 cc, has been quite high [31, 32]. Furthermore, the F-STEP is technically very challenging for obese patients, mainly because the distance between the abdominal incision and the prostate adenoma would be too long to perform finger dissection. On the other hand, the lower complication rate of the procedure in smaller glands does not justify the application of such a complex technique for a simple prostatectomy, while other well-established standard approaches are being used successfully. Further advances in surgical instruments and rapidly growing technologies of laparoscopic surgery may facilitate application of this type of surgery in the future and alleviate our current safety concerns.

Table 14.2 Single-port transvesical enucleation of the prostate: data from published series

			Mean (range)							
Reference	Year	Pts	BMI (kg/m^2)	Operative duration (min)	Estimated blood loss (cc)	Prostate volume (cc)	Resected tissue weight (g)	Hospitalization (days)	Catheterization (days)	Transfusion (%)
Desai et al. [32][a]	2009	34	26 (21–41)	116 (45–360)	460 (50–2,500)[b]	102.5 (50–247)	68 (17–212)	3 (1–10)	6 (4–13)	5 (15)
Oh et al. [33]	2011	32	–	109.42	176.54	73 (48.3–102.6)	48.35	3.02	5.31	2 (6.3)
Wang et al. [41][c]	2012	9	21.5	160.9 (130–210)	418.8 (100–900)	83.8 (60.2–116.9)	50.9 (42–76)	7 (5–11)	8.6 (6–14)	1 (11.1)
Lee et al. [42]	2012	7	–	189.3 (155–280)	600 (100–2,000)	100.8 (86–133.6)	57.40 (45–68)	3.14	5.29	2 (28.5)

[a]In four (12 %) cases, surgery was converted to open. Two patients underwent open surgery for managing complications (enterotomy 1, bleeding 1), and in two patients, the skin incision was minimally enlarged to facilitate finger enucleation of the apical adenoma

[b]There was one death of a Jehovah's Witness who refused transfusion of blood and blood products

[c]Conversion to open surgery in one case (11.11 %)

Robot-Assisted Laparoscopic Simple Prostatectomy

Robotic-assisted laparoscopic surgery and its added benefits over conventional laparoscopy, such as enhanced ergonomics and more dexterous instruments, have allowed surgeons to expand applications of the modern minimally invasive surgery techniques. In 2008, Sotelo et al. described the first series of robot-assisted simple prostatectomy (RASP) in seven patients [34]. The surgery was performed using four-arm da Vinci® Surgical System following the insertion of six transperitoneal ports, identical to robotic-assisted radical prostatectomy. Then through a horizontal incision proximal to the junction of the bladder and prostate, adenoma was reached and dissected. The mean prostate volume was 77.6 cc on preoperative transrectal ultrasound study, and the average operative time was 195 min (range: 120–300 min). The mean estimated blood loss was 298 mL (range: 60–800 mL) with the transfusion rate of 14.2 % (one patient). Recently, Matei et al. applied a similar technique in 35 men and reported encouraging functional outcome at the final follow-up [35]. The mean intraoperative blood loss was as low as 121 cc with 0 % transfusion rate, while authors reported practically no blood loss in ten patients. They were also able to resect 81.2 % of the prostate tissue, using RASP. Through their retrospective review of patients' charts, they showed that RASP resection volume was higher than the amount of tissue removed through open (75.6 %) and transurethral (70.4 %) approach.

Robotic platform allows precise complex movements of surgical arms and optimum visualization of the surgical field. This allows surgeons to step up their surgical techniques and tackle more complex cases, while improving their functional outcomes and minimize the complications.

Accordingly, Coelho et al. described a modified RASP technique aiming to decrease perioperative blood loss, shorten the hospital stay, and eliminate the need for postoperative continuous bladder irrigation [36]. In this technique following standard adenomectomy, during the reconstructive part of the procedure, instead of performing the classical "trigonization" of the bladder neck and closure of the prostatic capsule, authors offer three modified surgical steps: (1) plication of the posterior prostatic capsule, (2) a modified van Velthoven continuous vesicourethral anastomosis, and finally (3) suture of the anterior prostatic capsule to the anterior bladder wall (Fig. 14.4). In this series of six patients, the mean estimated blood loss was 208 mL and the mean operative time was 90 min. As the main advantage of the surgical technique, all patients were discharged on postoperative day 1 without the need for continuous bladder irrigation at any time after surgery.

Recently, Clavijo et al. has described robot-assisted intrafascial simple prostatectomy (IF-RSP) [37]. In this technique, intrafascial plane (the plane between the prostate capsule and prostatic fascia) was dissected in order to perform total excision of the prostate tissue along with complete preservation of the neurovascular bundles. This was demonstrated by near-identical prostate volumes measured by TRUS and reported by pathologist, as well as 96 % decrease in serum PSA levels postoperatively (mean PSA level, 0.2 ng/mL; range, 0.00–0.84 ng/mL). In addition to excellent functional outcome, authors believe that using this technique helps to eliminate the risk of residual or future prostate cancer, without interrupting patients' potency or continence.

More recently, Fareed et al. published their experience with a novel technique of robotic single-port suprapubic transvesical enucleation of the prostate (R-STEP) for management of the large-size benign prostate [38]. The surgical procedure included an initial transurethral incision of the prostatic apex. Subsequently, a cystotomy was created and a GelPort® laparoscopic system was placed in the bladder. The robotic operating system was docked through the GelPort® platform, and enucleation of the adenoma was performed (Fig. 14.5). Mean operative time was 3.8 h and the mean EBL was 584 mL (>1 L in

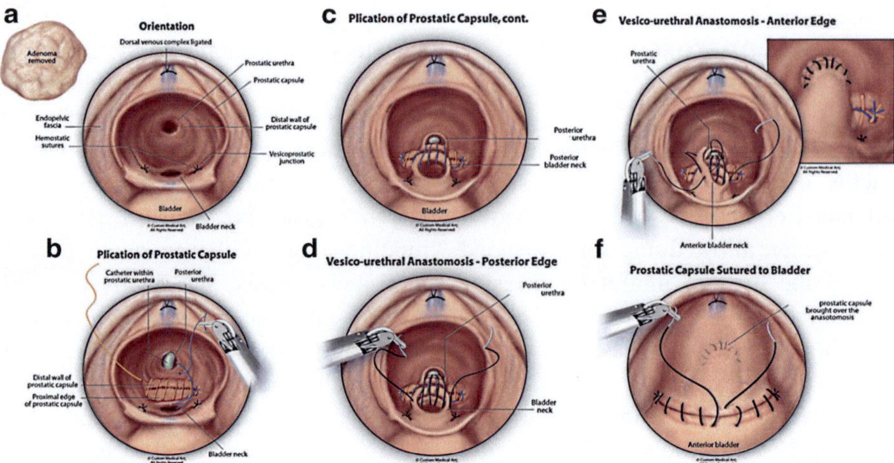

Fig. 14.4 Modified technique of robotic-assisted simple prostatectomy. (**a**) After removal of the adenoma, two 2–0 monocryl sutures, in a figure of eight, are placed at 5 and 7 o'clock positions, in the vesicoprostatic junction, for additional hemostasis. (**b**) Plication of the prostatic capsule: the proximal edge of the capsule was approximated to the distal capsule using one arm of a continuous 3–0 monocryl suture. (**c**) The posterior bladder neck is sutured to the posterior urethra using the other arm of the continuous 3–0 monocryl suture. This suture approximates the bladder to the urethral stump, allowing subsequently tension-free vesicourethral anastomosis. (**d**) Continuous modified van Velthoven vesicourethral anastomosis: the posterior part of the anastomosis is performed with one arm of a 3–0 continuous monocryl suture, in a clockwise direction, from the 5 to 9 o' clock position. (**e**) The posterior bladder neck is sutured to the posterior urethra using the other arm of the continuous 3–0 monocryl suture. This suture approximates the bladder to the urethral stump, allowing subsequently tension-free vesicourethral anastomosis. (**f**) Continuous modified van Velthoven vesicourethral anastomosis: the posterior part of the anastomosis is performed with one arm of a 3–0 continuous monocryl suture, in a clockwise direction, from the 5 to 9 o' clock position (From Coelho et al. [36]. Reprinted with permission from John Wiley and Sons)

three patients). Two patients received an intraoperative blood transfusion, and two patients required digital rectal assistance for complete enucleation. Despite acceptable functional outcome, it seems the procedure still carries a high risk of complications. It seems that further evolution of the R-STEP is likely to be strictly dependent on the development of appropriate instrumentation. Thus, its role in the surgical armamentarium of BPH remains to be determined. A summary of published data on RASP has been shown in Table 14.3.

From surgical cost standpoint, we could not find any published comprehensive study in our literature review. However, one study from Venezuela in a very small series of patients showed about $1,500 higher cost of RASP comparing to the LSP [34]. In contrast, another report from Italy revealed that RASP was on average about $1,600 cheaper than open simple prostatectomy, principally due to the costs of longer hospitalization in open surgeries. Interestingly, the same study also revealed similar costs for RASP and TURP [35]. Meanwhile, it has been demonstrated by several studies that the number of surgeries that have been done by a robot in a single center is a major index in the evaluation of the economy of robotic surgeries. Robot-assisted laparoscopic surgery comes at a high cost, but it can become cost-effective in mostly high-volume centers with high-volume surgeons [39]. Moreover, the indirect benefits of robotic surgery including decreased length of hospital stay and return to work are considerable and must be measured when evaluating its cost-effectiveness.

Surgeons aimed to combine the benefits of open simple prostatectomy with potential advantages of a minimally invasive approach by describing laparoscopic simple prostatectomy. Although

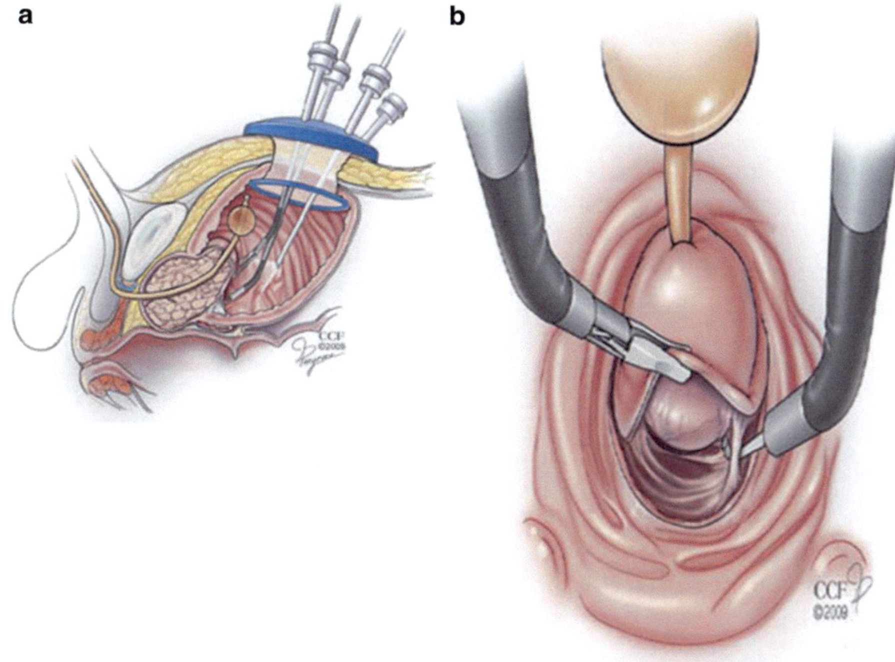

Fig. 14.5 (**a**) Illustration of robotic single-port suprapubic transvesical enucleation of the prostate. GelPort inserted in the superior aspect of the bladder with the da Vinci robot 12 mm scope and 5 mm robotic ports introduced through the gel platform. The 30° lens angled upwards is used to reduce instrument clashing. An additional 5 mm port is placed lateral and cephalad to the right robotic hand instrument port to assist with suction and retraction. (**b**) Illustration depicting adenoma enucleation. A flexible grasper in the left hand and flexible monopolar cautery in the right hand were used. The inner ring of the GelPort TM was used to isolate the Foley balloon away from the surgical field (From Fareed et al. [38]. Reprinted with permission from John Wiley and Sons)

it is proven to be feasible, the technical challenges of this surgical procedure have prevented the widespread adoption of LSP by most urological surgeons. The evolution of robot-assisted laparoscopy was able to overcome most of LSP limitations. In terms of long learning curve for LSP, it seems that RASP is easier to perform, learn, and teach; therefore, it is more likely to popularize this surgical technique. In addition, robotic platform allows the procedure to be performed without the need for special devices due to the advantages provided by the EndoWrist® technology of the robotic arms and precise 3D vision. The global access to da Vinci® robot and limited worldwide penetration of this technology, along with the surgical costs and economic aspects of the treatment, are critical issues that need to be addressed in future studies before any general recommendation could be made.

The exact indication of laparoscopic or robotic-assisted prostatectomy is still evolving. While the introduction of sophisticated surgical devices promise a less invasive procedure (compared to open simple prostatectomy), at the same time transurethral surgical procedures are evolving. The advent of new energy sources and endoscopic equipment has allowed surgeons to tackle larger prostates with acceptable surgical outcomes. The two approaches, i.e., transabdominal versus transurethral, compete to gain popularity among surgeons for large prostate sizes. We believe the procedure that promises a shorter learning curve, less morbidity, and lower cost will be the one that will win the contest.

Table 14.3 Robot-assisted simple prostatectomy: data from published series

			Mean (range)							
Reference	Year	Pts	BMI (kg/m²)	Operative duration (min)	Estimated blood loss (cc)	Prostate volume (cc)	Resected tissue weight (g)	Hospitalization (days)	Catheterization (days)	Transfusion (%)
Sotelo et al. [34]	2008	7	–	195 (120–300)	381.6 (60–800)	77.66 (40–106)	50.48 (40–64.5)	1.33 (1–2)	7.5 (6–10)	1 (14.3)
John et al. [43]	2009	13	26 (23–31)	210 (150–330)	500 (100–1,100)	100 (90–180)	82 (50–150)	6 (5–15)	6 (3–15)	0
Coelho et al. [36][a]	2011	6	28.1	90 (75–120)	208 (100–300)	157 (90–300)	145 (84–186)	1	4.8 (4–6)	0
Sutherland et al. [44][b]	2011	9	–	183 (148–278)	206 (50–500)	136.5 (86–265)	112 (53–220)	1.3 (0.8–3)	13 (12–14)	0
Vora et al. [45]	2012	13	–	179.4 (90–270)	219.4 (50–500)	163 (110–220)	127 (100–165)	2.78 (1–8)	8.89 (5–14)	0
Matei et al. [35]	2012	35	–	186 (134–300)	121 (10–700)	96.2 (37–240)	87.04 (26–189)	3.2 (2–9)	7.4 (5–14)	0
Clavijo et al. [37]	2013	10	–	106 (60–180)	375 (150–900)	81 (47–153)	81 (50–150)	1 (0–3)	8.9 (6–14)	1 (10)

[a]All patients were discharged on postoperative day 1 without the need of continuous bladder irrigation at any time after RASP
[b]One case converted to open surgery

References

1. Freyer P. Total enucleation of the prostate. Br Med J. 1912;2(2702):999.
2. Millin T. The surgery of prostatic obstructions. Ir J Med Sci. 1947;257:185–9.
3. Nesbit RM. A history of transurethral prostatectomy. Rev Mex Urol. 1975;35:249–62.
4. Lu-Yao GL, Barry MJ, Chang CH, Wasson JH, Wennberg JE. Transurethral resection of the prostate among Medicare beneficiaries in the United States: time trends and outcomes. Prostate Patient Outcomes Research Team (PORT). Urology. 1994;44(5):692–8; discussion 698–699.
5. McNicholas TA. Management of symptomatic BPH in the UK: who is treated and how? Eur Urol. 1999;36 Suppl 3:33–9. 52347 [pii] 52347.
6. Gordon NS, Hadlow G, Knight E, Mohan P. Transurethral resection of the prostate: still the gold standard. Aust N Z J Surg. 1997;67(6):354–7.
7. McVary KT, Roehrborn CG, Avins AL, Barry MJ, Bruskewitz RC, Donnell RF, Foster Jr HE, Gonzalez CM, Kaplan SA, Penson DF, Ulchaker JC, Wei JT. Update on AUA guideline on the management of benign prostatic hyperplasia. J Urol. 2011;185(5): 1793–803. doi:10.1016/j.juro.2011.01.074. S0022-5347(11)00224-2 [pii].
8. Oelke M, Bachmann A, Descazeaud A, Emberton M, Gravas S, Michel MC, N'Dow J, Nordling J, de la Rosette JJ. EAU guidelines on the treatment and follow-up of non-neurogenic male lower urinary tract symptoms including benign prostatic obstruction. Eur Urol. 2013;64(1):118–40. doi:10.1016/j.eururo.2013.03.004. S0302-2838(13)00228-5 [pii].
9. Souverein PC, Erkens JA, de la Rosette JJ, Leufkens HG, Herings RM. Drug treatment of benign prostatic hyperplasia and hospital admission for BPH-related surgery. Eur Urol. 2003;43(5):528–34. S0302283803000897 [pii].
10. Vela-Navarrete R, Gonzalez-Enguita C, Garcia-Cardoso JV, Manzarbeitia F, Sarasa-Corral JL, Granizo JJ. The impact of medical therapy on surgery for benign prostatic hyperplasia: a study comparing changes in a decade (1992–2002). BJU Int. 2005; 96(7):1045–8.doi:10.1111/j.1464-410X.2005.05735.x. BJU5735 [pii].
11. Suardi N, Gallina A, Salonia A, Briganti A, Deho F, Zanni G, Abdollah F, Naspro R, Cestari A, Guazzoni G, Rigatti P, Montorsi F. Holmium laser enucleation of the prostate and holmium laser ablation of the prostate: indications and outcome. Curr Opin Urol. 2009;19(1):38–43. doi:10.1097/MOU.0b013e32831a700800042307-200901000-00009 [pii].
12. Rajbabu K, Chandrasekara SK, Barber NJ, Walsh K, Muir GH. Photoselective vaporization of the prostate with the potassium-titanyl-phosphate laser in men with prostates of >100 mL. BJU Int. 2007;100(3):593–8. doi:10.1111/j.1464-410X.2007.06985.x. BJU6985 [pii]; discussion 598.
13. Zhou LY, Xiao J, Chen H, Zhu YP, Sun YW, Xuan Q. Extraperitoneal laparoscopic adenomectomy for benign prostatic hyperplasia. World J Urol. 2009; 27(3):385–7. doi:10.1007/s00345-008-0359-8.
14. Porpiglia F, Terrone C, Renard J, Grande S, Musso F, Cossu M, Vacca F, Scarpa RM. Transcapsular adenomectomy (Millin): a comparative study, extraperitoneal laparoscopy versus open surgery. Eur Urol. 2006; 49(1):120–6.doi:10.1016/j.eururo.2005.09.017.S0302-2838(05)00666-4 [pii].
15. Yun HK, Kwon JB, Cho SR, Kim JS. Early experience with laparoscopic retropubic simple prostatectomy in patients with voluminous Benign Prostatic Hyperplasia (BPH). Korean J Urol. 2010;51(5):323–9. doi:10.4111/kju.2010.51.5.323.
16. van Velthoven R, Peltier A, Laguna MP, Piechaud T. Laparoscopic extraperitoneal adenomectomy (Millin): pilot study on feasibility. Eur Urol. 2004;45(1):103–9. S0302283803004202 [pii]; discussion 109.
17. Oktay B, Koc G, Vuruskan H, Danisoglu ME, Kordan Y. Laparoscopic extraperitoneal simple prostatectomy for benign prostate hyperplasia: a two-year experience. Urol J. 2011;8(2):107–12. 1020/546 [pii].
18. Mariano MB, Tefilli MV, Graziottin TM, Morales CM, Goldraich IH. Laparoscopic prostatectomy for benign prostatic hyperplasia – a six-year experience. Eur Urol. 2006;49(1):127–31. doi:10.1016/j.eururo.2005.09.018. S0302-2838(05)00667-6 [pii]; discussion 131–122.
19. Sotelo R, Spaliviero M, Garcia-Segui A, Hasan W, Novoa J, Desai MM, Kaouk JH, Gill IS. Laparoscopic retropubic simple prostatectomy. J Urol. 2005; 173(3):757–60. doi:10.1097/01.ju.0000152651.27143.b0. S0022-5347(05)60328-X [pii].
20. Mariano MB, Graziottin TM, Tefilli MV. Laparoscopic prostatectomy with vascular control for benign prostatic hyperplasia. J Urol. 2002;167(6):2528–9. S0022-5347(05)65025-2 [pii].
21. Porpiglia F, Fiori C, Cavallone B, Morra I, Bertolo R, Scarpa RM. Extraperitoneoscopic transcapsular adenomectomy: complications and functional results after at least 1 year of follow-up. J Urol. 2011;185(5): 1668–73. doi:10.1016/j.juro.2010.12.047. S0022-5347(10)05389-9 [pii].
22. Baumert H, Ballaro A, Dugardin F, Kaisary AV. Laparoscopic versus open simple prostatectomy: a comparative study. J Urol. 2006;175(5):1691–4. doi:10.1016/S0022-5347(05)00986-9. S0022-5347(05)00986-9 [pii].
23. McCullough TC, Heldwein FL, Soon SJ, Galiano M, Barret E, Cathelineau X, Prapotnich D, Vallancien G, Rozet F. Laparoscopic versus open simple prostatectomy: an evaluation of morbidity. J Endourol. 2009;23(1):129–33. doi:10.1089/end.2008.0401.
24. Garcia-Segui A, Gascon-Mir M. Comparative study between laparoscopic extraperitoneal and open adenomectomy. Actas Urol Esp. 2012;36(2):110–6. doi:10.1016/j.acuro.2011.09.002. S0210-4806(11)00373-1 [pii].
25. Barret E, Bracq A, Braud G, Harmon J, Almeida D, Rozet F, Cathelineau X, Vallancien G. The morbidity

of laparoscopic versus open simple prostatectomy. Eur Urol Suppl. 2006;5:274.
26. Desai MM, Berger AK, Brandina R, Aron M, Irwin BH, Canes D, Desai MR, Rao PP, Sotelo R, Stein R, Gill IS. Laparoendoscopic single-site surgery: initial hundred patients. Urology. 2009;74(4):805–12. doi:10.1016/j.urology.2009.02.083. S0090-4295(09)00522-6 [pii].
27. Jung YW, Kim YT, Lee DW, Hwang YI, Nam EJ, Kim JH, Kim SW. The feasibility of scarless single-port transumbilical total laparoscopic hysterectomy: initial clinical experience. Surg Endosc. 2010;24(7):1686–92. doi:10.1007/s00464-009-0830-7.
28. Desai MM, Rao PP, Aron M, Pascal-Haber G, Desai MR, Mishra S, Kaouk JH, Gill IS. Scarless single port transumbilical nephrectomy and pyeloplasty: first clinical report. BJU Int. 2008;101(1):83–8. doi:10.1111/j.1464-410X.2007.07359.x. BJU7359 [pii].
29. Hong TH, You YK, Lee KH. Transumbilical single-port laparoscopic cholecystectomy : scarless cholecystectomy. Surg Endosc. 2009;23(6):1393–7. doi:10.1007/s00464-008-0252-y.
30. Sotelo RJ, Astigueta JC, Desai MM, Canes D, Carmona O, De Andrade RJ, Moreira O, Lopez R, Velasquez A, Gill IS. Laparoendoscopic single-site surgery simple prostatectomy: initial report. Urology. 2009;74(3):626–30. doi:10.1016/j.urology.2009.03.039. S0090-4295(09)00504-4 [pii].
31. Desai MM, Aron M, Canes D, Fareed K, Carmona O, Haber GP, Crouzet S, Astigueta JC, Lopez R, de Andrade R, Stein RJ, Ulchaker J, Sotelo R, Gill IS. Single-port transvesical simple prostatectomy: initial clinical report. Urology. 2008;72(5):960–5. doi:10.1016/j.urology.2008.06.007. S0090-4295(08)00702-4 [pii].
32. Desai MM, Fareed K, Berger AK, Astigueta JC, Irwin BH, Aron M, Ulchaker J, Sotelo R. Single-port transvesical enucleation of the prostate: a clinical report of 34 cases. BJU Int. 2009;105(9):1296–300. doi:10.1111/j.1464-410X.2009.09106.x. BJU9106 [pii].
33. Oh JJ, Park DS. Novel surgical technique for obstructive benign prostatic hyperplasia: finger-assisted, single-port transvesical enucleation of the prostate. J Endourol. 2011;25(3):459–64. doi:10.1089/end.2010.0453.
34. Sotelo R, Clavijo R, Carmona O, Garcia A, Banda E, Miranda M, Fagin R. Robotic simple prostatectomy. J Urol. 2008;179(2):513–5. doi:10.1016/j.juro.2007.09.065. S0022-5347(07)02567-0 [pii].
35. Matei DV, Brescia A, Mazzoleni F, Spinelli M, Musi G, Melegari S, Galasso G, Detti S, de Cobelli O. Robot-assisted simple prostatectomy (RASP): does it make sense? BJU Int. 2012;110(11 Pt C):E972–9. doi:10.1111/j.1464-410X.2012.11192.x.
36. Coelho RF, Chauhan S, Sivaraman A, Palmer KJ, Orvieto MA, Rocco B, Coughlin G, Patel VR. Modified technique of robotic-assisted simple prostatectomy: advantages of a vesico-urethral anastomosis. BJU Int. 2011;109(3):426–33. doi:10.1111/j.1464-410X.2011.010401.x.
37. Clavijo R, Carmona O, De Andrade R, Garza R, Fernandez G, Sotelo R. Robot-assisted intrafascial simple prostatectomy: novel technique. J Endourol. 2013;27(3):328–32. doi:10.1089/end.2012.0212.
38. Fareed K, Zaytoun OM, Autorino R, White WM, Crouzet S, Yakoubi R, Haber GP, White MA, Kaouk JH. Robotic single port suprapubic transvesical enucleation of the prostate (R-STEP): initial experience. BJU Int. 2012;110(5):732–7. doi:10.1111/j.1464-410X.2012.10954.x.
39. Liberman D, Trinh QD, Jeldres C, Zorn KC. Is robotic surgery cost-effective: yes. Curr Opin Urol. 2012;22(1):61–5. doi:10.1097/MOU.0b013e32834d543f.
40. Chlosta PL, Varkarakis IM, Drewa T, Dobruch J, Jaskulski J, Antoniewicz AA, Borowka A. Extraperitoneal laparoscopic Millin prostatectomy using finger enucleation. J Urol. 2011;186(3):873–6. doi:10.1016/j.juro.2011.04.080. S0022-5347(11)03861-4 [pii].
41. Wang L, Liu B, Yang Q, Wu Z, Yang B, Xu Z, Cai C, Xiao L, Chen W, Sun Y. Preperitoneal single-port transvesical enucleation of the prostate (STEP) for large-volume BPH: one-year follow-up of Qmax, IPSS, and QoL. Urology. 2012;80(2):323–8. doi:10.1016/j.urology.2012.02.064. S0090-4295(12)00418-9 [pii].
42. Lee JY, Han JH, Moon HS, Yoo TK, Choi HY, Lee SW. Single-port transvesical enucleation of the prostate for benign prostatic hyperplasia with severe intravesical prostatic protrusion. World J Urol. 2012;30(4):511–7. doi:10.1007/s00345-011-0758-0.
43. John H, Bucher C, Engel N, Fischer B, Fehr JL. Preperitoneal robotic prostate adenomectomy. Urology. 2009;73(4):811–5. doi:10.1016/j.urology.2008.09.028. S0090-4295(08)01581-1 [pii].
44. Sutherland DE, Perez DS, Weeks DC. Robot-assisted simple prostatectomy for severe benign prostatic hyperplasia. J Endourol. 2011;25(4):641–4. doi:10.1089/end.2010.0528.
45. Vora A, Mittal S, Hwang J, Bandi G. Robot-assisted simple prostatectomy: multi-institutional outcomes for glands larger than 100 grams. J Endourol. 2012;26(5):499–502. doi:10.1089/end.2011.0562.

15 Laparoscopic/Robotic Simple Prostatectomy

Rao S. Mandalapu, Adnan Ali, Sailaja Pisipati, and Ashutosh K. Tewari

Introduction

The normal prostate gland is composed of fibromuscular stromal cells, glandular elements, and smooth muscle cells. Benign prostatic hyperplasia (BPH) is characterized by prostatic stromal and epithelial cell hyperplasia in the periurethral region of the prostate. Though the adenomatous growth of the prostate begins at the age of 30, an estimated 90 % of men have histologic evidence of BPH by the age of 80 years. Approximately 40 % of men will have clinically significant BPH after the age of 50 years [1, 2]. Benign prostatic hyperplasia is the most common benign neoplasm in American men, affecting nearly 6.5 million men aged 50–79 years in the United States [3, 4]. The treatment options for clinically significant benign prostatic hyperplasia have been dramatically changed in the recent past with the development of minimally invasive procedures and advanced medical therapies. However, open prostatectomy remains the surgery of choice in selected patients. Several contemporary series have reported objective improvement in urinary symptoms after open prostatectomy [5, 6].

In an attempt to reduce the length of hospital stay and morbidity associated with the open prostatectomy, minimally invasive approaches have evolved. Mariano et al. first reported their experience of laparoscopic simple prostatectomy (LSP) in 2002 [7]. Contemporary studies have shown that LSP was associated with prolonged operative time, less blood loss, reduced length of hospital stay, and shorter period of catheterization [8, 9]. However, LSP has not gained wider acceptance due to the technical difficulty, restricted range of movements, two-dimensional views, and a steep learning curve.

Robot-assisted simple prostatectomy (RASP) holds potential for improving perioperative outcomes following simple prostatectomy. Sotelo et al. first reported RASP in 2008 and contemporary series demonstrated feasible and reproducible outcomes with an acceptable complication rate [10–14]. Subsequent publications have suggested that RASP is a safe and feasible option for clinically significant benign prostatic hyperplasia in select patients with larger prostates.

Indications

The indications of simple prostatectomy include a large prostate gland with an estimated weight of more than 80 g with moderate to severe lower urinary tract symptoms (LUTS) and/or with

R.S. Mandalapu, M.D. • A. Ali, M.B.B.S. • S. Pisipati, M.D., FRCS (Urol) • A.K. Tewari, M.B.B.S., M.Ch. (✉)
Department of Urology, Icahn School of Medicine at Mount Sinai, Mount Sinai Hospital, 1425 Madison Avenue, 6th Floor, New York, NY 10029, USA
e-mail: raomsmd@gmail.com; dr.adnanali@hotmail.com; sailaja13in@yahoo.com; ashtewari@mountsinai.org

B. Chughtai et al. (eds.), *Treatment of Benign Prostatic Hyperplasia: Modern Alternative to Transurethral Resection of the Prostate*, DOI 10.1007/978-1-4939-1587-3_15,

significantly bothering symptoms which are refractive to medical management, bladder outlet obstruction with acute urinary retention, recurrent gross hematuria of prostatic origin, recurrent urinary tract infections associated with bladder diverticulum secondary to bladder outlet obstruction, bladder calculi secondary to urinary retention and bladder outlet obstruction, and pathophysiological changes in the upper tracts due to benign prostatic hyperplasia and outlet obstruction. Those who have developed complications of BPH, such as bladder diverticulum, and large bladder calculi are particularly benefited by combining diverticulectomy and/or bladder stone removal along with simple prostatectomy.

Patients with history of hypospadias and urethral stricture diseases are considered for open simple prostatectomy to avoid further trauma to the urethra by transurethral procedures.

Simple prostatectomy should also be considered in patients with severe ankylosis of the hip/knee joints that limits lithotomy position for transurethral resection of the prostate or any other minimally invasive procedures performed in lithotomy position.

The choice of surgical approach depends on the patient's presenting characteristics and also surgeon's expertise in minimally invasive procedures and/or robotic surgery.

Contraindications

Contraindications to simple prostatectomy include a small fibrous prostate gland, carcinoma of the prostate, and prior pelvic surgery or radiation in which the planes are obliterated to approach the prostate gland.

Preoperative Evaluation

Men with clinically significant BPH who are the candidates for surgery will have the International Prostate Symptom Score (IPSS) questionnaire completed prior to surgery. They will have a peak urinary flow rate (Qmax) determination, and post-void residual (PVR) urine volume will be documented prior to surgery. Cystoscopy evaluation was indicated in patients with hematuria, suspected bladder diverticulum, and urethral stricture disease. Prostate cancer should be ruled out in all men by a digital rectal examination and a serum prostate-specific antigen determination. Prostate biopsy is performed if indicated.

The upper urinary tract should be evaluated preoperatively in men with history of hematuria, recurrent urinary tract infections, and a hydronephrosis with computed tomography (CT urogram) in patients with normal renal functions or with renal ultrasonography and/or magnetic resonance imaging (MRI). Renal function assessment is indicated in all patients who had urinary retention secondary to bladder outlet obstruction due to BPH. All the patients should undergo a thorough medical evaluation and/or be medically cleared for surgery. The type of anesthesia to be administered and the risks associated are thoroughly discussed with the patient and his family by an attending anesthesiologist. The patient is kept NPO after midnight on the day before the scheduled surgery. Patients are advised to have self-administered Fleet enema the night before surgery.

Surgical Technique

Robot-Assisted Simple Prostatectomy

The da Vinci Surgical System provides better visualization with 3-D high-resolution operative field and precision with exceptional dexterity to facilitate technically demanding simple prostatectomy procedure. Though the functional outcomes of RASP are comparable to open simple prostatectomy, RASP demands technical skills and expertise. RASP has been described in three different approaches, suprapubic, transvesical, and retropubic approach depending on the surgeon's preference.

Instrumentation

Port Access

1. Versaport Plus bladeless 5–12 mm-trocar (Covidien)
2. Versaport bladeless optical 5 mm trocar (Covidien)

3. ENDOPATH dilating tip trocar and housing 10/12 mm
4. Trocars with dilating tip (Cardinal Health, Inc.)

Robotic Instruments

1. da Vinci Surgical System (Intuitive Surgical Inc., Sunnyvale, CA)
2. InSite Vision System, da Vinci robotic system with zero-degree and 30-degree scopes (Intuitive Surgical Inc., Sunnyvale, CA)
3. EndoWrist Maryland bipolar forceps (Intuitive Surgical Inc., Sunnyvale, CA)
4. EndoWrist curved monopolar scissors (Intuitive Surgical Inc., Sunnyvale, CA)
5. EndoWrist ProGrasp forceps (Intuitive Surgical Inc., Sunnyvale, CA)
6. EndoWrist needle drivers (Intuitive Surgical Inc., Sunnyvale, CA)
7. New robotic fourth arm and accessories
8. Karl Storz robotic urology instrument tray

Conventional Instruments (Disposable)

1. Hydroline trumpet valve with Pulse Wave cassette (Cardinal Health, Inc.)
2. Weck Hem-o-lok clips (Teleflex Medical)
3. Endoscopic needles – Polysorb (Covidien)
4. BIOSYN sutures (Cardinal Health, Inc.)
5. Endo Catch Gold (10 mm) (Covidien)
6. Endo Shears (5 mm) (Covidien)
7. V-Loc 26-mm sutures (Covidien)
8. Chromic Gut V-20 (26 mm) (Covidien)
9. Sofsilk cutting suture (26 mm) (Covidien)
10. Maxon sutures (40 mm) (Covidien)

Suprapubic Approach

Positioning

After induction of general anesthesia, the patient is placed in Trendelenburg position with legs secured in stirrups and arms tucked and padded at the sides. Foley catheter is placed under strict aseptic precautions and secured. Orogastric tube is placed to decompress the stomach.

Port Placement

A pneumoperitoneum is created by insufflation using a Veress needle inserted supraumbilically. After adequate insufflation, a 12 mm trocar is placed supraumbilically for the placement of stereoscopic endoscope. Five trocars, three for robotic arms and two for assistants, are placed. First, two 8 mm pararectus trocars for the robotic arms are placed on the right and the left side for the second and third robotic arms. Another 8 mm trocar is placed in the left lumbar region for the fourth arm or the robot. Additionally, 12 and 5 mm assistant ports are placed on the patient's right side to provide retraction, suction, and irrigation and for passing clips and sutures. Following the placement of trocars, the da Vinci robot is placed between the patient's legs and the robotic arms are brought above the patient and docked.

Surgical Technique

After gaining abdominal access with zero-degree scope, thorough inspection of the pelvic structures will be carried out with particular focus on adhesions. Adhesions, if any, are lysed with sharp and blunt dissection to free up pelvis access. Medial umbilical ligaments are identified; peritoneal incision is made using monopolar cautery lateral to the medial umbilical ligaments starting at the vas deferens on either side; a wide inverted U-shaped dissection will be carried out through the urachus in the midline. Flimsy connective tissue in the space of Retzius is dissected using monopolar electrocautery and blunt dissection. These maneuvers will drop down the bladder. After periprostatic fat clearance anteriorly, superficial dorsal venous plexus is secured with cauterization/suture ligation.

The prostatovesical junction is identified by bimanual bladder neck pinch using blunt robotic instruments. The bladder neck is incised in the midline using hot shears and Maryland bipolar forceps. Appropriate plane of dissection should be followed carefully to identify mucosa of the bladder neck. Once the bladder lumen is entered anteriorly at the bladder neck, stroma of the prostate identified and a figure-of-eight traction suture using 0 silk is placed. Median lobe of the prostate is identified, if present, and mobilized by anterior traction applied using the third arm of the robot to provide posterior exposure. An incision is made using monopolar electrocautery in the posterior portion of the bladder neck, and the plane between the adenoma (transition zone) and the peripheral zone is developed. This plane is carefully followed distally towards apex of the prostate. The urethra is transected proximal to the external urinary sphincter at the apex of the prostate. Hemostasis is secured using electrocautery and Hem-o-lok clips (Teleflex Medical). Bladder neck is advanced distally to achieve mucosa-to-mucosa anastomosis between the bladder neck and the distal urethra using Chromic Gut V-20 (Covidien) suture. A 20-F Foley catheter is advanced through the anterior urethra into the bladder under direct vision during the anastomosis. After the Foley catheter is secured, gentle traction was applied temporarily for the hemostasis.

Transvesical Approach

After bladder drop-down is performed as described in suprapubic approach, vertical midline cystotomy incision is made starting at the dome of the bladder to gain access to the prostate transvesically. Vicryl stay sutures are used to maintain cystotomy access to the prostate. Adenoma of the prostate is identified and secured with a traction suture to facilitate dissection. An incision is made through the bladder mucosa overlying prostatic adenoma and proceeds through the plane between the prostate capsule and the adenoma. Using traction and monopolar electrocautery dissection, the entire adenoma is enucleated. Hemostasis is secured with electrocautery and suture ligation in the prostatic fossa.

If hemorrhage is persistent, prostate pedicles are ligated using Chromic suture near the bladder neck at 5 o' clock and 7 o' clock positions. Intravenous indigo carmine dye may be given to aid in the visualization of the ureteral orifices to avoid incorporation of the ureters in the suture ligation of the prostatic pedicles. The prostate capsule is closed after placing a 20-F Foley catheter into the bladder through the anterior urethra and prostatic fossa. The Foley catheter is secured with 30 cc of sterile water in the balloon. Cystotomy is closed in layers with 2–0 V-Loc sutures (Covidien). We prefer gentle traction applied to Foley catheter temporarily for hemostasis.

Retropubic Approach

After bladder drop-down as described in suprapubic approach, the anterior periprostatic area is defatted; superficial dorsal venous plexus is secured with cauterization/suture ligation. A transverse incision is made through the prostatic capsule approximately 2 cm distal to the bladder neck. Adenoma of the prostate is identified and the plane between the adenoma (transition zone) and the peripheral zone is developed. The adenoma is dissected further using blunt dissection and electrocautery to secure hemostasis. The urethra is transected proximal to the external urinary sphincter and distal to the verumontanum. The bladder neck mucosa is advanced to the urethral mucosa, and anastomosis completed using 2–0 Chromic Gut (Covidien) suture. A 20-F Foley catheter is inserted through the anterior urethra into the bladder and secured, gentle traction applied temporarily for the hemostasis.

Several contemporary series have demonstrated objective improvement in urinary symptoms after RASP [10–20].

Table 15.1 shows preoperative and perioperative characteristics and postoperative outcomes.

We analyzed our experience with robot-assisted simple prostatectomy (Tewari et al., unpublished data); the mean age was 73 years (range, 64–82); preoperative PSA was 17.8 ng/ml (range 12.8–21.2); mean operative time was 172 min (range, 117–245); blood transfusion rate was 0 %; mean resected prostate weight was

Table 15.1 Preoperative and perioperative characteristics and functional outcomes

	Preoperative characteristics				Perioperative characteristics									Outcomes					
	No. of pts, n	Mean age, yrs	Mean PSA, ng/ml	Mean prostate volume on TRUS, ml	TP/EP approach	TV/SP/RP	Mean operative time, min	Mean length of stay, days	Mean Foley catheter duration, days	Mean blood loss, ml	Transfusion, n (%)	Mean resected prostate weight, g	Conversion to open	Pre-op IPSS	Post-op IPSS	Pre-op Qmax, ml/s	Post-op Qmax, ml/s	Pre-op QoL	Post-op QoL
Sotelo et al. 2008 [10]	7	64.7	12.5	77.7	TP	TV	195	1.3	7.5	382	1 (14.3)	50.5	0	22	7.3	17.8	55.5	3.8	2.3
Yuh et al. 2008 [14]	3	76.7	25.2	323	TP	RP	211	1.3	NR	558	1 (33)	301	0	17.7	NR	NR	NR	NR	NR
John et al. 2009 [11]	13	70[a]	NR	100[a]	EP	TV	210[a]	6[a]	6[a]	500[a]	0	82[a]	0	NR	NR	NR	23[a]	NR	NR
Uffort et al. 2010 [20]	15	65.8	5.2	70.9	EP	SP	128.8	2.5	4.6	139.3	0	46.4		23.9	8.1	NR	NR	4.9	2.2
Sutherland et al. 2011 [15]	9	68	17.4	136.5	TP	RP	183	1.3	13	206	0	112	1	17.9	7.8	NR	NR	NR	NR
Coelho et al. 2011 [16]	6	69	7	157	TP	SP	90	1	4.8	208	0	145	0	19.8	5.5	7.8	19	NR	NR
Vora et al. 2012 [13]	13	67.1	12.3	163.3	TP	SP	179.4	2.8	8.9	219.4	0	121.1	0	18.2	5.3	4.4	19.1	NR	NR
Matei et al. 2012 [12]	35	65.2	5.4	106.6	TP	SP	186	3.2	7.4	121	0	87	0	28	7	6.6	18.9	NR	NR
Clavijo et al. 2013 [17]	10	71.7	5.8	81	TP	SP	106	1	8.9	375	1 (10)	81	0	18.8	1.7	12.4	33.5	3.7	0.5
Banapour et al. 2014 [18]	16	68.4	12.8	141.8	TP	SP & RP	228	1.3	8[a]	197	0	94.2		22[a]	7[a]	NR	NR	4[a]	2[a]
Leslie et al. 2014 [19]	25	72.9	9.4	149.6	TP	TV	214	4	9	143	1 (4)	88	0	23.9	3.6	11.3	20	NR	NR

IPSS International Prostatic Symptom Score, *Qmax* maximum flow rate, *QoL* quality of life, *NR* not reported
[a]Median; *TRUS* transrectal ultrasound, *TP* transperitoneal, *EP* extraperitoneal, *TV* transvesical, *SP* suprapubic, *RP* retropubic

172.2 g (range, 108.5–243); mean estimated blood loss was 213 ml (range, 150–300); conversion to open simple prostatectomy was 0 %; potency was preserved in all patients and continence was preserved in all but one patient.

Postoperative Management

The postoperative management of robotic simple prostatectomy mirrors that of most major surgical procedures. Patients are encouraged early ambulation. The Jackson-Pratt drain output and intake/output fluid status are monitored. Patients will be on clear liquid diet postoperatively and advanced as tolerated. Most patients will be discharged home on the first postoperative day after the drain is removed, and Foley catheter management with leg bag will be taught to the patient and his family. Patient will return to outpatient setting for Foley catheter removal and a voiding trial in a week's time. Pathology is reviewed and follow-up examinations are done in order to exclude prostate cancer. PSA and DRE are monitored as the risk of prostate cancer development still remains.

Complications

The reported case series complications are shown in Table 15.1. The complications reported below are exfoliated from the simple prostatectomy series.

Early Complications

Hemorrhage

A wide range of perioperative bleeding events has been reported in the literature for simple prostatectomy [21]. Published peer-reviewed data report blood loss between 50 and 500 ml. Blood transfusion rate is almost zero in most series. Sotelo et al. reported that one patient required blood transfusion in their series of seven patients [10]. Yuh et al. reported a case series of three patients with a mean blood loss of 558 ml, and one patient required blood transfusion [14]. These two case series are reported as an early experience with robotic simple prostatectomy. Apart from these early reports, no perioperative blood transfusions have been reported in subsequent series (Table 15.1).

This variability is mostly attributed to differences in transfusion thresholds, autologous blood banking, and surgeon's experience. Delayed bleeding (>2 weeks postoperatively) is rare and should be managed initially with bladder irrigation, Foley catheter traction, and reoperation if needed.

Infection

Epididymitis, wound infection and urinary tract infections are not uncommon following open prostatectomy. The rates of UTI or epididymitis are comparable to rates after minimally invasive procedures. Risk factors include long-term indwelling Foley catheters, history of epididymitis, and chronic UTI. Surgical site infections have been reported to occur in 2.5–4.3 % of patients [21–23].

Incontinence

Incontinence is an uncommon complication; the reported rates of urinary incontinence in a large series of 1,804 open prostatectomies were 3.7 % and 1.2 % for early and late urinary incontinence, respectively [24]. This usually results from perforation and partial avulsion of the prostatic capsule or avulsion of the urethra at the apex. Sharply excising the urethra at the apex can help minimize the trauma to the external sphincter. Less than 9 % of cases report urge incontinence due to bladder instability; this is generally transient and resolves within 8 weeks following surgery.

Late Complications

Bladder Neck Contracture

Bladder neck contracture occurs in around 7.6 % of cases. The etiology of contractures remains unclear and is unrelated to adenoma size. But, the incidence is found to be higher following suprapubic prostatectomy than after retropubic prostatectomy [25]. Bladder neck contractures may initially be managed by dilation, while recurrent contractures require urethrotomy. Reconstruction of bladder neck for refractory contractures is rarely required.

Erectile and Sexual Dysfunction

Retrograde ejaculation is common following simple prostatectomy, and the incidence is found to be similar to that seen after transurethral resection of the prostate. This is due to resection or disruption of the internal sphincter allowing the ejaculate to pass in retrograde direction into the bladder. A 1994 publication estimated the rate of erectile dysfunction after open prostatectomy to be 16–32 % depending on the approach used [26]. Meanwhile the recent guidelines by the American Urological Association (AUA) state that given the lack of data, an estimate of the risk could not be made.

Other Complications

Rectal injury is a rare occurrence. Pubic osteitis is a rare complication following prostatectomy, with patients presenting 4–6 weeks postoperatively with severe pelvic and lower abdominal pain along with low-grade fever. This condition is usually self-limited. Analgesics and anti-inflammatory drugs provide symptomatic relief.

Cardiovascular and thromboembolic events are the two leading causes of mortality following prostatectomy. Large series have reported the mortality rates to be 0.06–0.2 % [24, 27]. Patients are encouraged to ambulate early following surgery.

Summary

Robot-assisted simple prostatectomy is a feasible alternative in patients with clinically significant BPH and in selected patients with large prostate. Contemporary case series report with minimal blood loss, shorter hospital stay, less postoperative morbidity, and minimal surgical complications when compared to open simple prostatectomy. The reports demonstrate good perioperative outcomes with excellent symptomatic and functional improvements following robotic simple prostatectomy.

Though the robot-assisted simple prostatectomy series are small non-comparative case series, additional prospective studies would validate these results.

Disclosure

Dr. Ashutosh Tewari discloses that he is the principal investigator on research grants from Intuitive Surgical, Inc. (Sunnyvale, California, USA) and Boston Scientific Corporation; he is a non-compensated director of the Prostate Cancer Institute (Pune, India) and Global Prostate Cancer Research Foundation; he has received research funding from the Prostate Cancer Foundation, the LeFrak Family Foundation, Mr. and Mrs. Paul Kanavos, Craig Effron & Company, Charles Evans Foundation, and Christian and Heidi Lange Family Foundation.

References

1. Berry SJ, Coffey DS, Walsh PC, Ewing LL. The development of human benign prostatic hyperplasia with age. J Urol. 1984;132:474–9.
2. Park T, Choi JY. Efficacy and safety of dutasteride for the treatment of symptomatic benign prostatic hyperplasia (BPH): a systematic review and meta-analysis. World J Urol. 2014;32(4):1093–105.
3. Wei JT, Calhoun E, Jacobsen SJ. Urologic diseases in America project: benign prostatic hyperplasia. J Urol. 2005;173:1256–61.
4. Wei JT, Calhoun E, Jacobsen SJ. Urologic diseases in America project: benign prostatic hyperplasia. J Urol. 2008;179:S75–80.
5. Gacci M, Bartoletti R, Figlioli S, et al. Urinary symptoms, quality of life and sexual function in patients with benign prostatic hypertrophy before and after prostatectomy: a prospective study. BJU Int. 2003; 91:196–200.
6. Varkarakis I, Kyriakakis Z, Delis A, Protogerou V, Deliveliotis C. Long-term results of open transvesical prostatectomy from a contemporary series of patients. Urology. 2004;64:306–10.
7. Mariano MB, Graziottin TM, Tefilli MV. Laparoscopic prostatectomy with vascular control for benign prostatic hyperplasia. J Urol. 2002; 167:2528–9.
8. Baumert H, Ballaro A, Dugardin F, Kaisary AV. Laparoscopic versus open simple prostatectomy: a comparative study. J Urol. 2006;175:1691–4.

9. McCullough TC, Heldwein FL, Soon SJ, et al. Laparoscopic versus open simple prostatectomy: an evaluation of morbidity. J Endourol. 2009;23:129–34.
10. Sotelo R, Clavijo R, Carmona O, et al. Robotic simple prostatectomy. J Urol. 2008;179:513–5.
11. John H, Bucher C, Engel N, Fischer B, Fehr JL. Preperitoneal robotic prostate adenomectomy. Urology. 2009;73:811–5.
12. Matei DV, Brescia A, Mazzoleni F, et al. Robot-assisted simple prostatectomy (RASP): does it make sense? BJU Int. 2012;110:E972–9.
13. Vora A, Mittal S, Hwang J, Bandi G. Robot-assisted simple prostatectomy: multi-institutional outcomes for glands larger than 100 grams. J Endourol/Endourol Soc. 2012;26:499–502.
14. Yuh B, Laungani R, Perlmutter A, et al. Robot-assisted Millin's retropubic prostatectomy: case series. Can J Urol. 2008;15:4101–5.
15. Sutherland DE, Perez DS, Weeks DC. Robot-assisted simple prostatectomy for severe benign prostatic hyperplasia. J Endourol/Endourol Soc. 2011;25: 641–4.
16. Coelho RF, Chauhan S, Sivaraman A, et al. Modified technique of robotic-assisted simple prostatectomy: advantages of a vesico-urethral anastomosis. BJU Int. 2012;109:426–33.
17. Clavijo R, Carmona O, De Andrade R, Garza R, Fernandez G, Sotelo R. Robot-assisted intrafascial simple prostatectomy: novel technique. J Endourol/ Endourol Soc. 2013;27:328–32.
18. Banapour P, Patel N, Kane CJ, Cohen SA, Parsons JK. Robotic-assisted simple prostatectomy: a systematic review and report of a single institution case series. Prostate Cancer Prostatic Dis. 2014;17:1–5.
19. Leslie S, de Castro Abreu AL, Chopra S et al. Transvesical robotic simple prostatectomy: initial clinical experience. Eur Urol. 2014;66(2):321–9.
20. Uffort EE, Jensen JC. Robotic-assisted laparoscopic simple prostatectomy: an alternative minimal invasive approach for prostate adenoma. J Robotic Surg. 2010;4:7–10.
21. Tubaro A, Carter S, Hind A, Vicentini C, Miano L. A prospective study of the safety and efficacy of suprapubic transvesical prostatectomy in patients with benign prostatic hyperplasia. J Urol. 2001;166:172–6.
22. Condie Jr JD, Cutherell L, Mian A. Suprapubic prostatectomy for benign prostatic hyperplasia in rural Asia: 200 consecutive cases. Urology. 1999;54: 1012–6.
23. Meier DE, Tarpley JL, Imediegwu OO, et al. The outcome of suprapubic prostatectomy: a contemporary series in the developing world. Urology. 1995;46:40–4.
24. Serretta V, Morgia G, Fondacaro L, et al. Open prostatectomy for benign prostatic enlargement in southern Europe in the late 1990s: a contemporary series of 1800 interventions. Urology. 2002;60:623–7.
25. Roos NP, Ramsey EW. A population-based study of prostatectomy: outcomes associated with differing surgical approaches. J Urol. 1987;137:1184–8.
26. McConnell JD, Barry MJ, Bruskewitz RC. Benign prostatic hyperplasia: diagnosis and treatment. Agency for Health Care Policy and Research. Clin Pract Guidel Quick Ref Guide Clin 1994;8:1–17.
27. Gratzke C, Schlenker B, Seitz M, et al. Complications and early postoperative outcome after open prostatectomy in patients with benign prostatic enlargement: results of a prospective multicenter study. J Urol. 2007;177:1419–22.

Transurethral Microwave Therapy 16

Ilija Aleksic, Vladimir Mouraviev, and David M. Albala

Introduction

In the treatment of symptomatic benign prostatic hyperplasia (BPH), there are many minimally invasive procedure options. Minimally invasive techniques for the treatment of BPH have been developed for those patients who do not respond to or cannot tolerate pharmacological therapy. This includes those who are high-risk patients or unwilling to undergo surgical therapy. The choice of a minimally invasive therapeutic option is determined by availability, surgeon's preference, experience, and efficacy.

Transurethral microwave thermotherapy (TUMT) was introduced as an office-based procedure. It involved placing a specially designed urinary catheter into the bladder, allowing a microwave antenna to be positioned within the prostate. It uses radiant heating to ablate prostate tissue. The microwave generator delivers energy to heat the prostate tissue between 45°°C and 55 °C. The heating process causes necrosis of the prostate tissue that is obstructing the urethra.

McCaskey used ultraviolet lamps to generate heat to treat prostatism in 1921. Corbus, in 1929, used diathermy probes for the same purpose. Yerushalmi and associates reintroduced microwave therapy in poor surgical candidates in 1985 with prostatic enlargement [1]. Over the last decade, high-energy TUMT was revived as an attractive alternative to standard prostatectomy, TURP as well as medical therapy for BPH with the advent of later generation devices (Fig. 16.1). According to a 2011 American Urological Association (AUA) update on BPH management [2], TUMT is effective in at least partially relieving lower urinary tract symptoms (LUTS) secondary to BPH and may be considered in men with moderate to severe symptoms. A 2012 systematic review of the literature identified 15 randomized control trials evaluating TUMT in a total of 1,585 men with symptomatic BPH [3]. The authors concluded that TUMT is an effective alternative to transurethral resection of the prostate (TURP). In addition, the EAU [4] recommends the use of TUMT for patients who are no longer responsive to medication and want to avoid surgical intervention; they further suggest that it has become the most popular minimally invasive treatment worldwide [5]. In fact, a steady

I. Aleksic, M.D.
Urology, Associated Medical Professionals of NY, Syracuse, NY, USA

V. Mouraviev, M.D.
Clinical Research, Urology, Associated Medical Professionals of NY, Syracuse, NY, USA

D.M. Albala, M.D. (✉)
Urology, Associated Medical Professionals of NY/ Crouse Hospital, 1226 E. Water St., Syracuse, NY, USA
e-mail: Dalbala@ampofny.com

B. Chughtai et al. (eds.), *Treatment of Benign Prostatic Hyperplasia: Modern Alternative to Transurethral Resection of the Prostate*, DOI 10.1007/978-1-4939-1587-3_16,

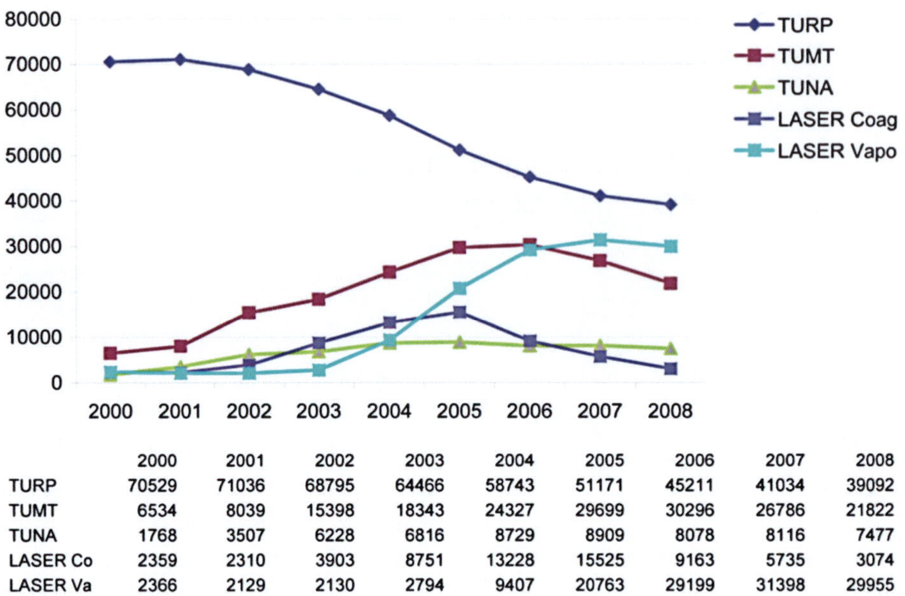

	2000	2001	2002	2003	2004	2005	2006	2007	2008
TURP	70529	71036	68795	64466	58743	51171	45211	41034	39092
TUMT	6534	8039	15398	18343	24327	29699	30296	26786	21822
TUNA	1768	3507	6228	6816	8729	8909	8078	8116	7477
LASER Co	2359	2310	3903	8751	13228	15525	9163	5735	3074
LASER Va	2366	2129	2130	2794	9407	20763	29199	31398	29955

Fig. 16.1 Number of BPH procedures by year for different BPH procedures in the USA (2000–2008) (From Malaeb, B.S., et al., National trends in surgical therapy for benign prostatic hyperplasia in the United States (2000–2008). Urology, 2012. 79(5): pp. 1111–6. Reprinted with permission from Elsevier Limited)

decrease in the number of TURPs has been reported in part due to increased utilization of minimally invasive techniques [6, 7].

Historical Consideration

Microwave therapy was initially developed in the 1980s for treatment of malignant disease, and then it was applied to the treatment of BPH [8]. The literature of the time coined the term "hyperthermia" to describe these therapies, as they produced lower temperatures than those required for tissue ablation. However, the original techniques failed because higher temperatures (>45 °C) were needed to ablate BPH tissue and the transrectal approach often used was inappropriate, as it treated the peripheral zone and not the transition zone [9]. In the early 1990s, transurethral hyperthermia was found to have little efficacy and a double-blinded, randomized study concluded that transrectal hyperthermia was not effective [10, 11]. So began the path to discovery of novel microwave therapies that can obtain desirable temperatures and can be delivered transurethrally. These therapies reach higher intraprostatic temperatures and are now referred to as "thermotherapy." Thermotherapy is defined as tissue temperature above 45 °C. Temperatures above 45 °C are thermotoxic for prostate tissue but also reach the thermal threshold for pain receptors localized in the urethral mucosa.

Thus, modifications to the technology first evolved to deliver more energy, yielding high enough temperatures to ablate BPH tissue. TUMT allowed higher temperatures to be reached deep into the lateral lobes of the prostate, causing coagulative necrosis of the adenomatous tissue and even ablation of some prostatic tissue. Further modifications included the development of urethral cooling mechanisms. However, debate has ensued on whether or not cooling was necessary as evidence of damage to the urethra was inconclusive and a perceived benefit of decreased pain was in question. Therefore, two kinds of microwave devices have been developed and a widely accepted classification of presently available systems is largely based on the presence or absence of a urethral cooling system. As such, it appears that no research has been published as to whether cooling or non-cooling devices differ in their clinical effectiveness.

Biophysics of TUMT

Transurethral microwave thermotherapy (TUMT) involves the insertion of a specially designed coude-type catheter into the bladder allowing a microwave antenna to be properly positioned within the prostatic fossa. The heat transferred to the prostatic tissue produces coagulative necrosis and subsequent relief of obstruction or lower urinary tract symptoms (LUTS) due to benign prostatic hyperplasia (BPH). The underlying principle of action is the electromagnetic radiation transmitted by the antenna at frequencies typically between 915 and 1,296 MHz. This is absorbed by molecules such as H_2O causing oscillation and energy transfer to tissue in the form of heat [9]. Usually, this therapy is delivered in a single 1-h session.

The main objective is to cause coagulative necrosis of prostatic tissue, the extent of which is reliant both on temperature attained and duration maintained [12]. Studies performed in vitro have delineated the thermal effect at the cellular level [13], illustrating that thermal damage follows an exponential temperature/time relationship predominantly driven by temperature. Small increases in thermal energy result in large increases in tissue necrosis [14, 15]. The histopathological net effect appears to be cell death rather than tissue contractility [16]. Additional proposed mechanisms include nerve ablation, denervation of α-receptors with a subsequent decrease in smooth muscle tone [17–19]. Brehmer et al. also demonstrated that thermotherapy increased the sensory threshold in the posterior urethra [20], possibly contributing to rapid alleviation of LUTS. Microwave penetration is defined as the tissue depth where the strength has decreased to 37 % of value at origin [21], most often a distance of 15 mm at the abovementioned frequencies [9]. Furthermore, it has been reported that a possible secondary mechanism of the cell death, such as an apoptosis in the areas of the prostate adjacent to the field of necrosis, occurs in later development [22]. Others have also illustrated that apoptosis may play a significant role in the treatment effect of even mild thermotherapy [23]. The clinical benefits of microwave thermotherapy are likely due to a multifactorial mechanism. It is, however, evident that the clinical response is dose dependent [24], bringing forth the development of devices that can cause tissue ablation, while protecting the urethra with cooling mechanisms.

Three Generations of TUMT Devices

The temperature in the prostate depends on three parameters: the microwave power (watts), which heats the tissue; the blood flow, which cools down the heated tissue; and heat conduction, which redistributes the heat. Of these, the microwave power and the blood flow are the most important factors to obtain therapeutic temperatures. Both cooled and non-cooled systems are in use. The newest generation microwave systems provide significantly more benefit to the patient, without the limitations of early microwave systems and interstitial therapies. Cooling allows generation of greater intraprostatic tissue temperatures (50–80 °C), preserves urethral mucosal tissue, and decreases morbidity. High tissue temperatures produce a large volume of necrosis in a short time. The coolant makes the procedure more comfortable for the patient and protects adjacent healthy tissue. With low-temperature, non-cooled treatment, the hottest point is at the urethra and diminishes rapidly.

The FDA-approved high-energy TUMT devices are as follows:

The **first generation of TUMT devices** includes the CoreTherm® (ProstaLund) which provides feedback treatment with a temperature monitoring probe that is inserted into the prostate from the catheter. The temperature probe contains multiple temperature transducers to map the temperature distribution in the prostate along the probe. The microwave power and the treatment time are varied according to these readings. Intraprostatic temperature monitoring allows control by the treating physician, who can estimate the prostate volume treated.

The **second-generation machine** Targis Cooled ThermoTherapyTM (Urologix) uses a dipolar impedance matched antenna in a 21-Fr catheter that effectively delivers heat in the 902–928 MHz range. It was one of the first anesthesia-free, minimally invasive BPH procedure designed for in-office use having proprietary microwave technology to precisely deliver targeted high energy deep to the BPH tissue while leaving other nontargeted areas intact. The low-temperature coolant protects the urethra and bladder neck during energy delivery, enhancing patient comfort and minimizing recovery time. The intermediate follow-up results (up to 5 years) demonstrated a high durability treatment effect. It can be performed in an office or outpatient setting in about 1 h. The urologist places the microwave delivery system, which is on the tip of the flexible catheter, into the bladder and inflates a standard urological balloon for positioning. The antenna is then positioned in the prostatic urethra. The coolant emitted from the catheter simultaneously protects the urethra.

The other second-generation machine TMX 2000TM (Thermatrx) provides the lowest energy but is not a cooled system. The antenna directs heat and energy to the appropriate target (periurethral tissue) but does not direct heat to sensitive tissues (bladder neck and external sphincter). Low energy and low power are required to achieve tissue necrosis without cooling, on average 6–7 W. A known and reproducible dose of heat is applied. Actual periurethral tissue temperature is continuously measured. Multiple treatment coil lengths are available to the urologist in order to ensure that the optimal dose of heat is applied to the appropriate size of the prostate. The TMX 2000 can treat prostatic lengths (bladder neck to verumontanum) of 2.5 cm and longer.

The **third-generation device** Prolieve® System (Boston Scientific) provides water-cooled balloon dilation TUMT. The treatment begins with intraurethral lidocaine 10 min prior to catheter placement, then proceeds to the inflation of a 46-Fr dilatation/prostatic compression balloon of the transurethral catheter. This system features a quick power ramp up to thermotherapy temperatures. Thermotherapy is delivered for about 45 min at a maximum of 50 W as heated fluid is circulated in the prostate balloon. During a 5-min cool down period, the prostate balloon remains inflated and the bladder is filled with 180 cc. The catheter is removed, and a voiding trial is begun.

The paradigms for treatment vary because thermotherapy is not created similarly in all devices. There are differences in power (maximum power: Thermatrx – 23 W, Prolieve – 50 W, Cooled ThermoTherapy – 75 W, CoreTherm – 80 W), delivery, urethral cooling, and the efficacy and safety profile. This is all reported in the published peer-review literature. Thermatrx has low power and no urethral cooling. CoreTherm has high power and intraprostatic temperature monitoring. Targis has high power and urethral cooling. At low blood flow rates, the CoreTherm adds safety by reducing the microwave power and avoiding a possible overtreatment. At high blood flow, the CoreTherm adds efficacy by increasing the microwave power.

Clinical Implications

TUMT is performed on an outpatient basis and commonly takes between 30 and 60 min. Postoperative catheterization times can range from a few days to several weeks. Although all TUMT devices are designed to deliver microwave energy to the prostate in a similar manner, contemporary devices differ in a variety of technical details. The main differentiating feature between TUMT devices is the design of the microwave antenna and urethral catheter [25]. Other differences include treatment duration and therapy monitoring systems.

The major distinction used to group TUMT devices is the presence or absence of a cooling mechanism, which is a widely accepted classification. To our knowledge, there are no studies currently on whether a cooling mechanism has an effect on clinical outcome. A similar question exists for the level of achieved intraprostatic temperature and whether it influences treatment efficacy. Details on target temperatures are scarce, and there are no trials that address their effect on clinical outcomes after TUMT. Beyond assuring that treatment temperatures reach a necrosis threshold of 45 °C, there is a paucity of evidence that there is any correlation between therapeutic prostate temperature and clinical outcomes.

Multiple trials suggest safety and efficacy, with improvement in flow rates and I-PSS both in the short and long term [26–29]. The Cooled Thermocath system is a third-generation device that uses a 28.5-min treatment protocol at higher temperatures. The major advancement by the design lies in the efficiency of the cooling mechanism [9]. The first trial for the device showed comparable efficacy with the Targis 60-min trial [30]. At 5-year follow-up, durability and efficacy was demonstrated when compared to the Targis system (see Table 16.2), indicating successful progression of TUMT technology [38].

Device-specific contraindications for TMx-2000 include previous radiation therapy to the pelvic region [9]. A study of TMx-2000 effectiveness demonstrated similar results of the other systems [39]. Interestingly, the study was done with only intraurethral lidocaine and oral anti-inflammatories and anxiolytics with no prostatic block, which may be in part attributed to temperature monitoring optimized by the device for patient tolerance. A follow-up study demonstrated maintenance of subjective improvement [32]. All devices use a rectal probe with thermocouplers for continuous monitoring of rectal-wall temperatures. However, there is no conclusive evidence to support one device over another.

Treatment Outcomes

Multiple studies have demonstrated that various modalities of TUMT have short- and long-term improvement in subjective score measures and quantitative parameters such as Qmax (Tables 16.1 and 16.2) [9].

Table 16.1 Short-term results of TUMT trials (≤2 years)

References	Device	Sample size	Baseline		Follow-up change		F/U length (mos)
			Qmax	*IPSS*	*Qmax*	*IPSS*	
Huidobro et al. [30]	CTC 28.5	40	9.4	21.2	15.1	8.6	12
Albala et al. [39]	TMx-2000	125	22.2	8.9	14	12.8	24
Albala et al. [32]	TMx-2000	200	23	8.4	17.8	3	24
Wagrell et al. [40]	PLFT	103	21	7.6	13.3	7	12
Laguna et al. [41]	Prostatron 2.5/3.5	388	19.1	9.4	14.6	19.1	12
Gravas et al. [42]	PLFT	41	21.9	7.7	12.6	7.1	12
Djavan et al. [43]	Targis	51	19	6	13	7.5	18
Shore et al. [44]	Prolive	16	10.1	21.2	0.1	13.3	6
	Targis	14	10.5	22.9	3.1	12	6

Table 16.2 Long-term results of trials (≥2 years)

References	Device	Sample size	Baseline		Follow-up changes		F/u length (years)
			I-PSS	*Qmax*	*I-PSS*	*Qmax*	
Kaplan et al. [27]	Targis	345	21	7.5	13	10.5	5
D'Ancona et al. [31]	Prostatron 2.5	31	13.3[a]	9.3	5.8[a]	15.1	2.5
Albala et al. [32]	TMx-2000	125	22.5	9.2	12.4	11.9	4
Francisca et al. [33]	Prostatron 2.5	78	21	8.3	12	10.7	3
Floratos et al. [34]	Targis	78	20	9.2	9.4	16.5	5
Selvaggio et al. [35]	Urologix-30	140	18.5	8.5	5.9	12.1	4
Laguna et al. [36]	Prostatron	213	20.3	NA	12.1	NA	4
Mattiason et al. [37]	CoreTherm	102	21	7.6	13.8	5.7	5
Mynderse et al. [38]	CTC 28.5	66	20.8	8.3	12.2	5	5
	Targis	125	20.8	7.8	10.3	2	5

[a]Madsen symptom score

There is limited data on long-term follow-up. Short- and intermediate-term follow-up studies suggest that both energy levels are comparably efficacious. Five sham-controlled trials enrolling 674 patients have evaluated TUMT devices that employed a urethral cooling mechanism [45–49]. All of the trials were randomized and found the treatment to be significantly more effective than the sham control in terms of symptoms and physiological measures. In one randomized control trial involving non-cooled TUMT, there appeared to be statistically significant improved symptom score and flow rate data when compared to sham treatment [32]. An international pooled report demonstrated that TUMT was associated with significant changes (about 50 %) in IPSS, QOL, and Qmax up to 4 years after the procedure, with improvement diminishing slightly between 24 and 48 months [50]. Most recently, a 2013 study evaluated the use of TUMT in patients with bladder outlet obstruction (BOO) who are unsuitable for surgery and found that 77 % were relieved of their catheter [51].

To date, the study with the longest follow-up for TUMT is 11 years. It was conducted in patients with BOO, illustrating the durability of the therapy with only 7 % of patients requiring secondary intervention [52]. Other studies cite retreatment rates between 5.9 % and 9.1 %, with follow-up between 18 and 60 months [37, 38, 43]. It is important to note that the vast majority of long-term studies on the durability and efficacy of TUMT are subject to selection bias because they consist of patients who remained in the study that may overrepresent those responding to treatment.

A 5-year follow-up of patients undergoing TUMT demonstrated that their IPSS showed sustained subjective improvement despite a decrease of Qmax after 24 months. One must consider these results in the context of a 36 % retreatment rate (medical or surgical) after an average of 2.67 years [53]. When using urodynamic parameters to evaluate the patient postoperatively, it has been shown that after 8 years' follow-up, TUMT outcomes persisted in patients [54]. For those patients with moderate to severe obstruction, TURP had better outcomes when evaluating IPSS and QOL indices. The need for additional treatments was 11 % for TURP and 28 % for TUMT during the 8-year follow-up period. When considering treatment costs, TUMT proved to be less expensive than TURP in several evaluations [55]. This fact may be primarily due to TUMT being an office procedure.

Finally, the available efficacy data of thermotherapies have been criticized for a number of issues, including a concern over the quality of comparative controls, domination of positive data from single-center studies rather than multicenter studies, issues of sham versus true effects within the efficacy parameters, appropriate direct comparator issues, technology changes occurring faster than clinical experience accumulated, no significant effect on PSA cut-off or prostate volume, high or unreported retreatment rates, and inability to predict which patients would benefit.

The first multicenter, randomized head-to-head comparison of second-generation Targis system versus third-generation Prolieve thermodilatation system was conducted recently assessing objective and subjective measures in the short term [44]. The results demonstrated the superiority of third-generation versus second-generation technique. Thirty men with symptomatic BPH were treated either with Prolieve or Targis system and then followed for 6 months. Fifteen from sixteen (94 %) Prolieve patients remained catheter-free compared with 3 of 14 (21 %) Targis patients ($p=0.0001$). Foley catheter indwelling time was 58.8 h for one Prolieve patient compared with 103.9 h for the Targis-treated nine patients. Mean AUA scores for Prolieve improved from 21.2 at baseline to 12.3 and 7.9 at week 2 and month 6, respectively; for Targis improvement was less impressive – from 22.9 at baseline to 17.9 and 10.9, respectively ($p>0.05$). Overall, the incidence of device-related events was 31 % for Prolieve patients compared with 64 % for Targis patients ($p>0.05$). The most common events were urinary retention, dysuria, and hematuria.

Adverse Effects

Morbidities of TUMT are in concordance with other heat delivering therapies of the prostate. These include hematuria, urinary retention, dysuria/urgency, urinary tract infections, retrograde ejaculation, erectile dysfunction, and stricture [3].

A systemic review of randomized trials expressed the retreatment rate as events per person per year of follow-up. This study showed that surgical intervention for stricture for TUMT patients was 0.63/100 and for TURP patients was 5.85/100 person years [3, 56]. Furthermore, the incidence of hospitalization, hematuria, clot retention, blood transfusions, TUR syndrome, and urethral strictures was significantly higher with TURP than TUMT, whereas the inverse was true with catheterization time, dysuria, and urinary retention [3, 38]. Data has also shown that TUMT may have less impact on sexual function than TURP [33, 57, 58].

The systematic literature review also revealed that TUMT had shorter hospital stays when compared to TURP at <1 day versus 5 days, respectively. However, a longer catheterization period for TUMT over TURP of 7–15 days versus 2–4 days was noted, respectively [3]. Also, patients undergoing TUMT were more likely to require retreatment when compared to TURP (relative risk 10.0), although they required less surgical retreatment for strictures. Mean reduction in IPSS after 12 months was greater for TURP (77 % vs. 65 %), as was the increase in Qmax (119 % vs. 70 %). Lastly, TURP was found to be associated with a greater incidence of retrograde ejaculation (58 % vs. 22 %) and an increased need for transfusion (6 % vs. 0 %) when compared to TUMT [3].

Contraindications to TUMT include implanted pacemakers or defibrillators, penile prosthesis, urinary sphincters, metal in the pelvic/hip region, urethral stricture, peripheral arterial disease with intermittent claudication or Leriche's syndrome, prostatic ball-valve median lobe, and evidence of prostate or bladder cancer [9].

Conclusion

BPH is the most common age-related abnormality of the prostate. TUMT has established itself as a safe and effective alternative to TURP. This procedure is continually evolving toward delivering better outcomes that are more tolerable to the patient and are more likely to be done in the outpatient setting by the urologist. A relatively low rate of morbidity and the absence of anesthesia from the treatment protocol make TUMT a true outpatient procedure [59]. Predictive parameters for unfavorable outcome with TUMT include low energy levels, small prostate volume, mild to moderate BOO, and advanced age [60]. When compared to other minimally invasive modalities such as laser vaporization, TUMT is far less invasive and is therefore associated with a lower need for anesthesia and a shorter hospital stay [61]. With a better understanding of the various treatment options available to patients, clinicians can offer minimally invasive treatments to patients who fail medications or are high-risk surgical candidates.

References

1. Yerushalmi A, et al. Localized deep microwave hyperthermia in the treatment of poor operative risk patients with benign prostatic hyperplasia. J Urol. 1985;133(5):873–6.
2. McVary KT, et al. Update on AUA guideline on the management of benign prostatic hyperplasia. J Urol. 2011;185(5):1793–803.
3. Hoffman RM, et al. Microwave thermotherapy for benign prostatic hyperplasia. Cochrane Database Syst Rev. 2012;9, CD004135.
4. de la Rosette JJ, et al. EAU guidelines on benign prostatic hyperplasia (BPH). Eur Urol. 2001;40(3): 256–63; discussion 264.
5. Madersbacher S, et al. EAU 2004 guidelines on assessment, therapy and follow-up of men with lower urinary tract symptoms suggestive of benign prostatic obstruction (BPH guidelines). Eur Urol. 2004;46(5):547–54.
6. Yu X, et al. Practice patterns in benign prostatic hyperplasia surgical therapy: the dramatic increase in minimally invasive technologies. J Urol. 2008;180(1): 241–5; discussion 245.
7. Malaeb BS, et al. National trends in surgical therapy for benign prostatic hyperplasia in the United States (2000–2008). Urology. 2012;79(5):1111–6.
8. Laguna MP, Muschter R, Debruyne FM. Microwave thermotherapy: historical overview. J Endourol. 2000; 14(8):603–9.
9. Walmsley K, Kaplan SA. Transurethral microwave thermotherapy for benign prostate hyperplasia: separating truth from marketing hype. J Urol. 2004; 172(4 Pt 1):1249–55.

10. Abbou CC, et al. Transrectal and transurethral hyperthermia versus sham treatment in benign prostatic hyperplasia: a double-blind randomized multicentre clinical trial. The French BPH hyperthermia. Br J Urol. 1995;76(5):619–24.
11. Le May C. First Canadian clinical study of transurethral hyperthermia in benign prostatic hyperplasia. Assessment of 220 patients. Eur Urol. 1992;21(3):184–6.
12. Wagrell L, et al. Aspects on transurethral microwave thermotherapy of benign prostatic hyperplasia. Tech Urol. 2000;6(4):251–5.
13. Bhowmick S, Swanlund DJ, Bischof JC. Supraphysiological thermal injury in Dunning AT-1 prostate tumor cells. J Biomech Eng. 2000;122(1):51–9.
14. Bhowmick S, et al. Evaluation of thermal therapy in a prostate cancer model using a wet electrode radiofrequency probe. J Endourol. 2001;15(6):629–40.
15. Bolmsjo M, et al. Cell-kill modeling of microwave thermotherapy for treatment of benign prostatic hyperplasia. J Endourol. 2000;14(8):627–35.
16. Corvin S, et al. Effect of heat exposure on viability and contractility of cultured prostatic stromal cells. Eur Urol. 2000;37(4):499–504.
17. Brehmer M, Baba S. Transurethral microwave thermotherapy: how does it work? J Endourol. 2000;14(8):611–5.
18. de la Rosette JJ, D'Ancona FC, Debruyne FM. Current status of thermotherapy of the prostate. J Urol. 1997;157(2):430–8.
19. Brehmer M, Hilliges M, Kinn AC. Denervation of periurethral prostatic tissue by transurethral microwave thermotherapy. Scand J Urol Nephrol. 2000;34(1):42–5.
20. Brehmer M, Nilsson BY. Elevation of sensory thresholds in the prostatic urethra after microwave thermotherapy. BJU Int. 2000;86(4):427–31.
21. Bolmsjo MB, Vrba T. Microwave applicators for thermotherapy of benign prostatic hyperplasia: a primer. Tech Urol. 2000;6(4):245–50.
22. Brehmer M. Morphological changes in prostatic adenomas after transurethral microwave thermotherapy. Br J Urol. 1997;80(1):123–7.
23. Brehmer M, Svensson I. Heat-induced apoptosis in human prostatic stromal cells. BJU Int. 2000;85(4):535–41.
24. Devonec M, et al. Clinical response to transurethral microwave thermotherapy is thermal dose dependent. Eur Urol. 1993;23(2):267–74.
25. Bolmsjo M, et al. The heat is on–but how? A comparison of TUMT devices. Br J Urol. 1996;78(4):564–72.
26. Miller PD, et al. Cooled thermotherapy for the treatment of benign prostatic hyperplasia: durability of results obtained with the Targis system. Urology. 2003;61(6):1160–4; discussion 1164–5.
27. Kaplan SA, Blute M, Bruskewitz RC, Larson TR, Utz W, Ugarte R, Mayer R. Long term efficacy and durability in 345 patients treated with transurethral microwave thermotherapy for benign prostatic hyperplasia: five year results. J Urol. 2002;167(Suppl):297.
28. Berger AP, et al. Transurethral microwave thermotherapy (TUMT) with the Targis system: a single-centre study on 78 patients with acute urinary retention and poor general health. Eur Urol. 2003;43(2):176–80.
29. Thalmann GN, et al. Transurethral microwave therapy in 200 patients with a minimum followup of 2 years: urodynamic and clinical results. J Urol. 2002;167(6):2496–501.
30. Huidobro C, Cabezas J, Cote E, Mynderse L, Partin A, Preminger G. Results of a new advancement in high temperature cooled thermotherapy (TUMT) for benign prostatic hyperplasia (BPH). J Urol. 2003;169(Suppl):390.
31. D'Ancona FC, et al. Transurethral resection of the prostate vs high-energy thermotherapy of the prostate in patients with benign prostatic hyperplasia: long-term results. Br J Urol. 1998;81(2):259–64.
32. Albala DM, Andriole G, Davis BE, Eure GR, Kabalin JN, Lingeman JE. Transurethral microwave thermotherapy (TUMT) using the Thermatrx TMX-2000: durability exhibited in a study comparing TUMT with a Sham procedure in patients with benign prostatic hyperplasia (BPH). J Urol. 2003;169(Suppl):465.
33. Francisca EA, et al. Sexual function following high energy microwave thermotherapy: results of a randomized controlled study comparing transurethral microwave thermotherapy to transurethral prostatic resection. J Urol. 1999;161(2):486–90.
34. Floratos DL, et al. Long-term followup of randomized transurethral microwave thermotherapy versus transurethral prostatic resection study. J Urol. 2001;165(5):1533–8.
35. Selvaggio O, Ditonno P, Battaglia M, Bettocchi C, Saracino A, Palazzo S. Long term results (4 years) of high-energy transurethral microwave. Eur Urol. 2003;2:102.
36. Laguna P, van Hest P, Smelov V, Gravas S, Kiemeney B, de la Rosette JJ. Efficacy and durability of the 30 minutes high energy TUMT protocol in 213 patients. J Endourol. 2002;15(Suppl):38.
37. Mattiasson A, et al. Five-year follow-up of feedback microwave thermotherapy versus TURP for clinical BPH: a prospective randomized multicenter study. Urology. 2007;69(1):91–6; discussion 96–7.
38. Mynderse LA, et al. Results of a 5-year multicenter trial of a new generation cooled high energy transurethral microwave thermal therapy catheter for benign prostatic hyperplasia. J Urol. 2011;185(5):1804–10.
39. Albala DM, et al. Office-based transurethral microwave thermotherapy using the TherMatrx TMx-2000. J Endourol. 2002;16(1):57–61.
40. Wagrell L, et al. Feedback microwave thermotherapy versus TURP for clinical BPH–a randomized controlled multicenter study. Urology. 2002;60(2):292–9.
41. Laguna MP, et al. Baseline prostatic specific antigen does not predict the outcome of high energy transurethral

microwave thermotherapy. J Urol. 2002;167(4): 1727–30.
42. Gravas S, Laguna MP, de la Rosette JJ. Efficacy and safety of intraprostatic temperature-controlled microwave thermotherapy in patients with benign prostatic hyperplasia: results of a prospective, open-label, single-center study with 1-year follow-up. J Endourol. 2003;17(6):425–30.
43. Djavan B, et al. Targeted transurethral microwave thermotherapy versus alpha-blockade in benign prostatic hyperplasia: outcomes at 18 months. Urology. 2001;57(1):66–70.
44. Shore ND, Sethi PS. A controlled, randomized, head-to-head comparison of the Prolieve thermodilatation system versus the Targis system for benign prostatic hyperplasia: safety, procedural tolerability, and clinical results. J Endourol. 2010;24(9):1469–75.
45. Trachtenberg J, Roehrborn CG. Updated results of a randomized, double-blind, multicenter sham-controlled trial of microwave thermotherapy with the Dornier Urowave in patients with symptomatic benign prostatic hyperplasia. Urowave Investigators Group. World J Urol. 1998;16(2):102–8.
46. Larson TR, et al. A high-efficiency microwave thermoablation system for the treatment of benign prostatic hyperplasia: results of a randomized, sham-controlled, prospective, double-blind, multicenter clinical trial. Urology. 1998;51(5):731–42.
47. Blute ML, et al. Transurethral microwave thermotherapy v sham treatment: double-blind randomized study. J Endourol. 1996;10(6):565–73.
48. Francisca EA, et al. Quality of life assessment in patients treated with lower energy thermotherapy (Prostasoft 2.0): results of a randomized transurethral microwave thermotherapy versus sham study. J Urol. 1997;158(5):1839–44.
49. Nawrocki JD, et al. A randomized controlled trial of transurethral microwave thermotherapy. Br J Urol. 1997;79(3):389–93.
50. Trock BJ, et al. Long-term pooled analysis of multicenter studies of cooled thermotherapy for benign prostatic hyperplasia results at three months through four years. Urology. 2004;63(4):716–21.
51. Aagaard MF, et al. Transurethral microwave thermotherapy treatment of chronic urinary retention in patients unsuitable for surgery. Scand J Urol. 2013; 48:290–4.
52. Vesely S, et al. Transurethral microwave thermotherapy: clinical results after 11 years of use. J Endourol. 2005;19(6):730–3.
53. Tan AH, et al. Long-term results of microwave thermotherapy for symptomatic benign prostatic hyperplasia. J Endourol. 2005;19(10):1191–5.
54. Vesely S, et al. TURP and low-energy TUMT treatment in men with LUTS suggestive of bladder outlet obstruction selected by means of pressure-flow studies: 8-year follow-up. Neurourol Urodyn. 2006;25(7):770–5.
55. Nickel JC. BPH: costs and treatment outcomes. Am J Manag Care. 2006;12(5 Suppl):S141–8.
56. Djavan B, Kazzazi A, Bostanci Y. Revival of thermotherapy for benign prostatic hyperplasia. Curr Opin Urol. 2012;22(1):16–21.
57. de la Rosette JJ, et al. Transurethral microwave thermotherapy: the gold standard for minimally invasive therapies for patients with benign prostatic hyperplasia? J Endourol. 2003;17(4):245–51.
58. Norby B, Nielsen HV, Frimodt-Moller PC. Transurethral interstitial laser coagulation of the prostate and transurethral microwave thermotherapy vs transurethral resection or incision of the prostate: results of a randomized, controlled study in patients with symptomatic benign prostatic hyperplasia. BJU Int. 2002;90(9):853–62.
59. D'Ancona FC, et al. Results of high-energy transurethral microwave thermotherapy in patients categorized according to the American Society of Anesthesiologists operative risk classification. Urology. 1999; 53(2):322–8.
60. D'Ancona FC, et al. High energy transurethral thermotherapy in the treatment of benign prostatic hyperplasia: criteria to predict treatment outcome. Prostate Cancer Prostatic Dis. 1999;2(2):98–105.
61. Djavan B, et al. Durability and retreatment rates of minimal invasive treatments of benign prostatic hyperplasia: a cross-analysis of the literature. Can J Urol. 2010;17(4):5249–54.

17 Transurethral Needle Ablation

Ciara S. Marley and Matthew P. Rutman

Abbreviations

BPH	Benign prostatic hyperplasia
I-PSS	International prostate symptom score
LUTS	Lower urinary tract symptoms
MTOPS	Medical therapy of prostate symptoms
Pdet	Detrusor pressure
PFR	Peak flow rate
PVR	Post void residual
Qmax	Max flow rate
QOL	Quality of life
RF	Radiofrequency energy
TRUS	Transrectal ultrasound
TUMT	Transurethral microwave thermotherapy
TUNA	Transurethral needle ablation of the prostate
TURP	Transurethral resection of prostate

Benign prostatic hyperplasia (BPH) is a nonmalignant growth of the prostate gland that can lead to a constellation of symptoms in the aging male known as lower urinary tract symptoms (LUTS). Longitudinal studies have shown that the prevalence of moderate to severe LUTS resulting from BPH negatively impacts mental and physical aspects of health [1]. Clinical evidence also demonstrates that if left untreated, bladder outlet obstruction can lead to serious complications including acute urinary retention, recurrent urinary tract infections, and bladder calculi. Medical therapy with alpha-receptor blockade and/or 5 alpha reductase inhibition is often the first-line treatment approach. These medications have well-established efficacy profiles [2]. However, not all patients on medication experience significant improvement in voiding symptoms. Some men experience intolerable side effects and others prefer a definitive approach that does not involve lifelong medication. Many attempts have been made to develop a method of treating BPH that is minimally invasive, efficacious, and cost-effective. One of the major advantages to transurethral needle ablation of the prostate (TUNA) is it can be performed in the office under topical anesthesia. With recent advances in technology, TUNA can now be used to create extremely precise microscopic and macroscopic lesions within the prostate.

C.S. Marley, M.A., M.D.
Department of Urology, Columbia University Medical Center, 161 Fort Washington Ave., New York, NY 10032, USA
e-mail: cmarleymd@gmail.com

M.P. Rutman, M.D. (✉)
Department of Urology, Columbia University College of Physicians and Surgeons, 11th Floor, HIP, 161 Ft. Washington Ave., New York, NY 10032, USA
e-mail: mr2423@columbia.edu

Transurethral Needle Ablation of the Prostate (TUNA)

Over the last decade, several minimally invasive therapies have been developed for the treatment of benign prostatic hyperplasia in men who are

B. Chughtai et al. (eds.), *Treatment of Benign Prostatic Hyperplasia: Modern Alternative to Transurethral Resection of the Prostate*, DOI 10.1007/978-1-4939-1587-3_17,

unwilling to remain on medication, in whom medical therapy has failed, who are unsuitable candidates for surgery, and in men who are concerned about the side effects of transurethral resection of prostate (TURP). Most thermal techniques involve hyperthermia (temperatures between 42 °C and 45 °C). Above 70 °C, thermal ablation of the treated tissue is achieved. TUNA therapy uses low-level radiofrequency energy to heat prostatic tissue and create a controlled localized necrotic lesion. Tissue is then selectively ablated with temperatures exceeding 60 °C while preserving the prostatic urothelium.

Delivery of Radiofrequency (RF) Energy

RF energy in TUNA is delivered directly into the prostate through a catheter device outfitted with adjustable needles which are placed in selected tissue areas. RF heat has been used effectively in the past to ablate accessory atrioventricular bundles in the Wolff-Parkinson-White syndrome [3]. In TUNA, low-level monopolar RF (490 kHz) waves allow for a deeper penetration and a more uniform temperature distribution than microwaves.

Experimental Studies

Early studies using a dog animal model and ex vivo human prostates demonstrated TUNA could generate 1 cm intra-prostatic necrotic lesions without causing damage to the rectum, bladder base, or prostatic urethra [4]. Schulman et al. demonstrated that necrosis was maximal at 7 days with the development of fibrosis at 15 days [5].

Schulman and Zlotta were the first to report the feasibility of the TUNA procedure in men with LUTS resulting from BPH. They concluded that this procedure was safe to perform in an outpatient setting and it was effective for improving symptomatic BPH [6].

Zlotta and colleagues then went on to publish a neurohistochemical study where they removed prostates from patients scheduled to undergo prostatectomy at 1–46 days after TUNA. They showed the maximal lesion size ranged from 10×7 to 20×10 mm and that the lesions were accurately positioned 0.3–1.0 cm from the urethra, which remained undamaged. Interestingly, 24 h after TUNA treatment, lesions did not stain for prostate-specific antigen, smooth muscle actin, or alpha adrenergic tissue [7].

Instruments

The TUNA system (Medtronic, Inc., Minneapolis, MN) consists of a specifically designed TUNA catheter called the ProVu system which is connected to a radiofrequency generator. The ProVu system has excellent visual optics allowing for direct visualization of needle placement. The catheter tip contains two needles that deploy at an unfixed angle. With previous generations of the TUNA catheter, needles were configured at an acute fixed angle with the catheter which made treatment of a high bladder neck or a median lobe difficult.

The needles can be withdrawn into Teflon shields, ensuring the treatment area is deep inside the prostatic lobes and away from the urethra. The power generator currently in use is computer driven and it adjusts its power output automatically based on the tissue temperature and impedance. As a result, tissue is heated faster and evenly and the procedure can be completed overall in shorter time (3 min per site). The latest hand piece has a temperature sensor at the needle tip instead of at the insulating sheath as in previous models. The sensor demonstrates consistent heating of 100C to 110 C at the core of each lesion.

Treatment

The patient is placed in dorsal lithotomy position and 2 % intraurethral lidocaine is injected into the meatus. A penile clamp can then be applied for 10 min, and IV sedation may be given. Spinal, general, or local anesthesias are all options. A grounding pad is placed over the sacrum.

adverse outcomes lies in the proper positioning of the needles with depth perception made possible with TRUS and placement of needles under direct vision. In the short term, the majority of patients have subjective (symptomatic) and objective (Qmax) improvements, even when presenting symptoms are severe. Roughly 14 % of patients will need to be treated by some other modality within 2 years.

References

1. Chute GG, Panser LA, Girman CJ, Oesterling JE, Guess HA, Jacobsen SJ, et al. The prevalence of prostatism: a population-based survey of urinary symptoms. J Urol. 1993;150:85.
2. McConnell JD, Roehrborn CG, Bautista OM, Andriole GL, Dixon CM, Kusek JW, et al. The long-term effect of doxazosin, finasteride, and combination therapy on the clinical progression of benign prostatic hyperplasia. N Engl J Med. 2003;349:2387.
3. Calkins H, Sousa J, El-Atassi R. Diagnosis and cure of the Wolff-Parkinson-White syndrome or paroxysmal supraventricular tachycardias during a single electrophysiologic test. N Engl J Med. 1991;324:1612.
4. Goldwasser B, Ramon J, Engelberg S. Transurethral needle ablation (TUNA) of the prostate using low-level radiofrequency energy: an animal experimental study. Eur Urol. 1993;24(3):400–5.
5. Schulman CC. Vandenbossche (TURF) Transurethral radiofrequency heating for benign prostatic hyperplasia at various temperatures with Thermex II: clinical experience. Eur Urol. 1993;23(2):302–6.
6. Schulman C, Zlotta A. Transurethral needle ablation of the prostate (TUNA): pathological, radiological and clinical study of a new office procedure for treatment of benign prostatic hyperplasia using low-level radiofrequency energy. Arch Esp Urol. 1994;47(9):895–901.
7. Zlotta AR, Raviv G, Peny MO, Noel J, Schulman C. Possible mechanisms of action of transurethral needle ablation of the prostate on benign prostatic hyperplasia symptoms: a neuro histochemical study. J Urol. 1997;157:894.
8. Hill B, Belville W, Bruskewitz R, Naslund M. Transurethral needle ablation versus transurethral resection of the prostate for the treatment of symptomatic benign prostatic hyperplasia: 5-year results of a prospective, randomized multicenter clinical trial. J Urol. 2004;171:2336–40.
9. Zlotta AR, Giannakopoulos X, Maehlum O, Ostrem T, Schulman C. Long-term evaluation of transurethral needle ablation of the prostate (TUNA) for treatment of symptomatic benign prostatic hyperplasia: clinical outcome up to five years from three centers. Eur Urol. 2003;44(1):89–93.
10. Boyle P, Robertson C, Vaughan ED, Fitzpatrick JM. A meta-analysis of trials of transurethral needle ablation for treating symptomatic benign prostatic hyperplasia. BJU Int. 2004;94(1):83–8.
11. American Urological Association Guideline: Management of Benign Prostatic Hyperplasia (BPH) 2010
12. Campo B, Bergamaschi F, Corrada P, Ordesi G. Transurethral needle ablation (TUNA) of the prostate: a clinical and urodynamic evaluation. Urology. 1997;49(6):847–50.
13. Steele GS, Sleep DJ. Transurethral needle ablation of the prostate: a urodynamic based study with 2-year follow-up. J Urol. 1997;158:1834–8.
14. Vaughan ED. Medical management of benign prostatic hyperplasia—are two drugs better than one? N Engl J Med. 2003;349:2449.
15. Naslund M, Carlson AM, Williams MJ. A cost comparison of medical management and transurethral needle ablation for treatment of benign prostatic hyperplasia during a 5-year period. J Urol. 2005;173:2090–3.
16. Schulman CC, Zlotta AR. Transurethral needle ablation of the prostate for treatment of benign prostatic hyperplasia: early clinical experience. Urology. 1995;45(1):28–33.

18 Prostatic Tissue Approximation (Urolift)

Henry H. Woo

The Urolift (Neotract, California, USA) is a novel, minimally invasive device for the treatment of lower urinary tract symptoms (LUTS) due to benign prostatic hyperplasia (BPH). It received Food and Drug Administration (FDA) approval as a treatment for LUTS in September 2013. The device is also approved for sale in the USA, European Union, Australia, New Zealand, Canada, Serbia, and Turkey.

Although the Urolift refers to the actual commercial product name, it is also used to describe the procedure performed – the prostatic urethral lift (PUL). The correct terminology would therefore be the use of the Urolift to perform the PUL procedure.

The Urolift differs from the great majority of minimally invasive surgical treatments for BPH/LUTS because it is mechanically based and does not involve the destruction or physical removal of prostatic tissue. It differs from other mechanically based treatments such as prostatic urethral stents because it does not attempt to conform to the anatomy of the prostatic urethra. Furthermore, through spot selective areas of deployment (as discussed below), the prosthesis becomes incorporated into the prostate and is covered by the urothelium.

H.H. Woo, M.B.B.S., FRACS (Urol) (✉)
Sydney Adventist Hospital Clinical School,
University of Sydney, San Clinic, Suite 406, 185 Fox Valley Road, Wahroonga, NSW 2076, Australia
e-mail: hwoo@urologist.net.au

In brief, PUL is performed under endoscopic guidance and Urolift prostheses are deployed with the aim of retracting the prostatic urethra towards the prostate capsule to open the prostatic urethral space. A metal tab on the prostatic urethral side is joined by a nonabsorbable suture to a metal tab that is deployed to anchor outside the prostate capsule; when the suture is placed under tension, the prostatic urethra is mechanically pulled open (Fig. 18.1).

The Urolift System

The Urolift implant deployed into the prostate is constructed from a nitinol capsular tab and a stainless steel urethral tab (Fig. 18.2). During deployment, the urethral tab can be placed at the desired position along a size 0 polyethylene terephthalate (PET) nonabsorbable monofilament suture, which is then automatically cut to the appropriate length by the device.

Currently, each delivery system (Fig. 18.3) is preloaded with only one Urolift implant. When multiple implants are to be deployed, a number of delivery systems must be used. The disposable delivery system is compatible with existing lower urinary tract endoscopic equipment and is placed with a 20 F cystoscope sheath. Through the delivery device, a 0° 2.9 mm diameter cystoscope lens enables the deployment of the implants to be visualized. The delivery device

B. Chughtai et al. (eds.), *Treatment of Benign Prostatic Hyperplasia: Modern Alternative to Transurethral Resection of the Prostate*, DOI 10.1007/978-1-4939-1587-3_18,

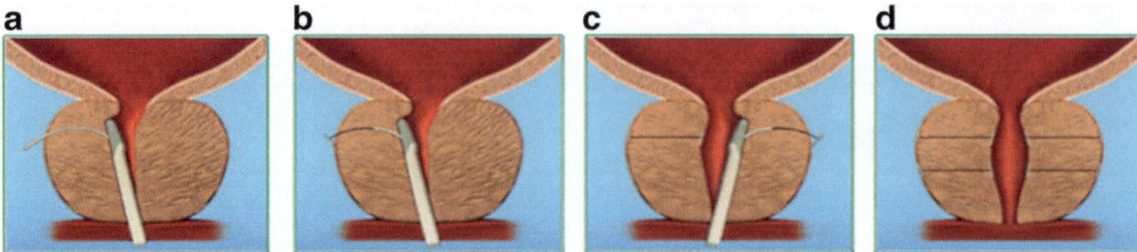

Fig. 18.1 Urolift system and delivery sequence. The prostatic urethral lift is a mechanical approach achieved by transurethrally deploying a needle beyond the prostate capsule (**a**) and delivering suture-based implants that are placed under tension (**b**, **c**) that mechanically retract the prostatic lobes (**d**) (Used with permission from NeoTract, Inc.)

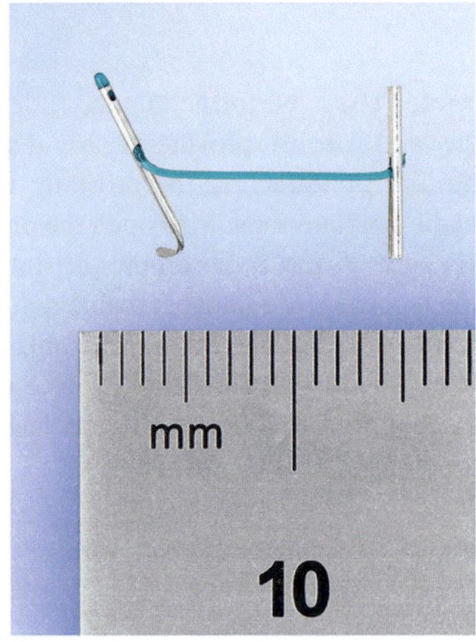

Fig. 18.2 Urolift implant (Used with permission from NeoTract, Inc.)

enables the assembled system to be grasped by the surgeon in a similar manner to a resectocope. There is a safety lock on the trigger, which once removed allows the surgeon to pull the trigger towards his or her hand in a purposeful motion. This leads to the deployment of a curved 19 gauge needle that will pass beyond the external boundaries of the prostatic capsule. At the end of this hollow needle, a distal nitinol tab has been preloaded. With the second pull of the trigger, the needle is completely retracted, while releasing, anchoring, and leaving the nitinol tab outside of the prostate capsule and simultaneously placing the suture under tension. The button on the outside edge of the delivery device handle is then pressed using the thumb of the hand holding the device; this simultaneously tensions the suture, fixes the stainless steel urethral tab on the PET suture, and cuts the suture flush.

Prostatic Urethral Lift Procedure

The PUL procedure can be performed under an anesthetic of the surgeon's and patient's preference. Procedures may be performed under local anesthetic block (urethrally instilled lidocaine jelly), variations of locally injected prostatic anesthetic blocks or general anesthesia (Fig. 18.4).

The patient is placed in the dorsal lithotomy position common for rigid cystoscopy. Following initial cystoscopic examination, the delivery device is introduced into the 20 F cystoscope sheath. With aim of creating an anterior channel in the prostatic urethra, the handle of the delivery device is rotated under visual guidance to a position that allows for anterolateral deployment of the implant into the lateral lobes of the prostate. It is important to not lean too heavily into the prostate in order to avoid inadvertent bone strike with the pubic bone. Once the desired position for deployment has been identified, the surgeon should employ a more gentle rotational movement, pivoting on tip of the delivery device where it contacts tissue. After the trigger is pulled, the suture will be in view. The delivery device should then be straightened and placed in vertical alignment with the urethra, followed by a slow and gentle forward advancement of the delivery unit until light reflects off the suture. This reflection

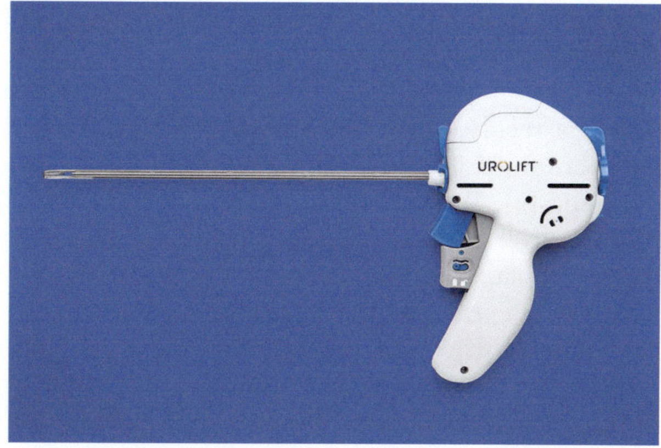

Fig. 18.3 Urolift delivery system (Used with permission from NeoTract, Inc.)

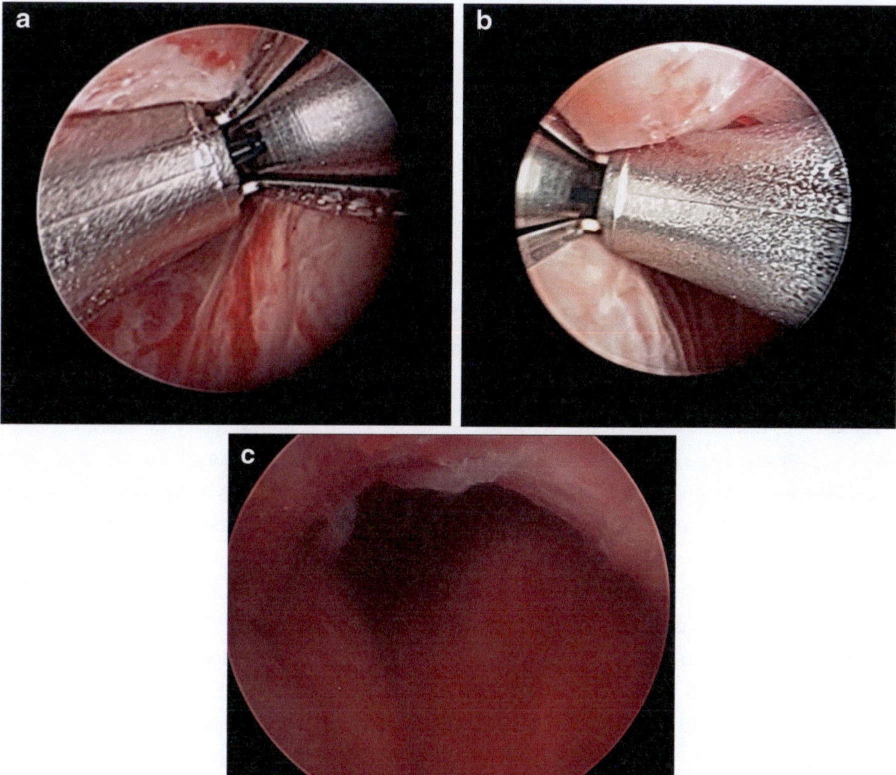

Fig. 18.4 (**a**–**c**) Deployment of the device (Used with permission from NeoTract, Inc.)

(referred to as the "Lamson sign" – Fig. 18.4b) indicates when the final button to complete the implant deployment should be depressed. Reports of technique similar to this description have been published [1, 2].

At first, an implant is deployed on each side and resultant distraction of the anterior part of the lateral lobes assessed. Further implants are deployed in order to create a visually apparent anterior channel.

Australian Multicenter Data

The first reported experience using the Urolift was performed in a bi-institutional study from Australia [3]. Two different prototype versions of the delivery device, neither of which are the current commercialized version, were utilized. This proof of principle study was able to confirm feasibility of deploying implants that traversed prostatic tissue between the prostatic urethra and the prostate capsule. These initial 19 patients had PUL procedures that were meticulously monitored under transrectal ultrasound and fluoroscopic guidance as well as visual endoscopic guidance. Given that the endoscopic deployment of the implants was indeed feasible, subsequent procedures no longer necessitated the use of imaging for guidance or confirmation of position. Two different prototypes of the delivery system were used during this series. This study confirmed the technical feasibility of the device to place tensioned implants between the prostatic urethra and the prostatic capsule as well as a favorable safety profile to justify further studies.

An expanded Australian multicenter study involving six sites evaluated 64 patients with follow-up out to 2 years [4]. During the first 25 cases, three different versions of the delivery system were used and the operative technique evolved. From case 26 onwards, the technique that is currently recommended was adopted for all remaining cases and the delivery system was consistent and the same as used for cases 20–25. Follow-up intervals were at 2 and 6 weeks and then at 3, 6, 12, and 24 months.

At the 2-week follow-up, the IPSS had fallen from a mean baseline of 22.6 ± 5.4 to 13.2 ± 6.3 (down 42 %). This reduction in symptoms scores was well sustained out to 2-year follow-up (IPSS = 12.6 ± 7.2).

Peak flow rate improvements were modest. On paired analysis, the peak flow improved from 8.3 ± 2.2 mL/s at baseline to 12.0 ± 7.6 at 2 weeks and for the 2-year follow-up, from a baseline of 7.4 ± 2.2 to 10.3 ± 4.1 at 2 years. The QOL index and BPH Impact Index demonstrated commensurate improvements that were seen at 2 weeks and sustained out to 2 years. There was no statistically or clinically relevant change in post residual volumes across all follow-up points in time.

Retreatment was necessary in 13 of the 64 men treated (20 %). Of these re-treatments, 12 were with either photoselective vaporization of the prostate or transurethral resection of the prostate; one patient elected to have re-treatment using the Urolift. When procedures were categorized as being procedures 1–25 and 26–64, the numbers retreated were 10 and 3, respectively. This clarification is important given that the 26th case represented a significant change in the manner in which the procedure was performed.

Randomized Controlled Trial: LIFT Study Data

Acceptance of new minimally invasive surgical therapies (MISTs) hinges on outcomes in randomized controlled studies. A transurethral resection of the prostate (TURP) is considered the "gold standard" for surgical intervention for LUTS due to BPH, and is generally considered to be the first comparator that should be studied. When drugs undergo comparative studies, they are usually tested against placebo; however, we know that MISTs lie in between drugs and cavitating surgery such as a TURP in terms of indications and outcome objectives.

For the first randomized control study evaluating the efficacy of PUL, sham treatment was selected as the comparator [5]. The precedent for using a sham procedure as a comparator for MISTs has been well established, particularly with studies on transurethral microwave treatment. Prior to proceeding with any such a study with PUL versus sham treatment, the trial protocol was pre-approved by the US Food and Drug Administration, Health Canada, and the Therapeutic Goods Administration (Australia).

The "Luminal Improvement Following Prostatic Tissue Approximation for the Treatment

Table 18.1 Comparison of mean change in outcomes at 3 months

	Mean, SD (no. responses) prostatic urethral lift (ITT)			Mean, SD (no. responses) control (ITT)			
Outcome measure	Baseline	3 months	Change	Baseline	3 months	Change	P value (2-sample 1 test)
AUASI	22.2, 5.48 (140)	11.2, 7.65 (140)	−11.1, 7.67 (140)	24.4, 5.75 (66)	18.5, 8.59 (66)	−5.9, 7.66 (66)	0.003
Qmax (ml/s)	8.02, 2.43 (126)	12.29, 5.40 (126)	4.28, 5.16 (126)	7.93, 2.41 (56)	9.91, 4.29 (56)	1.98, 4.88 (56)	0.005
QOL	4.6, 1.1 (140)	2.4, 1.7 (140)	−2.2, 1.8 (140)	4.7, 1.1 (66)	3.6, 1.6 (66)	−1.0, 1.5 (66)	<0.001
BPHII	6.9, 2.8 (140)	3.0, 3.1 (140)	−3.9, 3.2 (140)	7.0, 3.0 (66)	4.9, 3.2 (66)	−2.1, 3.3 (66)	<0.001
MSHQ-EjD	8.7, 3.1 (94)	10.9, 3.2 (94)	2.2, 2.5 (94)	8.8, 3.1 (50)	10.5, 3.5 (50)	1.7, 2.6 (50)	0.283
MSHQ-Bother	2.4, 1.7 (117)	1.6, 1.7 (117)	−0.8, 1.5 (117)	2.2, 1.7 (60)	1.5, 1.7 (60)	−0.7, 1.6 (60)	0.595
IIEF-5	13.3, 8.4 (132)	13.4, 9.2 (132)	0.1, 5.8 (132)	13.7, 8.5 (65)	15.2, 8.5 (65)	1.5, 6.4 (65)	0.139
PVR (ml)	85.5, 69.2 (140)	75.8, 83.9 (140)	−9.7, 85.5 (140)	85.6, 70.8 (65)	63.4, 64.0 (65)	−22.2, 70.7 (65)	0.306

From Roehrborn et al. [5]. Reprinted with permission from Elsevier Limited

of LUTS secondary to BPH" study (LIFT study) is a multicenter, randomized, controlled, blinded study performed in 19 centers across the United States, Canada, and Australia. A total of 206 men were randomized 2:1 into receiving PUL or sham treatment. The principle inclusion criteria required men aged ≥50 years of age, IPSS ≥ 13, Qmax ≤12 mL/s, and prostate volume between 30 and 80 cc inclusive.

At 3 months following treatment, the procedure type was unblinded to subjects and those allocated a sham procedure were invited to cross over to active treatment if they desired. The primary end point was to demonstrate that there was at least a 25 % greater reduction in symptoms score (AUA-SI) compared to the sham procedure on an intention to treat basis. The results of this analysis are summarized in Table 18.1. The primary efficacy objective was clearly reached.

Men treated with PUL were followed to one year and the results remarkably similar to the Australian studies.

A total of 53 of the 66 men who had been treated with the sham procedure elected to cross over to PUL. At 3 months following the PUL procedure, this provided a unique opportunity to compare these 3-month outcomes in a paired manner against their 3-month outcomes following the sham procedure [6] (Fig. 18.5). Improvements of a similar magnitude as observed with previous studies.

Other Published Data

An initial French experience of treating four men found the PUL to have a median procedural time of 11 min (range 6–11 min) [7]. One patient experienced no improvement in his urinary function while the remainder had improvements of the magnitude seen in earlier studies.

Another small study of 20 patients was reported that had a less restrictive entry criteria for treatment than was allowed compared to the Australian and LIFT studies [8]. Prostate sizes ranging from 19 to 109 cc were treated and men under the age of 50 years were also offered treatment. Again similar results to earlier pivotal studies were observed.

A larger series of 51 men where the same inclusion criteria and data instruments were used as the LIFT study again found almost identical results to the pivotal studies in terms of symptom improvement, flow rate, and sexual function.

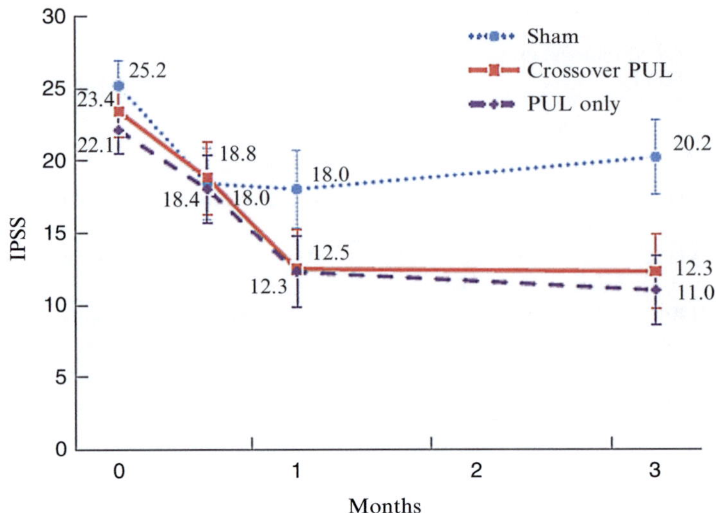

Fig. 18.5 Comparison of the IPSS from baseline to 3-month follow-up for patients who underwent sham procedure and later crossover PUL procedure. Also plotted are the "blinded" and randomized results from Woo et al. [3] on PUL-only patients. Crossover PUL IPSS improvement is significantly greater than that of sham and closely mimics prior published results. Values shown are the mean absolute IPSS; error bars represent the 95 % CI (From Cantwell et al. [6]. Reprinted with permission from John Wiley and Sons)

Indications

Suitable patients for treatment are those men who are considered to have LUTS due to BPH. Prior failed pharmacotherapy or failed PUL procedure is not a contraindication.

Clinical trials have described limitations to suitability predominantly on the basis of prostate anatomy. Large glands (>80 cc) or those with prominent middle lobes, for example, have not been included in clinical trials. However, clinical trials have not been performed that demonstrated potential efficacy or lack of efficacy for men with larger prostates or prominent middle lobes.

The safety of the Urolift has not been reported in clinical trials. It has however been tested under conditions representative of standard clinical use and in the manufacturers' instruction for use document, it is classified as "MR conditional."

Adverse Events

PUL seems to have significantly lower morbidity than other current surgical treatments for LUTS due to BPH. The documented adverse events associated with the Urolift have included hematuria, dysuria, and bladder spasms; these complications are minor and short lived. There have not been any serious adverse events in clinical outcomes reported to date.

Sexual Function

An interesting outcome from clinical trials has been the absence of significant sexual dysfunction. Almost all other treatments for BPH/LUTS report a measurable level of sexual dysfunction, whether they be pharmacotherapy, other MISTs, or cavitating surgery. The impact of the PUL on sexual function has been carefully evaluated in the pivotal clinical trials with established validated instruments.

Two papers have specifically addressed sexual function. The Australian multicenter study measured at baseline the Sexual Health Inventory for Men (SHIM) and Male Sexual Health Questionnaire for Ejaculatory Dysfunction (MSHQ-EjD) function score and these repeated at 6 weeks and 3, 6, and 12 months following the procedure [9]. Utilizing these instruments, this

Table 18.2 Ejaculatory function in the LIFT study. Male sexual health questionnaire for ejaculatory dysfunction (MSHQ-EjD) change from baseline after prostatic urethral lift

	1 month	3 months	6 months	12 months
Question 1 [Frequency]: How often have you been able to ejaculate or "cum" when having sexual activity?				
N (paired)	77	80	84	75
Baseline	4.08 ± 1.06	4.04 ± 1.06	4.02 ± 1.11	4.05 ± 1.06
Follow-up	4.25 ± 1.07	4.38 ± 1.01	4.35 ± 0.95	4.23 ± 1.03
Change [95 %CI]	0.17 [–0.06–0.39]	0.34 [0.15–0.52]	0.33 [0.11–0.54]	0.18 [–0.05–0.40]
P value	.109	<0.001	<0.001	0.038
Question 2 [Intensity]: How would you rate the strength or force of your ejaculation?				
N (paired)	77	80	84	75
Baseline	2.57 ± 1.22	2.56 ± 1.22	2.58 ± 1.21	2.59 ± 1.21
Follow-up	3.56 ± 1.34	3.45 ± 1.29	3.30 ± 1.32	3.18 ± 1.31
Change [95 %CI]	0.99 [0.70–1.29]	0.89 [0.62–1.15]	0.72 [0.48–0.95]	0.59 [0.33–0.84]
P value	<0.001	<0.001	<0.001	<0.001
Question 3 [Volume]: How would you rate the amount of volume of semen or fluid when you ejaculate?				
N (paired)	77	80	84	75
Baseline	2.49 ± 1.32	2.47 ± 1.35	2.54 ± 1.37	2.56 ± 1.37
Follow-up	3.48 ± 1.35	3.40 ± 1.38	3.30 ± 1.43	3.12 ± 1.27
Change [95 %CI]	0.99 [0.67–1.30]	0.93 [0.67–1.18]	0.76 [0.50–10.2]	0.56 [0.30–0.82]
P value	<0.001	<0.001	<0.001	<0.001
Question 4 [Bother]: If you have had any ejaculation difficulties or have been unable to ejaculate, have you been bothered by this?				
N (paired)	77	80	84	75
Baseline	2.0 ± 1.6	2.0 ± 1.6	2.1 ± 1.6	2.0 ± 1.7
Follow-up	1.3 ± 1.4	1.0 ± 1.3	1.1 ± 1.1	1.2 ± 1.3
Change [95 %CI]	–0.7 [–1.0–0.4]	–1.0 [–1.3–.07]	–1.0 [–1.3–0.7]	–0.8 [–1.1–0.4]
P value	<0.001	<0.001	<0.001	<0.001

Each parameter is listed as mean ± standard deviation (SD), and the change is represented as average and 95 % confidence interval (CI). P values were obtained by fitting a generalized estimating equation to each parameter for all available subjects

From McVary et al. [10]. Reprinted with permission from John Wiley and Sons

study demonstrated an absence of degradation of erectile or ejaculatory function. In a similar manner, the same sexual function instruments were also applied to men participating in the LIFT study [10]. When ejaculatory function in the LIFT study was sub-analyzed using the MSHQ-EjD, it demonstrated a consistent improvement in ejaculatory function (Table 18.2).

Future Directions

A randomized controlled trial comparing the PUL and TURP in 100 men has completed recruitment and is currently in progress. This study is identified as the BPH6 study (ClinicalTrials.gov identifier: NCT01533038) and is novel because the primary objective outcome is the fulfillment of six outcomes criteria out to 1 year of follow-up. The six requisite domains requiring fulfillment are listed in the table below (Table 18.3). These parameters focus on the main outcome parameters of therapies treating LUTS due to BPH and include parameters of efficacy, safety, and quality of life outcomes such as sexual function and continence. Perhaps, this study will be incorporated as important outcome parameters for future studies of therapies to treat LUTS due to BPH.

With the increasing utilization of MR prostate imaging, clinical studies will be necessary to further clarify its safety with contemporary MR

Table 18.3 Outcome objectives of the BPH6 study, comparing PUL with TURP

Domain	Outcome
1. LUTS	≥30 % reduction in IPSS compared to baseline
2. Recovery experience	Return to preoperative activity levels by 1 month
3. Erectile function	Less than six-point reduction in SHIM compared to baseline
4. Ejaculatory function	Response on MSHQ-EjD that indicates emission of semen. This excludes the response "could not ejaculate"
5. Continence	ISI score of four points or less at all follow-up time points
6. Safety	No procedure-related adverse event greater than Grade I on the Clavien-Dindo classification system modified for TURP at any time during procedure or follow-up

prostate protocols as well as any impact the prosthesis might have on image interpretation.

Additional studies should be directed to longer term outcomes and the efficacy of the procedure in men who on the basis of prostate configuration were not suitable for entry into clinical trials performed to this point in time.

References

1. Barkin J, Giddens J, Incze P, Casey R, Richardson S, Gange S. UroLift system for relief of prostate obstruction under local anesthesia. Can J Urol. 2012;19: 6217–22.
2. McNicholas TA, Woo HH, Chin PT, et al. Minimally invasive prostatic urethral lift: surgical technique and multinational experience. Eur Urol. 2013;64:292–9.
3. Woo HH, Chin PT, McNicholas TA, et al. Safety and feasibility of the prostatic urethral lift: a novel, minimally invasive treatment for lower urinary tract symptoms (LUTS) secondary to benign prostatic hyperplasia (BPH). BJU Int. 2011;108:82–8.
4. Chin PT, Bolton DM, Jack G, et al. Prostatic urethral lift: two-year results after treatment for lower urinary tract symptoms secondary to benign prostatic hyperplasia. Urology. 2012;79:5–11.
5. Roehrborn CG, Gange SN, Shore ND, et al. The prostatic urethral lift for the treatment of lower urinary tract symptoms associated with prostate enlargement due to benign prostatic hyperplasia: the L.I.F.T. Study. J Urol. 2013;190:2161–7.
6. Cantwell AL, Bogache WK, Richardson SF, Tutrone RF, Barkin J, Fagelson JE, Chin PT, Woo HH. Multicentre prospective crossover study of the 'prostatic urethral lift' for the treatment of lower urinary tract symptoms secondary to benign prostatic hyperplasia. BJU Int. 2014;113:615–22.
7. Delongchamps NB, Conquy S, Defontaines J, Zerbib M, Peyromaure M. Intra-prostatic UroLift((R)) implants for benign prostatic hyperplasia: preliminary results of the four first cases performed in France. Progres en urologie: journal de l'Association francaise d'urologie et de la Societe francaise d'urologie. 2012;22:590–7.
8. Garrido Abad P, Coloma Del Peso A, Sinues Ojas B, Fernandez Arjona M. Urolift(R), a new minimally invasive treatment for patients with low urinary tract symptoms secondary to BPH. Preliminary results. Arch Esp Urol. 2013;66:584–91.
9. Woo HH, Bolton DM, Laborde E, et al. Preservation of sexual function with the prostatic urethral lift: a novel treatment for lower urinary tract symptoms secondary to benign prostatic hyperplasia. J Sex Med. 2012;9:568–75.
10. McVary KT, Gange SN, Shore ND, et al. Treatment of LUTS secondary to BPH while preserving sexual function: randomized controlled study of prostatic urethral lift. J Sex Med. 2014;11(1):279–87. doi:10.1111/jsm.12333. Epub 2013 Sep 30. PMID: 24119101 [PubMed – in process].

19 Prostatic Stents

Gina M. Badalato and Matthew P. Rutman

Introduction

Prostatic stents are tubes that can be endoscopically placed into the prostatic urethra, either permanently or temporarily, to tent open adenomatous tissue and thereby open the bladder outlet. They immediately eliminate obstructive symptoms attributable to benign prostatic hypertrophy (BPH). Placement and symptomatic improvement is contingent on an adequately functioning detrusor [1].

Alexis Carrel is credited with the original idea of using stents to restore the patency of obstructed viscera in 1912, when he published his work using glass and metal tubes coated with paraffin wax to stent canine thoracic aortae [2]. This idea was then modified by the vascular surgeon Charles Dotter, to restore the luminal integrity of atherosclerotic vessels in 1964 [3]. Fabian then adapted this idea in 1980 when he first described the "urological spiral" as a temporary device to treat bladder outlet obstruction (BOO). Since that time, this technology has evolved to incorporate permanent (epithelializing) and temporary or biodegradable stents for not only BPH but also for urethral stricture and detrusor sphincter dyssynergia (DSD), although this review focuses on applications pertaining to the former [4, 5].

Indications for Permanent Prostatic Stents

A significant number of men will fail maximal medical therapy for BPH and necessitate surgical intervention in the form of a bladder outlet reductive procedure. The vast majority of these patients would be recommended for a transurethral resection of the prostate (TURP), although this procedure carries a mortality and morbidity historically estimated at 0.2 % and 18 %, respectively [6]. More recent meta-analyses with regard to TURP outcomes have reported a 0.1 % mortality during the first 30 days after the procedure, TUR syndrome in 0.8 % (range 0–5 %), blood transfusion in 2 % (range 0–9 %), clot retention in 4.9 % (range 0–39 %), and urinary tract infection in 4.1 % (range 0–22 %) [7, 8]. Although these complication rates are relatively low, they may not be negligible in a select cohort of elderly men with significant comorbidities and thus increased operative risk. In fact, 10–15 % of elderly men with symptomatic BPH are deemed poor candidates for a TURP, with the age-adjusted morbidity and mortality rates after

G.M. Badalato, M.D.
Department of Urology, Columbia University Medical Center, 11th Floor, HIP, 161 Ft. Washington Ave., New York, NY 10032, USA
e-mail: gmb2107@columbia.edu

M.P. Rutman, M.D. (✉)
Department of Urology, Columbia University College of Physicians and Surgeons, 11th Floor, HIP, 161 Ft. Washington Ave., New York, NY 10032, USA
e-mail: mr2423@columbia.edu

B. Chughtai et al. (eds.), *Treatment of Benign Prostatic Hyperplasia: Modern Alternative to Transurethral Resection of the Prostate*, DOI 10.1007/978-1-4939-1587-3_19,

TURP estimated at upwards of 25 % and 0.2 %, respectively, in men over 80 years of age [6, 9].

Prostatic stents have been proposed as an alternative treatment modality in such high-risk candidates with a functioning detrusor who would otherwise be committed to clean intermittent catheterization, with the inherent risk of traumatic catheterization in the setting of known BPH or an indwelling Foley catheter.

Permanent Prostatic Stents

The UroLume

Prostatic stents can be either permanent or temporary, with the former promoting epithelialization and anchoring into the prostatic stroma and the latter prohibitive of tissue ingrowth and may be biodegradable or retrievable. The UroLume Wallstent (American Medical Systems, Minnetonka, Minnesota, USA) was one of the first permanent stents manufactured and consisted of a stainless steel alloy woven into a mesh of approximately 42 French [10]. In 2007, Armitage et al. reported a systematic review of 20 case series evaluating the efficacy of the UroLume stent in a total of 990 subjects with BPH [11]. These trials with variable follow-up reported significant symptomatic improvement: 84 % of patients who were catheter-dependent voided spontaneously after insertion; International Prostate Symptom Score (IPSS) decreased by 10 points to 12.4; and Qmax increased by 4.2 units to 13.1 cc/s. However, of the 606 patients who were evaluated at 1 year of follow-up, 104 (16 %) sustained stent failure, with the majority due to stent migration (38 cases, 37 %). Masood and colleagues went on to publish a 12-year outcome analysis on 22 and 11 patients who completed a 5- and 12-year respective follow-up term with the UroLume [9]. Twenty-one (34 %) patients died of causes unrelated to BPH with the stent in situ. A total of 29 (47 %) stents were removed, 18 in the first 2 years, due to inappropriate case selection or stent migration; 4 were removed as a result of patient dissatisfaction, and late stent removal was predominantly a result of recrudescence of symptoms. While the authors did demonstrate that the stent could produce a durable effect at up to 12 years of follow-up, as a corollary to the significant explantation rate, they emphasized that careful patient selection and experience was requisite.

Although hour-glass and bell-shaped nitinol stents were piloted approximately 5 years ago, the high migration rates made these products unsuitable for clinical use [12, 13].

Last, Memotherm (Angiomed, Germany) permanent stents are composed of titanium alloy and can expand to 42 Fr with the application of heat. In addition to the thermosensitivity, the stent is easy to remove, as it unravels by pulling on a single wire. Clinical usage of this stent, however, was hampered by reported inability to void up to 8 weeks after insertion and a relatively high complication rate including recurrent infections and urgency, urothelial hyperplasia, and urethral stricture [14, 15].

Permanent Prostatic Stent Removal

As evidenced in the aforementioned case series, stents may warrant removal due to misplacement, migration, intolerability, progression of symptoms, or encrustation. The removal of permanent stents can be difficult following encrustation, migration, or stromal ingrowths, necessitating procedures under general anesthesia, which may be effectively defeating the purpose of stent placement to begin within this high-risk patient population. For UroLume stent extraction, techniques have involved TUR of the prostatic stroma and stent with the rigid resectoscope, use of the holmium laser, and, in some cases, wire-by-wire extraction [10, 16–18].

Temporary Prostatic Stents

Temporary prostatic stents were developed primarily to address transient BOO, such as in the setting of recent brachytherapy to the prostate or a thermal reductive therapy such as transurethral microwave therapy (TUMT). The temporary stents are intended to remain in the prostatic urethra for short periods of time and as a result do not epithelialize into the urethral wall. They serve as an alternative to an indwelling Foley or suprapubic catheter, or intermittent catheterization. Although bioabsorbable modalities are the paradigm in this situation, development of such a device is limited by the variable degradation time in each individualized setting; furthermore, the smaller lumen of temporary models makes these stents more prone to obstruction [10].

First-Generation Spiral Stents

First-generation spiral stents such as the Urospiral (Porges) and the Prosta Kath (Pharma-Plast) were 21 Fr in size made of stainless steel, the latter being gold plated, and designed to remain in place no longer than 12 months. Despite the finite duration, significant complication rates including hematuria with clot retention (5 %), stent migration (15 %), recurrent urinary tract infections (10 %), and encrustation (4 %) were reported in several series [19].

The Memokath

Because permanent and first-generation spiral stents were subject to incomplete epithelialization and thus encrustation on the exposed surface area, a thermo-sensitive second-generation stent the Memokath (Engineers and Doctors A/s, Hrnbaek, Denmark) was developed. The Memokath is composed of nickel alloy and is pliant to mold to the contour of the surface area it touches. When flushed with hot irrigation, the lower section of the stent at the prostatic apex will expand to secure the stent in position; when cooled, the spiral becomes soft to facilitate removal [10, 20]. The best data on the performance of the Memokath stent comes from a 14 case series meta-analysis of 839 patients. Although symptoms were assessed at variable time points after stent insertion, the Memokath stent reduced IPSS by 11–19 points and resulted in a Qmax increase of 3–11 ml/s [21]. Follow-up in this series was insufficient to provide commentary on durability, although a smaller series of 15 patients reported 9 (60 %) being catheter-free at 1 year and the remaining three undergoing stent removal at a mean time of 9 months [22].

The thermo-pliability of the Memokath stent has facilitated extraction, with a report by Barber and colleagues reporting on a 93 patient series whereby the stent was removed with topical anesthesia (43/93, 46 %), general anesthesia 35/93, 38 %), regional anesthesia (13/93, 14 %), and without anesthesia (2/93, 2 %). The procedure was rated as "easy" in 59 patients and the mean duration of the case was 11 min (range 3–30 min) [23].

Polyurethane Stents

Polyurethane stents or intraurethral catheters constitute three types: the intraurethral catheter (Angiomed, Germany), the Barnes stent (CR Bard, Covington, GA), and the trestle stent (Microvasive, Boston Scientific, Natick MA). The intraurethral catheter is 16 Fr in size, has a proximal tip shaped like a Malecot catheter, and can be left in place for up to 6 months. The stent is placed endoscopically and can be repositioned and retrieved via its distal string; it has reported applications to prevent transient outlet obstruction following thermotherapy to the prostate. The Barnes stent has a similar design as the intraurethral catheter, but only a single, not a double, proximal Malecot head and comes in one length only. The trestle is 22 Fr in diameter and consists of two tubes with an interlocking thread. Small nonrandomized series have been published reporting relatively acceptable tolerance of polyurethane stents largely after prostate thermotherapy; however, this remains to be validated in larger series and the cost efficacy for this post-procedural use investigated further.

The Spanner

The Spanner (Abbey Moor Medical, Inc., Minnesota, USA) is a retrievable stent that can remain in place for a mean of 57 days. The device essentially constitutes the proximal 4–6 cm of a Foley catheter, with modifiable prostatic lengths, and the added advantage of the fact no tubing is traversing the anterior urethra/meatus. The original pilot study introducing the apparatus involved 30 patients and reported a mean baseline and post-insertion Qmax of 8.2 and 11.6 ml/s, respectively, representing a 42 % improvement; with a relative decline in IPSS scores from 22.3 to 7.1, representing a 68 % decrease. Lack of device migration was confirmed radiographically at 12 weeks [24].

The clinical applicability of the Spanner has since been reported in the post-brachytherapy and transurethral microwave thermotherapy (TUMT) settings. First, Henderson et al. recruited a cohort of five patients with severe lower urinary tract symptoms or retention after brachytherapy, who agreed to undergo stent insertion at a mean of 40 days post-procedure. Although all patients sustained significant improvements in IPSS after placement, two of the five requested stent removal at 1 week; the balance of the cohort maintained the device for 30 days with some degree of dysuria/pain being the major complaint [25]. Outcomes with the Spanner were more compelling in a recent cohort of 196 patients who were randomized to receive the stent (100) or standard of care (86) immediately following TUMT. The patients had a stent/Foley in pace for up to 8 weeks; the Spanner group reported greater improvements in quality of life with patient satisfaction exceeding 86 % in this cohort [26].

Biodegradable Stents

The concept of the biodegradable stent takes the use of the temporary stent one advancement further in that the stents do not need to be removed and dissolve in situ. The concept of the biodegradable stent was first developed in 1993 and used in rabbits after urethrotomy; further work expanded the usage of these devices to the human ureter [27]. In fact Petas and colleagues reported a randomized series whereby 72 patients undergoing laser ablation of the prostate were assigned to the following groups: (1) polyglycolic acid biodegradable spiral stent ($n=27$), (2) no device ($n=23$), and (3) indwelling catheter ($n=22$). The first group was able to void at a median of 1 day in the degradable stent group, and a median of 6 days for the remaining groups, the latter after Foley removal. However, the stent degraded into polymer debris and particulate matter was sloughed in the urine; this passage ultimately obstructed voiding at 3–4 weeks postoperatively [28]. The optimal design of these stents thus remains in the developmental phase.

Conclusions

Permanent prostatic stents have acceptable applications for elderly men who seek symptomatic improvement from severe BPH-related bladder outlet obstruction who are not candidates for a transurethral procedure secondary to significant perioperative risk. However, some of the difficulty involved in stent removal, particularly as it pertains to epithelializing stents, may confound widespread usage in this patient population. Retrievable prostatic stents are being introduced to temporize obstructive symptoms after a procedure that would result in edema to prostatic tissue, with biodegradable stents in development.

References

1. Oelke M, Bachmann A, Descazeaud A, Emberton M, Gravas S, Michel MC, et al. EAU guidelines on the treatment and follow-up of non-neurogenic male lower urinary tract symptoms including benign prostatic obstruction. Eur Urol. 2013;64(1):118–40. PubMed PMID: 23541338. Epub 2013/04/02. Eng.
2. Anjum MI, Chari R, Shetty A, Keen M, Palmer JH. Long-term clinical results and quality of life after insertion of a self-expanding flexible endourethral prosthesis. Br J Urol. 1997;80(6):885–8. PubMed PMID: 9439402, Epub 1998/01/24. eng.
3. Fabian KM. The intra-prostatic "partial catheter" (urological spiral) (author's transl)]. Urologe A. 1980;19(4):236–8. PubMed PMID: 7414771. Epub 1980/07/01. Der Intraprostatische "Partielle Katheter" (Urologische Spirale). ger.
4. Oesterling JE, Kaplan SA, Epstein HB, Defalco AJ, Reddy PK, Chancellor MB. The North American experience with the UroLume endoprosthesis as a treatment for benign prostatic hyperplasia: long-term

results. The North American UroLume Study Group. Urology. 1994;44(3):353–62. PubMed PMID: 7521091, Epub 1994/09/01. eng.
5. Juma S, Niku SD, Brodak PP, Joseph AC. Urolume urethral wallstent in the treatment of detrusor sphincter dyssynergia. Paraplegia. 1994;32(9):616–21. PubMed PMID: 7997341. Epub 1994/09/01. eng.
6. Mebust WK, Holtgrewe HL, Cockett AT, Peters PC. Transurethral prostatectomy: immediate and postoperative complications. A cooperative study of 13 participating institutions evaluating 3,885 patients. J Urol. 1989;141(2):243–7.
7. Madersbacher S, Marberger M. Is transurethral resection of the prostate still justified? BJU Int. 1999;83(3):227–37. PubMed PMID: 10233485. Epub 1999/05/08. eng.
8. Ahyai SA, Gilling P, Kaplan SA, Kuntz RM, Madersbacher S, Montorsi F, et al. Meta-analysis of functional outcomes and complications following transurethral procedures for lower urinary tract symptoms resulting from benign prostatic enlargement. Eur Urol. 2010;58(3):384–97. PubMed PMID: 20825758. Epub 2010/09/10. eng.
9. Masood S, Djaladat H, Kouriefs C, Keen M, Palmer JH. The 12-year outcome analysis of an endourethral wallstent for treating benign prostatic hyperplasia. BJU Int. 2004;94(9):1271–4. PubMed PMID: 15610103. Epub 2004/12/22. eng.
10. Vanderbrink BA, Rastinehad AR, Badlani GH. Prostatic stents for the treatment of benign prostatic hyperplasia. Curr Opin Urol. 2007;17(1):1–6. PubMed PMID: 17143103. Epub 2006/12/05. eng.
11. Armitage JN, Cathcart PJ, Rashidian A, De Nigris E, Emberton M, van der Meulen JH. Epithelializing stent for benign prostatic hyperplasia: a systematic review of the literature. J Urol. 2007;177(5):1619–24. PubMed PMID: 17437773. Epub 2007/04/18. eng.
12. van Dijk MM, Mochtar CA, Wijkstra H, Laguna MP, de la Rosette JJ. The bell-shaped nitinol prostatic stent in the treatment of lower urinary tract symptoms: experience in 108 patients. Eur Urol. 2006;49(2):353–9. PubMed PMID: 16426738. Epub 2006/01/24. eng.
13. van Dijk MM, Mochtar CA, Wijkstra H, Laguna MP, de la Rosette JJ. Hourglass-shaped nitinol prostatic stent in treatment of patients with lower urinary tract symptoms due to bladder outlet obstruction. Urology. 2005;66(4):845–9. PubMed PMID: 16230150. Epub 2005/10/19. eng.
14. Williams G, White R. Experience with the Memotherm permanently implanted prostatic stent. Br J Urol. 1995;76(3):337–40. PubMed PMID: 7551842.
15. Gesenberg A, Sintermann R. Management of benign prostatic hyperplasia in high risk patients: long-term experience with the Memotherm stent. J Urol. 1998;160(1):72–6. PubMed PMID: 9628608.
16. Ogiste JS, Cooper K, Kaplan SA. Are stents still a useful therapy for benign prostatic hyperplasia? Curr Opin Urol. 2003;13(1):51–7. PubMed PMID: 12490816. Epub 2002/12/20. eng.
17. Shah DK, Kapoor R, Badlani GH. Experience with urethral stent explantation. J Urol. 2003;169(4):1398–400. PubMed PMID: 12629371. Epub 2003/03/12. eng.
18. Wilson TS, Lemack GE, Dmochowski RR. UroLume stents: lessons learned. J Urol. 2002;167(6):2477–80. PubMed PMID: 11992061. Epub 2002/05/07. eng.
19. Thomas PJ, Britton JP, Harrison NW. The Prostakath stent: four years' experience. Br J Urol. 1993; 71(4):430–2. PubMed PMID: 7684649.
20. Poulsen AL, Schou J, Ovesen H, Nordling J. Memokath: a second generation of intraprostatic spirals. Br J Urol. 1993;72(3):331–4. PubMed PMID: 7693295. Epub 1993/09/01. eng.
21. Armitage JN, Rashidian A, Cathcart PJ, Emberton M, van der Meulen JH. The thermo-expandable metallic stent for managing benign prostatic hyperplasia: a systematic review. BJU Int. 2006;98(4):806–10. PubMed PMID: 16879446. Epub 2006/08/02. eng.
22. Lee G, Marathe S, Sabbagh S, Crisp J. Thermo-expandable intra-prostatic stent in the treatment of acute urinary retention in elderly patients with significant co-morbidities. Int Urol Nephrol. 2005;37(3):501–4. PubMed PMID: 16307329. Epub 2005/11/25. eng.
23. Barber NJ, Roodhouse AJ, Rathenborg P, Nordling J, Ellis BW. Ease of removal of thermo-expandable prostate stents. BJU Int. 2005;96(4):578–80. PubMed PMID: 16104913. Epub 2005/08/18. eng.
24. Corica AP, Larson BT, Sagaz A, Corica AG, Larson TR. A novel temporary prostatic stent for the relief of prostatic urethral obstruction. BJU Int. 2004; 93(3):346–8. PubMed PMID: 14764134. Epub 2004/02/07. eng.
25. Henderson A, Laing RW, Langley SE. A Spanner in the works: the use of a new temporary urethral stent to relieve bladder outflow obstruction after prostate brachytherapy. Brachytherapy. 2002;1(4):211–8. PubMed PMID: 15062169. Epub 2004/04/06. eng.
26. Dineen MK, Shore ND, Lumerman JH, Saslawsky MJ, Corica AP. Use of a temporary prostatic stent after transurethral microwave thermotherapy reduced voiding symptoms and bother without exacerbating irritative symptoms. Urology. 2008;71(5):873–7. PubMed PMID: 18374395. Epub 2008/04/01. eng.
27. Kemppainen E, Talja M, Riihela M, Pohjonen T, Tormala P, Alfthan O. A bioresorbable urethral stent. An experimental study. Urol Res. 1993;21(3):235–8. PubMed PMID: 8342257.
28. Petas A, Talja M, Tammela TL, Taari K, Valimaa T, Tormala P. The biodegradable self-reinforced poly-DL-lactic acid spiral stent compared with a suprapubic catheter in the treatment of post-operative urinary retention after visual laser ablation of the prostate. Br J Urol. 1997;80(3):439–43. PubMed PMID: 9313664.

Prostatic Artery Embolization

20

Roger Valdivieso O'Donova, Pierre-Alain Hueber, Naeem Bhojani, Quoc-Dien Trinh, and Kevin C. Zorn

Introduction

Benign prostatic hyperplasia (BPH) affects a significant proportion of men and its prevalence increases with age. An enlarged prostatic gland can cause lower urinary tract symptoms (LUTS) by obstructing the bladder outlet and by increasing smooth muscle tone of the gland in reaction to an augmented resistance. Moreover, epidemiologic and pathophysiologic associations have been established between LUTS/BPH and erectile dysfunction (ED) [1]. Moderate or severe LUTS will occur in approximately one quarter of men in their 50s and in approximately half of all men 80 years or older [2]. If patients experiencing LUTS are bothered by their symptoms (i.e., they interfere with their quality of life and daily activities), they are advised to undergo medical treatment as indicated by the American Urological Association (AUA) and the European Association of Urology (EAU) guidelines [3, 4]. Relief of LUTS can be achieved medically by means of alpha-blockers or 5-alpha reductase inhibitors. A recent study showed that a phosphodiesterase type 5 inhibitor (PDE5-I) such as a tadalafil could be used as well to control LUTS caused by BPH [5]. Medical therapy is indicated for patients with moderate LUTS with no absolute surgical indications [6]. When medical control of symptoms fails, and/or complications occur, a surgical procedure can be attempted. Transurethral resection of the prostate (TURP), initially described in 1932, has long been considered the unopposed gold standard for interventional BPH treatment of smaller (60–80 cm^3) prostates and open prostatectomy is typically performed on patients for larger prostates. However, novel minimally invasive techniques (MIT) have been introduced in recent years with the aim of reducing complications, costs, and length of stay, while equaling or bettering the functional outcomes of conventional TURP [7].

R.V. O'Donova, M.D.
Urology Department, University of Montreal Hospital Center (CHUM), Laval, QC, Canada
e-mail: valdivieso.roger@gmail.com

P.-A. Hueber, M.D., Ph.D.
Section of Urology, Department of Surgery, Centre Hospitalier de l'Université de Montréal, CHUM, Montreal, QC, Canada
e-mail: pahueber@gmail.com

N. Bhojani, M.D., FRCSC
Urology Department, School of Medicine, University of Montreal, Montreal, QC, Canada
e-mail: naeem.bhojani@gmail.com

Q.-D. Trinh, M.D.
Surgery Department, Brigham and Women's Hospital, Boston, MA, USA
e-mail: trinh.qd@gmail.com

K.C. Zorn, M.D. (✉)
Robotic Surgery, Section of Urology, University of Montreal Health Center (CHUM), 235, boul. René-Levesque Est, suite 301, Montreal, QC H2X 1N8, Canada
e-mail: kevin.zorn@gmail.com

B. Chughtai et al. (eds.), *Treatment of Benign Prostatic Hyperplasia: Modern Alternative to Transurethral Resection of the Prostate*, DOI 10.1007/978-1-4939-1587-3_20,

The most common minimally invasive techniques are intraprostatic stents, transurethral needle ablation, transurethral microwave therapy, and laser vaporization. However, none of these minimally invasive techniques have been shown to be superior to TURP from a cost-versus-benefit standpoint. As such, TURP remains the standard treatment for BPH [8].

Embolization of iliac arterial branches has been successfully used to manage severe prostatic hemorrhage secondary to prostate cancer or BPH for over 30 years [9–12]. The first published case in which it was recognized that prostatic arterial embolization (PAE) could have a therapeutic effect on BPH was in 2000 by DeMeritt et al. [11]. PAE has only recently started to be used for primary control of LUTS related to BPH after feasibility and safety from trials in dogs and pigs were established [13–15]. The first intentional treatment of BPH with PAE in humans was done by Carnevale et al. in June 2008 and published in 2010. They performed PAE for patients with acute urinary retention (AUR) due to BPH who were waiting for surgery. Since the first PAE, different authors have published their initial results with PAE to assess the efficacy, durability, and adverse event rates of PAE in symptomatic patients.

Prostatic Anatomy and Vascular Supply

Prostate Zonal Anatomy

The contemporary description of the prostate anatomy is based on the work of McNeal in 1981 that defined four basic anatomic regions upon the analysis of 500 prostate specimens [16]. Each zone harbors specific embryologic and histologic features and are anatomically defined according to their spatial relationship to the prostatic urethra.

The prostatic urethra serves as a reference point and runs through the entire length of the prostate slightly closer to its anterior surface. A urethral crest projects inward from the posterior midline with prostatic sinuses on each side that drained the glandular periurethral ducts [17].

At the level of its midportion, the urethra bends forward to form an anterior angle of approximately 30° (varying from 0 to 90), which divides the prostatic urethra into a proximal (preprostatic) and a distal (prostatic) segment [17].

In the proximal segment, circular smooth muscles are thickened to form the involuntary internal urethral (preprostatic) sphincter [17]. At the angle of the urethra the ducts of the transition zone connect passing beneath the preprostatic sphincter to travel on its lateral and posterior side [17]. Duct development is limited in this region possibly because of their intimate relationship with the smooth muscle sphincter. Just distal to this angulation the urethral crest widens and protrudes from the posterior wall to form the verumontanum. At the apex of the verumontanum the utricle, a 6 mm müllerian vestigial remnant can be found flanked on each side of its orifice by the two small openings of the ejaculatory ducts. Around the openings of the ejaculatory ducts arise circumferentially the ducts of the central zone [17].

Hence, the prostate has been divided into four zones according to the location of their ducts in the urethra, their histology, and their embryologic origin. This zonal anatomy is also consistent with the type of pathologic lesion that they develop [16–18]. These four zones are:

1. The central zone (CZ)
2. The transition zone (TZ)
3. The peripheral zone (PZ)
4. The anterior fibromuscular stroma

The Central Zone (CZ)

The CZ represents 25 % of the glandular prostate. Its ducts arise close to the ejaculatory duct orifices and follow these ducts proximally, branching laterally near the prostate base. Its lateral border fuses with the proximal peripheral zone border, completing in continuity with the peripheral zone, a full disc of secretory tissue oriented in a coronal plane. Marked histologic differences between central and peripheral zones suggest important biologic differences [16, 18, 19].

The Transition Zone (TZ)

From endodermal origin (urogenital sinus) this zone surrounds the prostatic urethra proximal to the verumontanum. Normally, the transition zone accounts for 5–10 % of the glandular tissue of the prostate and includes two lateral lobes on either side [16, 18, 19]. A median lobe can also develop located between the two ejaculatory ducts and the urethra. As age increases, the transition zone can become enlarged giving rise to benign prostatic hypertrophy (BPH) and commonly causing bladder outlet obstruction.

In addition approximately 20 % of adenocarcinomas of the prostate originate in this zone [18]. Cancers in the transition zone show clinical features that are different from those shown by cancers in the peripheral zone. Patients with transition zone cancers have higher mean prostate-specific antigen levels and higher tumor volume than patients with peripheral zone cancers [20, 21]. However they tend to have lower Gleason scores and a more favorable prognosis [21].

The Peripheral Zone (PZ)

The peripheral zone is of mesodermal (Wolffian duct) origin and constitutes the bulk (over 70 %) of the prostate gland. It encloses and covers the posterior and lateral aspect of the gland. Posteriorly, the peripheral zone lies against the rectum and is the region palpable by digital rectal examination (DRE). Its ducts radiate laterally from the urethra distal to the verumontanum. The majority (70 %) of prostatic adenocarcinoma arises in this zone [18]. In addition this zone is the region most commonly affected by chronic prostatitis [22].

The Anterior Fibromuscular Stroma (AFMS)

The AFMS forms a thick, nonglandular shield that extends from the bladder neck to the striated sphincter and covers the entire anterior surface of the prostate. This stroma is composed of smooth and striated muscles cells that secrete collagen and elastin fibers. The inner layer is fused with the underlying anterior portion of the gland and can be replaced by glandular tissue in adenomatous enlargement of the prostate. Its external surface is in continuity with the prostatic capsule, the anterior visceral fascia, and the anterior portion of the preprostatic sphincter [16].

Vascular Supply of the Prostate

Precise knowledge of prostate vascular supply is sine qua non of selective prostatic artery embolization (PAE) procedure.

At the beginning of the century, the unequivocal existence of a specific prostate artery was subject of debate in the literature [23]. Since then, original works from cadaveric studies and in patients using angiography imaging have confirmed and well established the presence of the prostate arteries [23, 24]. Nevertheless, to this day, lack of a strict nomenclature for prostate vascularization persists and may be explained both by its anatomical variations and the various terminologies used historically in the literature to describe prostatic vessels [23, 24].

According to cadaveric studies described by Clegg in 1955, the PA is a well-defined trunk with variable origins but a rather constant course [23]. Hence the PA passes obliquely downward, forward, and medially along the anteroinferior surface of the bladder toward the prostate. At the junction of the bladder and the prostate PA typically divides into two equal size prostatic pedicles:

1. The prostate-vesical group or anterolateral pedicle that supplies the bladder neck and the periurethral portion of the gland
2. The capsular group or posterolateral pedicle that supplies the caudal and the peripheric portion of the gland

PAs are relatively small-sized diameters arteries varying between 1 and 2 mm that can have a common or separate origin. In addition, considerable tortuosity and anastomoses exist between the two groups [24].

The Anterolateral PA Pedicle

These arteries branch off perpendicularly to the urethra at the prostato-vesical junction and then travel in a caudal direction parallel to the urethra in the anterolateral quadrants typically at the 11 o'clock (on the right side) and the 1 o'clock (on the left side) positions, respectively [23, 24].

By supplying the transition zone including the periurethral portion this group of urethral arteries represents the main blood supply of the adenomatous portion of the gland that is enlarged in benign prostatic hyperplasia (BPH). Bouissou and Talazac who compared the cadaveric prostate vascularization in 100 pelvic halves comparing normal BPH and prostate cancer gland observed that this pedicle was frequently more developed in patients with BPH [25]. Hence, in patients with BPH treated with PAE embolization, this anterolateral prostatic pedicle is generally the preferred artery to be embolized [24]. Not surprisingly, these vessels are also frequently encountered during transurethral resection of the prostate during which they potentially can be the source of significant bleeding [26].

The Posterolateral PA Pedicle

The second main branch of the PA gives rise to the capsular arteries. This group of arteries travels posterolaterally to the prostate usually at the 7 o'clock (on the right side) and the 5 o'clock (on the left side) positions and then penetrates the prostate perpendicularly supplying the peripheral glandular portion of the prostate. These capsular vessels including arteries and veins provide the scaffolding for the cavernous nerve forming together the neurovascular bundle [23, 24].

The posterolateral prostatic pedicle vascularizes most of the peripheral and caudal gland. In PAE for BPH treatment, this artery is only embolized when access into the anterolateral prostatic pedicle is unsuccessful. Sometimes the anterolateral prostatic pedicle can be a difficult artery to catheterize because of its tortuous trajectory and its tight angulations when it arises from the superior vesical artery. In addition, the presence of atherosclerotic changes close to the ostium of the superior vesical artery can make selective catheterization even more difficult. In these cases it can be sometimes possible to perform retrograde embolization of the other pedicle through intraprostatic interpedicular anastomoses [24].

Anatomic Variations

As previously mentioned variations in this region are not uncommon. First the site of origin of the PA is quite variable and has been described with different frequency of distribution. In a study by Ambrosio and colleagues on cadaveric specimens, the most common origin of the prostate artery was described from the inferior vesical artery in 41.5 %, internal pudendal 26.4 %, and from the umbilical artery in 15.1 % of the case [27]. It can also come from obturator (5.7 %), inferior gluteal (1.9 %), and internal iliac (9.4 %) arteries [27]. In contrast, in the most recent report by Bilhim et al. using computed tomography angiography, PAs most frequently arise from the internal pudendal artery (35 %), from a common origin with the superior vesical artery (20 %), from the common anterior gluteal-pudendal trunk (15 %), from the obturator artery (10 %), or from the common prostato-rectal trunk (10 %) [24]. Other possible but rare origins included from the inferior gluteal artery, superior gluteal artery, or from an accessory pudendal artery (10 %) [24]. In the same study, they have confirmed that two prostatic pedicles may arise from the same artery in patients with only 1 PA (found in 60 % of pelvic sides), or may arise independently in patients with two independent PAs (found in 40 % of pelvic sides) [24].

In the presence of two separate prostatic vascular pedicles, there is one anterolateral prostatic pedicle with a superior or proximal origin usually from the common anterior gluteal-pudendal trunk close to or with a common origin with the superior vesical artery. When there is a common arterial trunk with the vesical and the anterolateral PAs, it is advisable to advance the microcatheter tip distally to the vesical arteries [24].

The posterolateral prostatic pedicle has an inferior or distal origin generally from the internal pudendal or obturator artery above the sciatic notch. At this location it can have a close relationship with the rectal or anal branches. It is not uncommon to find a common trunk between the posterolateral vessels and the middle rectal artery that has to be avoided during catheterization [24].

When only 1 PA is present, it usually arises independently from the vesical arteries (from the internal pudendal, obturator, or common anterior gluteal-pudendal trunk) and after a variable length it bifurcates into the anterolateral and posterolateral prostatic pedicles. In these cases, embolization of both prostatic pedicles can be performed with the tip of the catheter before the PA bifurcation [24].

PA Imaging

As previously mentioned, PAs are relatively small vessels with frequent variations and thus can be sometimes difficult to identify. Hence visualization of prostatic arteries using pre-procedural imaging is advised in order to plan a successful intervention and to prevent complications resulting from untargeted embolization of the adjacent organs such as the bladder, rectum, and penis. According to Bilhim et al., preoperative computed tomography angiography (CTA) can depict the pelvic arterial anatomy with excellent correlation with digital subtraction arteriography (DSA) findings per procedure and therefore be used to guide PAE [24, 28].

Patient Selection

Pre-procedural clinical evaluation and patient selection for prostatic arterial embolization (PAE) are paramount to improve technical and clinical results. For this reason rigorous inclusion and exclusion criteria are applied. These criteria may vary from one group performing the procedure to the other. Here we describe the main criteria used by the leading groups performing PAE [20, 29–31].

Patient Evaluation

Initially, the urologist performs a clinical evaluation to determine the nature and severity of the disease. The evaluation includes the assessment of symptoms using validated questionnaires such as the International Prostate Symptom Score (IPSS) and quality of life (QoL) to determine their severity. At this stage a digital rectal examination (DRE) is performed in order to estimate prostate volume and detect concomitant cancer. In patients with larger prostates, a transrectal ultrasound (TRUS) is also performed to evaluate prostate volume more accurately. Prostate-specific antigen (PSA) is also assessed to detect the probability of disease progression (high risk patients) and of prostatic cancer, guiding the eventual need for prostatic biopsy if PSA > 4 ng/ mL.

Uroflow studies are also performed before and after PAE to examine maximum flow rate (Q_{max}) and post-void residual volume (PVR). If the Q_{max} is very low (<6–8 mL/s), a urethral stricture is to be excluded performing a urethrocystoscopy. Carnevale et al. [30] include a transrectal or suprapubic ultrasound and a pelvic MRI to establish a documented baseline for each patient. They also include a urodynamic evaluation despite its invasive nature in order to exclude patients that experience infravesical obstruction associated with other bladder disorders and detrusor hypocontractility.

Finally, if the patient is considered for PAE, a computed tomographic angiography (CTA) is performed to study the patient's pelvic arterial anatomy. In addition, an MRI and/or a transrectal/suprapubic ultrasound may also be performed to establish a baseline prostatic volume.

Inclusion Criteria

Perreiral et al. [29] suggest to include male patients aged > 40 years, with a prostate volume >30 cm^3 and diagnosis of BPH with moderate to severe LUTS (IPSS > 18 and/or QoL > 3) refractory to medical treatment for at least 6 months. Some authors also include patients that are intolerant to medical modalities of treatment [30]. Patients that are in acute urinary retention refractory to medical therapy are also considered. Carnevale et al. prefer to use a different threshold for LUTS severity (IPSS ≥ 8) for consideration of PAE.

Exclusion Criteria

The exclusion criteria include: malignancy (based on pre-embolization, DRE, and TRUS examination and PSA measurements with positive biopsy), large bladder diverticula, large bladder stones, bladder atonia, neurogenic bladder, urethral stricture, bladder neck contracture, chronic renal failure, tortuosity and advanced atherosclerosis of iliac or prostatic arteries on pre-procedural CTA, active urinary tract infection, and unregulated coagulation parameters. Patients with a smaller prostate (i.e., volume <30 cm^3) were also excluded because PAE is believed to work based on prostate volume reduction, which will be more limited in patients with almost normal-sized prostates. Keeping these criteria in mind, Perreira et al. have observed that only a third of patients seen initially on consultation meet the criteria to be selected for PAE [29] (Table 20.1).

Table 20.1 Inclusion and exclusion criteria for prostatic arterial embolization (PAE)

Inclusion criteria
1. Age > 40 years
2. Prostate volume > 30 cm3
3. Diagnosis of BPH
Refractory to medical therapy
>6 months of therapy
4. Moderate to severe LUTS
IPSS >18 and/or QoL > 3
5. Acute urinary retention
Exclusion criteria
1. Malignancy (prostate or bladder)
2. Bladder anomalies
Large diverticula
Large stones
Neurogenic bladder
Bladder neck contractures
Bladder atonia
3. Chronic renal failure
4. Active urinary infection
5. Unregulated coagulation parameters
6. Tortuosity and advanced atherosclerosis of:
Iliac arteries
Prostatic arteries

BPH benign prostatic hyperplasia, *LUTS* lower urinary tract symptoms, *IPSS* International Prostate Symptom Score, *QoL* quality of life

Embolization Technique

The technique requires a well-trained interventional radiologist beyond the learning curve because of the complexity of the vascular anatomy of the prostate as well as the possible complications that could arise in more difficult cases. It is very important to properly identify the vasculature of the prostate and the variants that may occur amongst patients. The technique may vary from one group to the other. Here we present the so far published PAE techniques [20, 30, 31].

Preparation

The intervention is done under local anesthesia and on an outpatient basis in the interventional radiology suite after the patient has signed the informed consent. A fluoroquinolone PO is usually administered prior the procedure as antibioprophylaxis. The antibiotic may be continued 7–10 days post-procedure depending on the authors. Non-opioid analgesia is provided as well as nonsteroidal anti-inflammatory medications before and after PAE.

A Foley catheter is inserted prior the procedure and the balloon is inflated with a mixture solution of iodine contrast and normal saline. This helps provide good orientation to the prostate site and related pelvic structure during the procedure [30].

Identification and Catheterization of Prostatic Arteries

Embolization is performed via either unilateral femoral approach; thus, femoral pulses should be examined before in order to choose the best puncture site. The angiography is started by introducing the catheter via the right common femoral artery to catheterize the left (or right) internal iliac artery. Then using a pump injection (20 mL; 10 mL/s) the iliac vessels and the prostatic arteries are identified and evaluated. To better assess the blood supply to the prostate, a 5-French vertebral catheter (12 mL; 4 mL/s) is advanced at the common internal iliac trunk and a selective digital subtraction arteriogram (DSA) of the internal iliac artery is performed using the ipsilateral oblique projection (35°) and caudal-cranial angulation (10°) for better visualization. This way omission of any artery arising from the anterior and posterior division of the iliac is avoided.

Carnevale et al. prefer to use the 25–55° ipsilateral oblique view as well as a caudal view (10–20°) to better identify the inferior vesical artery (IVA) and all possible accessory branches to the prostate. These views combined with the Foley's balloon filled with contrast help better understand the anatomy and all the branches that irrigate the prostatic gland. Under this ipsilateral oblique perspective, catheterization of the IVA is performed with a small (<2.3 Fr) hydrophilic microcatheter and 2–3 mL of contrast are injected manually. At this point the posterior-anterior view is used as it helps to identify some contralateral prostate lobe branches, and the parenchymal phase. The microcatheter is then introduced deeper into the IVA at the ostium of the prostatic arteries and embolization is performed under direct visualization.

Embolization

Numerous embolic agents can be used for embolization of prostatic arteries. Carnevale et al. prefer to use 100–300 and 300–500 μm microspheres (Embosphere®). A recent randomized prospective study by Bilhim et al. [17] showed that the use of 200 μm microspheres was associated with a greater prostate volume reduction; however, clinical outcomes were improved with smaller microspheres (100 μm). The embolization material (2 mL) is mixed in a 20 mL 50–50 saline/contrast solution adding up to 22 mL. Pisco et al. [32] use an 80 mL solution of 1 mL polyvinyl alcohol (PVA) particles and 50–50 contrast saline solution. This solution is injected slowly under direct fluoroscopy. It is estimated that embolization requires 10–15 min to reach end point. Some authors would change the particle size per procedure depending on the level of pain experienced by the patient to avoid untargeted embolization [32]. After 3–5 min of having injected the embolization product, a flush of normal saline should be injected to pack the microspheres inside the prostate. If continued forward flow is observed, more embolic agent may be injected. The end point is considered to be total stasis in the prostatic vessels with interruption of blood flow and prostatic gland opacification. In general a single syringe of 2 mL of microspheres is sufficient for bilateral PAE. After end point is reached, the microcatheter is retired to the origin of the IVA and a manual injection of contrast is performed for final control and to look for additional prostatic branches. Embolization is later performed on the contralateral side using the same technique.

Post-Procedure Management

Patients are to remain 4–6 h without moving the punctured leg to avoid bleeding complications. If a vascular closure device is used, resting time can be reduced. The Foley catheter is left in place to help voiding without straining which helps to reduce the risks of puncture site complications. The catheter is removed 2–4 h post-procedure if the patient is not in acute urinary retention (AUR) and then the patient is discharged. If patients with AUR had chronic use of indwelling catheter, they are asked to come back in 1 week and trials are attempted in 1-week intervals. A clinical failure is determined if the patient cannot spontaneously void in 1 month.

The most common symptom after the procedure is dysuria and frequent urination could last for 3–5 days. Patients are asked to stop prostatic medications just after PAE. All patients are seen in outpatient consult one month after the procedure.

Technical and Clinical Success

Technical success is achieved when main bilateral prostatic arteries are embolized and much prostatic ischemia is achieved. The main purpose of PAE is to achieve prostatic ischemia as it has been established that better long-term clinical and urodynamic results are correlated with prostate ischemia [30]. Clinical success is defined as either the removal of the Foley catheter in patients with AUR, improvement of symptoms as seen in an improvement of IPSS and QoL questionnaires and no sexual disorders or major adverse events after the procedure.

Published Outcomes

Table 20.2.
Table 20.3.

Complications

Similar to other visceral embolization procedures PAE is associated with common symptoms such as nausea, vomiting, and fever in the absence of infection. Other more specific symptoms are urethral burning, periprostatic or pelvic pain, and small amounts of blood mixed with stool and urine referred by Carnevale et al. as the "post-PAE syndrome" [30]. This collection of symptoms is believed to be the result of the migration of polyvinyl alcohol (PVA) particles through the anastomosis between the prostatic and the neighboring arteries [33]. This syndrome is usually self-limiting and requires no intervention. Pisco et al. [20] reported in their latest prospective study of 250 patients the following adverse events: urinary tract infections requiring antibiotics (7.6 %), transient hematuria (5.6 %), transient hematospermia (0.4 %), balanoprostatitis (1.6 %), and inguinal hematoma (7 %). Six patients (0.02 %) that underwent PAE had acute urinary retention and a temporary bladder catheter had to be placed for a couple of hours. One major complication was reported. One patient developed bladder wall ischemia resulting surgical management to remove the necrotic tissue. This was secondary to untargeted embolization of the bladder. They believe that this complication was due to a proximal and aggressive embolization of both prostatic and vesical arteries. In a prospective study of 11 patients with urinary retention due to BPH, Antunes et al. reported no major complications after PAE [31]. However, they observed that nine patients reported mild and transitory pain, three patients presented minimal rectal bleeding, and two had diarrhea lasting 24 h. One patient had a single episode of hematuria. No groups have reported sexual dysfunction as a complication post PAE.

Discussion

PAE technique has emerged as an interesting approach in the quest for a nonsurgical alternative to standard BPH treatment for patients that do not respond to medical treatment and are not well suited for surgery or minimally invasive intervention. Nevertheless, the research in this field remains preliminary. The paucity of data precludes its candidacy to FDA approval or mention in any current professional practice guidelines such as AUA or EAU guidelines.

So far, only three groups worldwide have reported on the usage of PAE for BPH treatment reflecting the very limited use of this technique.

Table 20.2 Published PAE studies

Author	Year	Type	Material (μm)	Number of subjects	AUR (%)	Age (mean)	Mean follow-up (months)	Time of embolization mean (min)	Technical success (%)	Clinical success (%)
Rio Tinto et al.[36]	2012	Retrospective	100–200 PVA, non-spherical	103	15	66.8	N/A	83	97	89
Antunes et al. [31]	2013	Prospective	300–500, microspheres	11	100	68.5	N/A	197	100	91
Pisco et al. [20]	2013	Prospective	200, PVA non-spherical	255	13	65.5	10	73	98	72

PVA polyvinyl alcohol, *AUR* acute urinary retention

Table 20.3 Published follow-up outcomes

Author	IPSS						QoL						Prostate volume (mL)						Qmax (mL/s)					
	0	1	3	6	12	24	0	1	3	6	12	24	0	1	3	6	12	24	0	1	3	6	12	24
Rio Tinto et al.[36]	22.8	11.7	10.3	10.8	11.2	9.3	4.1	2.3	2.0	2.0	2.0	2.0	88	68.7	67	67.8	68	76	8.7	11.6	12.7	12.6	12.9	14.4
Antunes et al. [31]	N/A	7.1	N/A	N/A	2.8	N/A	N/A	N/A	N/A	N/A	N/A	N/A	69.7	N/A	N/A	N/A	N/A	N/A	0	11.9	N/A	N/A	N/A	N/A
Pisco et al. [20]	24	12.2	11	11.5	10.4	9	4.4	2.5	2.2	2.3	2.0	1.8	83.5	66.8	68.3	66.6	69.9	72	9.2	11.9	12.4	12	12.8	13.9

IPSS International Prostate Symptom Score, *QOL* quality of life, *Qmax* maximal urinary flow rate

BPH treatment with PAE requires a well-trained interventional radiologist. Prostatic vascularization is complex and highly variable demanding very precise knowledge of prostate vascular supply.

Most of the clinical data on the techniques comes from three cohorts (the largest including 255 patients) treated by Pisco and Bilhim et al. in Lisbon (Portugal) [20]. Other small cohorts have been reported including 11 patients described by Carnevale et al. in Sao Paulo (Brazil) [31] and another cohort of 15 patients reported by Bagla et al. in Alexandria VA in the USA [34].

In terms of safety, PAE is associated with low morbidity and no irritative urinary symptoms or ejaculatory dysfunction. A post-PAE syndrome has been defined with symptoms consisting of nausea, vomiting, fever in the absence of infection and pelvic pain that lasts 2–3 days post-PAE.

In the vast majority of cases, only minor complications such as UTI, transient hematuria, hematospermia, and inguinal hematomas have been reported [32]. However, the risk of complications secondary to off-target embolization to adjacent organs is present and can potentially be serious. For example, at least one patient had bladder wall ischemia that required surgical management [32]. Similarly one case report described ischemic rectitis resulting from rectal nontarget embolization [35]. Understandably the use of pre-procedural computed tomographic angiography is key both to plan successful intervention and limit the potential for serious complications.

Overall, short-term outcomes at 12 months showed approximately a 50 % decrease in IPSS from a mean score of 23–24 to a mean of 10.4–11.2. This improvement in IPSS was associated with mean Qmax increases of about 50 % while two points of QoL improvements were observed from 4 to 2. Globally these results suggest that PAE may be more effective than medical therapy but most likely inferior to most minimally invasive procedures including TUMT or TUNA. Similar results were observed at 24 months although only three studies reported midterm data for a total of 33 patients. To date there is no long-term data available aside from a report on two patients at 4 years. Interestingly MRI imaging in these patients suggests signs of de novo prostate growth raising concern on the long-term efficacy of PAE [31].

Finally, there has been no trial comparing PAE with TURP or any other BPH procedures. It is worth mentioning that one clinical trial is currently recruiting patients in the USA, Brazil, and France aiming to compare PAE with TURP (NCT01789840).

Thus, despite interesting preliminary results, if PAE wants to compete with the multitude of minimally invasive procedures currently available, it still has to prove equivalency or less adverse effects in head-to-head comparison trials. Whether PAE may be considered for patients that are not candidates for minimally invasive procedures remains to be demonstrated. It is important to note that most of the patients included in PAE studies were also eligible for standard BPH treatment such as TURP. For example, in one study out of the 296 patients eligible for PAE, 108 patients chose PAE while 159 patients opted for TURP and 36 for laser therapy [32].

It is worth mentioning that in general about 10 % of patients eligible for PAE are excluded because of advanced atherosclerotic disease and tortuosity of the iliac and prostatic arteries based on pre-procedure imaging. In addition, the procedure can often not be completed in another 3–5 % of patients for the same reason [32].

This proportion represents 10–15 % of patients in which PAE is not technically possible in a population of standard patients eligible for all procedures. However, this proportion is likely significantly higher in a population of patients not suited for surgery that is typically older with a higher prevalence of significant atherosclerotic disease. This adds another potential limitation of PAE use in candidates unfit for minimally invasive procedures.

In conclusion, PAE is an emerging experimental technique. Although comparative studies are lacking, preliminary results suggest short-term outcomes better than medical therapy but likely inferior to minimally invasive therapy. Long-term outcomes remain unknown. Therefore, with the current body of literature, PAE cannot be recommended for BPH management even as a treatment for patients refractory to medical therapy but not eligible for minimally invasive procedures. Upcoming results of trials comparing PAE with TURP will be interesting in order to determine whether PAE is intended to stay or not.

References

1. Andersson KE, et al. Tadalafil for the treatment of lower urinary tract symptoms secondary to benign prostatic hyperplasia: pathophysiology and mechanism(s) of action. Neurourol Urodyn. 2011; 30(3):292–301.
2. McVary KT. BPH: epidemiology and comorbidities. Am J Manag Care. 2006;12(5 Suppl):S122–8.
3. Madersbacher S, et al. EAU 2004 guidelines on assessment, therapy and follow-up of men with lower urinary tract symptoms suggestive of benign prostatic obstruction (BPH guidelines). Eur Urol. 2004; 46(5):547–54.
4. McVary KT, et al. Update on AUA guideline on the management of benign prostatic hyperplasia. J Urol. 2011;185(5):1793–803.
5. Oelke M, et al. Monotherapy with tadalafil or tamsulosin similarly improved lower urinary tract symptoms suggestive of benign prostatic hyperplasia in an international, randomised, parallel, placebo-controlled clinical trial. Eur Urol. 2012;61(5):917–25.
6. Burnett AL, Wein AJ. Benign prostatic hyperplasia in primary care: what you need to know. J Urol. 2006;175(3 Pt 2):S19–24.
7. Baazeem A, Elhilali MM. Surgical management of benign prostatic hyperplasia: current evidence. Nat Clin Pract Urol. 2008;5(10):540–9.
8. Varkarakis J, Bartsch G, Horninger W. Long-term morbidity and mortality of transurethral prostatectomy: a 10-year follow-up. Prostate. 2004;58(3): 248–51.
9. Mitchell ME, et al. Control of massive prostatic bleeding with angiographic techniques. J Urol. 1976;115(6):692–5.
10. Bischoff W, Goerttler U. Successful intra-arterial embolization of bleeding carcinoma of the prostate (author's transl). Urologe A. 1977;16(2):99–102.
11. DeMeritt JS, et al. Relief of benign prostatic hyperplasia-related bladder outlet obstruction after transarterial polyvinyl alcohol prostate embolization. J Vasc Interv Radiol. 2000;11(6):767–70.
12. Barbieri A, et al. Massive hematuria after transurethral resection of the prostate: management by intra-arterial embolization. Urol Int. 2002;69(4):318–20.
13. Jeon GS, et al. The effect of transarterial prostate embolization in hormone-induced benign prostatic hyperplasia in dogs: a pilot study. J Vasc Interv Radiol. 2009;20(3):384–90.
14. Sun F, et al. Transarterial prostatic embolization: initial experience in a canine model. AJR Am J Roentgenol. 2011;197(2):495–501.
15. Sun F, et al. Benign prostatic hyperplasia: transcatheter arterial embolization as potential treatment–preliminary study in pigs. Radiology. 2008;246(3): 783–9.
16. Bilhim T, et al. Prostatic arterial supply: anatomic and imaging findings relevant for selective arterial embolization. J Vasc Interv Radiol. 2012;23(11): 1403–15.
17. Bilhim T, et al. Does polyvinyl alcohol particle size change the outcome of prostatic arterial embolization for benign prostatic hyperplasia? Results from a single-center randomized prospective study. J Vasc Interv Radiol. 2013;24:1595–602.
18. Pereira JA, et al. Radiologic anatomy of arteriogenic erectile dysfunction: a systematized approach. Acta Med Port. 2013;26(3):219–25.
19. Pisco JM, et al. Erratum to: Embolisation of prostatic arteries as treatment of moderate to severe lower urinary symptoms (LUTS) secondary to benign hyperplasia: results of short- and mid-term follow-up. Eur Radiol. 2013;23(9):2573–4.
20. Pisco JM, et al. Embolisation of prostatic arteries as treatment of moderate to severe lower urinary symptoms (LUTS) secondary to benign hyperplasia: results of short- and mid-term follow-up. Eur Radiol. 2013;23(9):2561–72.
21. Pais D, et al. Sciatic nerve high division: two different anatomical variants. Acta Med Port. 2013;26(3): 208–11.
22. Bilhim T, et al. Middle rectal artery: myth or reality? Retrospective study with CT angiography and digital subtraction angiography. Surg Radiol Anat. 2013; 35(6):517–22.
23. Bilhim T, et al. Unilateral versus bilateral prostatic arterial embolization for lower urinary tract symptoms in patients with prostate enlargement. Cardiovasc Intervent Radiol. 2013;36(2):403–11.
24. Bilhim T, et al. Radiological anatomy of prostatic arteries. Tech Vasc Interv Radiol. 2012;15(4): 276–85.
25. Bouissou H, Talazac A. Arterial vascularization of the normal and the pathological prostate. Ann Anat Pathol (Paris). 1959;4(1):63–79.
26. Flocks RH. The arterial distribution within the prostate gland; its role in transurethral prostatic resection. J Urol. 1937;37:524–48.
27. Ambrosio JD, De Almeida JS, De Souza A. Origin of prostatic arteries in man. Rev Paul Med. 1980; 96(3–4):52–5.
28. Bilhim T, et al. Prostatic arterial supply: demonstration by multirow detector angio CT and catheter angiography. Eur Radiol. 2011;21(5): 1119–26.
29. Pereira JA, et al. Patient selection and counseling before prostatic arterial embolization. Tech Vasc Interv Radiol. 2012;15(4):270–5.
30. Carnevale FC, Antunes AA. Prostatic artery embolization for enlarged prostates due to benign prostatic hyperplasia. How i do it. Cardiovasc Intervent Radiol. 2013;36:1452–63.

31. Antunes AA, et al. Clinical, laboratorial, and urodynamic findings of prostatic artery embolization for the treatment of urinary retention related to benign prostatic hyperplasia. A prospective single-center pilot study. Cardiovasc Intervent Radiol. 2013;36(4):978–86.
32. Pisco J, et al. Prostatic arterial embolization for benign prostatic hyperplasia: short- and intermediate-term results. Radiology. 2013;266(2):668–77.
33. Fernandes L, et al. Prostatic arterial embolization: post-procedural follow-up. Tech Vasc Interv Radiol. 2012;15(4):294–9.
34. Bagla S, et al. Utility of cone-beam CT imaging in prostatic artery embolization. J Vasc Interv Radiol. 2013;24:1603–7.
35. Moreira AM, et al. Transient Ischemic rectitis as a potential complication after prostatic artery embolization: case report and review of the literature. Cardiovasc Intervent Radiol. 2013;36(6):1690–4.
36. Rio Tinto H, et al. Prostatic artery embolization in the treatment of benign prostatic hyperplasia: short and medium follow-up. Tech Vasc Interv Radiol. 2012; 15(4):290–3.

Ethanol Injection of Prostate

21

Alexander C. Small and Michael A. Palese

Introduction

Here's to alcohol: the cause of, and answer to, all of life's problems.
Matt Groening, creator of The Simpsons

Lower urinary tract symptoms (LUTS) secondary to benign prostatic hyperplasia (BPH) are extremely common in older men. It is estimated that 50 % of men over 50 years old, 75 % over 70, and 90 % over 80 suffer from BPH. BPH can significantly affect quality of life and also cause complications like urinary tract infections and permanent renal damage. Over the past few decades, treatment of this condition has rapidly evolved from major surgery consisting of simple prostatectomy to a multipronged approach consisting of medical therapies and minimally invasive surgical techniques. One technique is ethanol injection into the prostate as a method for chemoablation.

A.C. Small, M.D.
Department of Urology, New York Presbyterian Hospital, Columbia University Medical Center, New York, NY, USA
e-mail: alexcsmall@gmail.com

M.A. Palese, M.D. (✉)
Urology Department, The Mount Sinai Medical Center, One Gustave L. Levy Place, Box 1272, New York, NY 10029, USA
e-mail: michael.palese@mountsinai.org

Injectable therapies for BPH are a particularly appealing strategy to treat BPH [1, 2]. Theoretically, these procedures are minimally invasive, can be performed quickly in the office, do not require anesthesia, and promise fewer side effects (Table 21.1). With the introduction of new strategies and the widespread use of alpha-adrenergic blockers, the use of transurethral resection of the prostate (TURP) has declined significantly since 2000 [1]. Simultaneously, there has been a shift toward minimally invasive and office-based procedures. While there was much excitement in the early 2000s surrounding prostatic ethanol injection, subsequent trials have not lived up to the initial promise. Experts now have varied opinions on this approach – some suggest chemoablation is still in its "renaissance," while others write that ethanol ablation has not survived the test of time [3, 4]. Overall, early studies showed promising results, but variable outcomes and lack of standard techniques have hindered the widespread adoption of ethanol ablation. In this chapter, we will review the techniques and evidence for this approach.

Historical Perspectives

In the early 1900s, surgeons first described several approaches to access the prostate for relief of obstruction and treatment of inflammatory conditions including early transperineal,

B. Chughtai et al. (eds.), *Treatment of Benign Prostatic Hyperplasia: Modern Alternative to Transurethral Resection of the Prostate*, DOI 10.1007/978-1-4939-1587-3_21,

Table 21.1 Advantages and disadvantages of ethanol injection of the prostate

	Advantages	Disadvantages
Candidates	Can be performed on high-risk patients who are not surgical candidates	Not ideal for very large glands
Procedure	Does not require general anesthesia	Usually requires catheterization post-op
	Fast operative time	
	Can be done outpatient	
Efficacy	Satisfactory short- and intermediate-term outcomes	High re-treatment rates (0–41 %)
Adverse effects	Uncommon post-op complications	Procedure can be painful
	Reduced sexual side effects compared to TURP	Rare risk of bladder necrosis

transrectal, and transurethral techniques [5]. British surgeon Sir James Roberts is credited for first using intraprostatic injection therapy to treat obstructive symptoms [6]. From 1909 to 1916, Sir Roberts served as the physician for the Viceroy of India, who suffered from lower urinary tract symptoms. Sir Roberts injected a mixture of carbolic acid, glacial acetic acid, glycerin, and distilled water transperineally into the prostate under digital guidance in an effort to alleviate his patient's obstructive symptoms. In the 1930s, two surgeons, Lower and Johnston, injected a variety of agents including alcohol into the prostates of dogs. While they showed significant size reduction, there was significant mortality of the animals [5].

In 1966, Talwar and Pande published the first systematic study of prostatic injection therapy. One hundred and eighty-eight patients with urinary retention underwent transperineal injection of carbolic acid, glacial acetic acid, and glycerin [7]. They described favorable results and several advantages of injection therapy over traditional open prostatectomy including high rates of symptom relief (78 % of patients alleviated of retention), reduced cost over major surgery, reduced mortality from the procedure, ability to operate on high risk candidates and ability to pursue more invasive options if injection fails [5]. Over the next 50 years, these initial principles guided subsequent studies of prostatic injection therapy.

Ethanol injection has simultaneously been adopted in other fields of medicine to treat a wide range of conditions including atrial fibrillation, esophageal varices, renal cysts, parathyroid adenomas, hepatocellular carcinomas, and other tumors [8]. Outcomes in these other diseases have been well studied and are generally favorable. The locally destructive properties of ethanol make it a potentially appealing tool for urologic surgeons.

Mechanisms of Action

Ethanol (in the 95–98 % anhydrous form) injected into prostatic parenchyma destroys tissue by several mechanisms to provide relief of LUTS. It immediately creates inflammation, endothelial cell dehydration, and protein denaturation. These changes lead to the formation of fibrous tissue, small vessel thrombosis, coagulation necrosis, lysis of intraprostatic nerves, and finally subsequent atrophy of prostatic tissue [9–11].

Animal models have demonstrated severe effects of ethanol injection. In the first study in 1988, Littrup et al. injected seven dog prostates with ethanol. Although 71 % ($n = 10$) showed the desired outcome of pathologic intraglandular hemorrhagic necrosis, extraprostatic leakage and unintentional organ damage were unacceptably common. Three subjects experienced external sphincter necrosis and four had periurethral tissue necrosis [12]. After this study, the need to minimize leakage of ethanol and maintain the prostatic capsule was clear. Subsequent animal models showed that injection therapy could be safe and efficient when the mechanism of delivery and dosage were controlled. Prostate volume reductions were achieved in all canines, but the lesion sizes were not consistent and dose–response relationships were not observed [13]. These models also demonstrated the importance of a superficial location of the injection to maximize cavity formation confluent with the urethra to maximize the lumen, compared to deep injections that resulted in subcapsular cavities [8].

Pathologic studies have highlighted several important considerations in the mechanisms of action of ethanol ablation. First, diffusion properties of ethanol vary depending on tissue type. Up to a third of injections result in significant intraprostatic diffusion and backflow along the needle tract, thereby creating highly variable lesions. Second, the degree of diffusion seems to correlate with intraglandular resistance suggesting differential flow into fibrous tissue versus excretory ducts. And third, the prostate capsule can act as a natural barrier to prevent injected substances from diffusing beyond the organ. Injection beyond this barrier can be devastating [14].

Techniques for Ethanol Injection

The safety and efficacy of prostatic ethanol injection in early case series and preclinical models led to human studies aiming to refine the techniques used for injection and further elucidate patient outcomes. The majority of these procedures have been performed outpatient under regional combined with local anesthesia or light general anesthesia via three main approaches [6].

The transperineal percutaneous approach first described by Roberts in 1909 and subsequently studied by Talwar and Pande in the 1960s remained the most popular form of prostatic injection through the end of the twentieth century. Preclinical models showed risk of extraprostatic tissue necrosis compared to the transurethral approach [10]. However in 2001 and 2003, an Italian and a Taiwanese group published their experiences with transperineal injection therapy using transrectal ultrasound (TRUS) guidance. Both studies were small, with 8 and 11 patients, respectively, but managed to show measurable improvements in symptom scores, post-void residual (PVR) volumes, and urinary flow rates at 6 months [15, 16]. In these cohorts, one patient experienced urinary retention requiring a TURP and one patient reported severe perineal pain and urge incontinence. This approach has the advantage of continuous visualization with TRUS during the procedure for needle localization, but the downside is possible backflow into the perineum.

The transurethral ethanol ablation of the prostate (TEAP) has become the predominant mechanism for injection therapy. Available access, technological improvements, and urologist comfort with cystoscopy have allowed for the most development using this approach. While there are several historical case series for transurethral injections, the modern feasibility trials of ethanol ablation were done in 1999 and 2002. These trials were conducted in Japan and the United States and had 10 and 13 patients, respectively [17, 18]. Both studies demonstrated measurable improvements in American Urological Association (AUA) symptom score and maximum urinary flow rate (Qmax), but Goya et al. were unable to show any decrease in gland volume.

Curved needle devices for TEAP were also introduced in the early 2000s by Ditrolio et al. (InjectTx device, InjectTx Inc., San Jose, California) and Plante et al. (original called the OPAL probe, ProSurg, Santa Barbara, California and later known as the ProstaJect system, American Medical Systems, Minneapolis, MN, USA) [18, 19]. The ProstaJect system was submitted to the FDA (investigational new drug IND 61337) in March 2002. These devices helped visualize the injection sites and measure advancement of the needle. Using these devices for TEAP, injections are placed at the 3 o'clock and 9 o'clock positions, with a variable third injection used for larger prostates (however some studies use up to eight injections). The dose of ethanol ranges from 5 to 26 mL and is often calculated based on the TRUS-measured prostate volume (15–40 % in studies). To overcome the limitations of uneven prostate diffusion, King et al. investigated a novel microporous hollow fiber catheter (MiHFC) (Twin Star Medical, Minneapolis, MN, USA) to inject ethanol into the prostate in an animal model. The new device increases the surface area compared to a traditional hollow bore needle to create flow into the interstitial space of the gland. They compared the MiHFC device to standard needles by injecting the prostates of individual dogs with both each instrument on opposite sides of the prostate. The lesions created with the MiHFC compared to the control needle were more uniform and significantly larger (0.83 +/− 0.31 cm^3 vs. 0.52 +/− 0.21 cm^3, $p=0.03$) [20].

Finally, transrectal ultrasound-guided ethanol injections were only recently studied. The potential advantages of this approach are that it minimizes urethral mucosal injury and hematuria due to multipoint punctures and alcohol spillage. There is a theoretical risk of urethrorectal fistula formation. Although there are no reported instances of this occurring, this complication has been observed in the microwave therapy literature [5]. In a trial from Li et al., the transrectal approach was shown to be safe and effective in 70 patients [11].

Major Clinical Studies of Ethanol Injection

The early clinical trials of ethanol injection showed promising results (Table 21.2). In 2004, Goya et al. in Japan recruited 34 patients for transurethral ethanol ablation and followed them for a median of 4.3 years [21]. The patients' mean age was 68 years and prostate volume was 49 mL. Patients were injected with 3–14 mL of ethanol in 2–10 sites, based on surgeon's discretion. After the procedure, 31 patients were discharged on the same day and 3 patients were hospitalized. All patients had catheters left in place for an average of 7.6 days (range 3–22 days). Patients experienced no major complications and several minor adverse affects including epididymitis ($n=1$), chronic prostatitis ($n=1$), bleeding ($n=1$), and meatal stenosis ($n=2$). At 1, 2, and 3 years, patient had subjective improvements in International Prostate Symptom Scores [IPSS] (21.8 to 9.6, 10.4, and 13.1, all $p<0.01$) and quality of life scores [QoL] (5.0 to 2.3, 2.4, and 2.8, all $p<0.01$). They also showed measurable improvements in peak flow rate (8.3–13.6 mL/s, 15.2 mL/s, and 12.7 mL/s, all $p<0.01$). Average prostate volume decreased significantly at 1 year (49 mL to 46, $p<0.01$) but increased at 2 years (49 mL) and 3 years (51 mL). Most notably, re-treatment rates in this cohort were very high – 13 % at 1 year, 26 % at 2 years, and 41 % at 3 years.

In the same year, the results of a large European prospective trial were released [22]. Grise et al. studied 115 symptomatic patients over 50 years old with BPH who they injected transurethrally with the ProstaJect device and followed for 1 year. In this study, ethanol treatment dosages were based on prostate volume, prostate length, and median lobe involvement, with an average of 14 mL ethanol injected (range 4–26 mL). Catheters were removed in 98 % of patients 4 days

Table 21.2 Major clinical studies of ethanol injection therapy since 2004

Study	Location	Access	N	Max follow-up time	Outcomes (% change) 12 months (*or 6 months)		Key findings
					IPSS	Qmax	
Grise 2004	International	TU	115	12 mo	−50 %	+35 %	Two patients with bladder necrosis requiring surgery
Plante 2007	Vermont	TU	79	6 mo	−52 %	+101 %	No ethanol dose effect
Li 2014	China	TR	70	24 mo	−67 %	+226 %	No complications with low-dose ethanol; 0 % re-treatment rate
Larson 2006	Brazil + Chile	TU, TR, TP	65	12 mo	−44 %	+33 %	Alcohol gel had lower rates of side effects
El-Husseiny 2011	UK	TU	56	54 mo	−37 %	+91 %	23 % re-treatment rate
Arslan 2014	Turkey	TU	52	12 mo	−42 %	+52 %	13.8 % re-treatment rate
Sakr 2009	Egypt	TU	35	50 mo	−71 %	+220 %	25 % re-treatment rate
Goya 2004	Japan	TU	34	4.3 years (median)	−35 %	+63 %	41 % re-treatment rate
Mutaguchi 2006	Japan	TU	21	16 mo	n/a	n/a	Effective for men in retention

TU transurethral, *TR* transrectal, *TP* transperineal
*At 6 months

after the procedure. This study also showed improvements at 1 year in IPSS (20.6 to 10.3, $p<0.01$), QoL (4.4 to 2.1, $p<0.01$), maximum flow rate (9.9–13.4 mL/s, $p<0.01$), and prostate volume (−16 %). Only 7 % of patients required re-treatment with TURP within the year. The most common adverse effects were irritative symptoms (26 %), hematuria (16 %), incontinence (3 %), and retrograde ejaculation (3 %). Two patients experienced the severe complication of bladder necrosis, one requiring urinary diversion and the other requiring ureteral reimplantation. While this study was strong in its large number of patients and multiple center involvement, the study findings are limited by follow-up of only 1 year. Their most important finding, however, was the low but very real risk of bladder necrosis associated with TEAP.

Plante et al. published results of an American multicenter phase I/II trial of TEAP in 2007 [23]. Their study randomized 79 men with BPH three different doses of ethanol based on prostate volume (15 % of volume, 25 % or 40 %) to be injected transurethrally with the ProstaJect device. The prostate was injected under direct vision up to 2 cm maximum depth. Patients were followed for 6 months. The patients had an average age of 64 years (range 50–79) with a mean prostate volume of 45 g. They were injected with an average of 14.0 mL (range 4–20 mL) and following the procedure, 98 % of patients had their catheter removed after 3 days. Published results were stratified by the three ethanol doses— in all groups, patients showed improvements from the baseline, but there were no significant differences between the groups. All primary outcome measures showed improvement including IPSS (23 to ~11), QoL (4.4 to ~2.0), maximum urinary flow (8.3 mL/s to 11.5–16.7 mL/s), and post-void residual (103 mL to 79–98 mL). Adverse events were mild or moderate including hematuria (42.9 %), irritative voiding (40.3 %), pain/discomfort (25.6 %), and urinary retention (22.1 %), and they did not vary by dosage group. All procedures were performed outpatient in an operating room (55 %), surgery center (22 %), or office (23 %) under regional (71 %) or local anesthesia (29 %). This study was the most rigorous trial to date evaluating safety and potential efficacy of TEAP. The strengths included comparing three doses of ethanol injection, rigorously defining the protocols for therapy, and looking at a large cohort for a phase II trial. However, there was no control group, and the authors did not report overall efficacy rates making it difficult to compare this study to others. Their finding that higher doses of ethanol are no better than lower doses has important clinical implications.

In 2003, Badlani and Desai presented an abstract at the AUA Annual Meeting on a randomized trial comparing TEAP with TURP for bladder outlet obstruction; however, these results have never been formally published [24]. In this study, 60 men were assigned to three groups—superficial ethanol injection (0.5 cm), deep ethanol injection (1–2 cm), and TURP ($n=20$ in each group)—and were followed for 6 months. They found that TURP resulted in a significantly great reduction in ultrasound-measured prostate volume than TEAP. There were also significant reductions in IPSS, QoL, and Qmax in all groups from baseline to 6 months, but no significant differences between groups. TEAP was converted to TURP in 12.5 % of patients.

Several other international studies of TEAP were subsequently published, showing similar results. Mutaguchi et al. in Japan studied TEAP in 21 "high risk" men in urinary retention due to BPH ($n=16$) or prostate cancer ($n=5$). After injection with a mean volume of 10.6 mL ethanol (22 % of prostate volume) and placement of a catheter for a mean of 12.4 days, 81 % of the men were able to void spontaneously. None of this cohort required re-treatment at 16-month mean follow-up, and they experienced significant improvements in PVR and prostate volume. No urodynamics were recorded [25]. Larson et al. recruited 65 patients in Brazil and Chile to undergo transrectal ($n=8$), transurethral ($n=36$), or transperineal ($n=21$) injection with a novel alcohol gel in an attempt to minimize complications associated with backflow of liquid ethanol. At 1 year of follow-up, patients showed statistically significant improvements in IPSS, QoL, and Qmax, with no differences identified between the three approaches. There were no adverse effects associated with treatment, and only 6 % ($n=4$) required re-treatment with TURP [26]. Sakr et al. in Egypt prospectively studied a cohort of 35 men with BPH for 50 months and showed durable results of TEAP. They injected 6–12 mL in 5–10 sites of the prostate. They showed improvements in IPSS, Qmax, PVR, and prostate size that were durable after 4 years; however, a quarter of patients required re-treatment by the end of the study. None of this cohort experienced intraoperative complications, but all patients had postoperative urinary retention requiring catheter placement for a mean of 6.7 days. Other adverse events were rare, with acute epididymitis, chronic prostatitis, and urethral stricture occurring in one patient each [27]. El-Husseiny et al. studied a similar group of medically high risk patients in the UK. Over 2 years, 56 men with symptomatic BPH were recruited and followed for 54 months after TEAP. This group used the ProstaJect system to inject the prostate up to six locations. Again, there were significant improvements in IPSS, QoL, Qmax, and PVR. Also consistent with prior studies, 23 % of patients in this cohort required alternative treatment (with repeat TEAP, TURP, or stenting). The authors did not report adverse events. Of note, only 25 % (14 of the original 54) of patients followed for the full study with the others dropping out due to death from non-TEAP-related causes, illness precluding attendance, and noncompliance [28]. The conclusions of this particular study must be viewed with skepticism due to the poor retention rate and non-reporting of adverse events. Finally, Arslan et al. published their initial results using ethanol injection in Turkey in 2014. This group studied 52 patients with LUTS over 1 year following TEAP. IPSS, Qmax, and prostate volume seemed to improve; however, the authors did not provide statistical analysis of their results. One patient experienced hematuria and another epididymoorchitis. There were no serious complications; however, 14 % of the patients required alternative treatment by 1 year with open prostatectomy ($n=4$) and TURP ($n=3$) [29]. While each of these studies has serious limitations, taken together these cohorts represent over 200 men who underwent TEAP with measurable improvements in symptoms and without major complications. A German review in 2013 evaluated 14 studies published on TEAP to date with 515 total patients. The authors showed that injection quantities varied widely from 2 to 26 mL resulting in unpredictable reductions in prostate volume from –4 to –45 %, post-void residual urine volume from –1 to –99 %, and Qmax from +32 to +186 %. All studies showed subjective improvements in IPSS ranging from –40 to –74 % [30].

Li et al. used TRUS-guided transrectal ethanol injection for BPH in the most recent study published in 2014 [11]. They studied 70 patients (45 with LUTS and 25 with complete retention requiring indwelling catheter) including patients with significant comorbidities like COPD and CHF. Under ultrasound guidance, ethanol was injected with a 21-gauge percutaneous transhepatic cholangiography needle in 2 or 3 sites. The first and second injections were made on both sides of the prostatic inner gland (0.5–1.0 cm from needle tip to bladder and 1.0–1.5 cm from needle to lower urinary tract) and the variable third injection was along sagittal plane when hyperplastic middle lobe protruded into bladder. The dose of ethanol was initially calculated as 1/3 of the volume of the prostatic inner gland and subsequently decreased to one fourth of the volume after several complications. Transrectal ethanol injection showed favorable clinical response at 24 months: prostate volume decreased 16.3 % (46.8 +/– 8.1 to 55.9 +/– 16.7 mL, $p<0$ .001), flow increased over 200 % (4.7 +/– 3.1 mL/s to 15.3 +/– 3.2 mL/s, $p<0.001$), and post-void residual volume decreased (30.8 +/– 71.5 mL to 25.9 +/– 12.0 mL $p<0.001$). Also subjective measures improved including IPSS (29.3 +/– 6.7 points pretreatment to 9.8 +/– 2.4 points post-treatment, $p=0.001$) and QoL (1.9 +/– 0.7 points post-treatment to 5.3 +/– 1.7 points pretreatment, $p<.001$). Treatment time was brief, averaging 7.3 min (range 5–9 min). In the 36 patients that received the higher dose of ethanol, 12 patients (33 %) had dysuria and 4 patients (11 %) had complications including cystitis ($n=2$) and urinary tract injury requiring long-term catheterization ($n=2$). In the subsequent 34 patients who received the lower dose of ethanol, 1 patient (3 %) had dysuria and no patients had complications. No patients experienced recurrence of symptoms and none required re-treatment at 2 years. Although there was no comparison group, this study showed similar results for transrectal ethanol injection to TEAP with an improved treatment time and satisfactory complication rates. In fact, this approach may contribute to the low rates of urethral mucosal injury and irritation compared to TEAP.

Complications and Adverse Effects Associated With Ethanol Injection

Adverse effects of ethanol injection are not uncommon, and severe complications have been reported in the literature (Table 21.3). The most common side effect of ethanol injection seems to be immediate postoperative urinary retention requiring Foley catheterization. Some studies report 100 % catheterization rates, while others report no patients requiring catheters. Other common adverse effects include dysuria (26–40 %), hematuria (2–43 %), and pelvic pain (0–26 %). Less frequent side effects include ureteral damage (5–6 %), epididymitis/cystitis/prostatitis (2–5 %), incontinence (3 %), and retrograde ejaculation (3 %).

In the early animal studies, associated morbidity of ethanol injections included necrosis of the external prostatic sphincter and mucosa of the urethra and bladder [12]. In later human studies, two cases of bladder necrosis were reported following TEAP [31]. Grise et al. reported two cases at two different centers of patients with bladder necrosis. One patient presented with recurrent urinary retention and was found to have a urinary leak requiring diversion. The other patient also had urinary retention requiring a TURP and underwent subsequent ureteral reimplantation of distal ureteral stenosis [22].

Table 21.3 Common complications from ethanol injection

Adverse effect	Incidence (%)
Urinary retention	0–100
Dysuria	26–40
Hematuria	2–43
Perineal/abdominal pain	0–26
Epididymitis/cystitis/prostatitis	2–5
Urethral stenosis/stricture/injury	5–6
Incontinence	0–3
Retrograde ejaculation	0–3

There is also one case report of an intravesical calculus formed from sloughed prostatic tissue following ethanol injection [32]. This 78-year-old man presented with irritative symptoms and hematuria 6 months after a TEAP procedure. Ultrasound revealed a 5-cm stone which required cystolithotomy. Examination of the stone showed components of prostatic hyperplastic glandular stroma with coagulative necrosis and peripheral calcification, suggesting that the dislodged prostatic mass acted as a nidus for peripheral calcification.

Most of these side effects are relatively minor and tolerable; however, the rare reports of bladder necrosis have affected the widespread adoption of ethanol ablation.

Future Directions

Despite early promising outcomes in ethanol chemoablation for BPH, the procedure has not caught on. The AUA 2010 guidelines for the management of BPH included ethanol injection in the preliminary literature search, but excluded it from the evidence review and guideline statement [33]. The European Association of Urology issued guidelines in 2013 for the treatment of LUTS and BPH, which stated, "intraprostatic ethanol injections are therefore regarded as experimental procedures and should only be used in trials. RCTs with long-term follow-up comparing ethanol injections with TURP, other minimally invasive procedures, or drugs are needed to judge adequately the value of this treatment modality" [34]. With neither professional organization recommending the procedure, ethanol ablation remains a niche treatment for BPH.

There are currently no clinical trials underway studying ethanol injection of the prostate (clinicaltrials.gov); however, it serves as a prototype for several new injectable therapies that are currently under development. Like ethanol, injection with botulinum toxin initially garnered excitement as a treatment for BPH. This toxin functions by inducing apoptosis in prostate epithelial and stromal cells leading to tissue atrophy. Thirteen small studies showed significant improvements in LUTS with variable durability from 3 to 30 months [34, 35]. However, the most recent and largest randomized, double-blind placebo-controlled study published in 2013 was negative, showing only modest symptom improvement with botulinum toxin and comparable placebo effects [36]. Two new compounds are currently undergoing clinical trials for BPH injection therapy—NX-1207 (Nymox Corporation, Hasbrouck Heights, NJ, USA), a novel apoptotic protein, and PRX302 (Sophiris Bio Inc., La Jolla, CA, USA), a pore-forming protein activated by prostate-specific antigen. NX-1207 has completed a phase 3 multicenter prospective randomized, double-blind placebo-controlled evaluation for BPH (NCT 00918983); however, results have not yet been published. Two other phase 3 trials are ongoing for re-injection with NX-1207 (NCT 01846793) and for use in combination with tamsulosin (NCT 02003742). PRX302 showed promising safety and efficacy in a phase 2 study published in 2013 [37]. A phase 3 randomized double-blind trial is ongoing to assess the efficacy of a single treatment of this compound (NCT 01966614). Ultimately success and adoption of these agents will be based on the outcomes of these trials, safety, availability, and cost.

Conclusions

Ethanol injection for chemoablation of the prostate for the treatment of benign prostatic hyperplasia is a concept first described in the early 1900s and subsequently earned considerable excitement and research over the last decade. Studies initially showed promising results, but variable outcomes and lack of standard techniques hindered the widespread adoption of ethanol ablation. Small cohorts and short follow-up times limited these open-label trials. Patients experienced satisfactory results at 1 year, but no predictive efficacy parameters (i.e., number or location of injections) or dose–response relationships have ever been shown. Injections result in highly uneven lesions and extraprostatic leakage can have devastating consequences.

Furthermore, re-treatment rates are high with one study suggesting 41 % at 3 years [21]. Several innovations like the micropore needle and ethanol gel injection have already been able to enhance the efficacy and decrease some side effects. Eventually, ethanol injection or injection with a novel prostate-targeted compound may eventually become a suitable option for high-risk patients with BPH; however, additional research with high-quality, multicenter, randomized trials is required before this technology can become widely adopted.

References

1. Malaeb BS, Yu X, McBean AM, Elliott SP. National trends in surgical therapy for benign prostatic hyperplasia in the United States (2000–2008). Urology. 2012;79(5):1111–7.
2. Ditrolio J, Lusuardi L, Patel P, Hruby S, Watson RA, Janetschek G, et al. New emerging technologies in benign prostatic hyperplasia. Curr Opin Urol. 2013;23(1):25–9.
3. Plante MK. Editorial comment. Urology. 2014; 83(3):591.
4. Kaplan SA. Re: transurethral ethanol ablation of the prostate for symptomatic benign prostatic hyperplasia: long-term follow-up. J Urol. 2012;187(1):211–2.
5. Plante MK, Folsom JB, Zvara P. Prostatic tissue ablation by injection: a literature review. J Urol. 2004; 172(1):20–6.
6. Buchholz NNP, Andrews HO, Plante MK. Transurethral ethanol ablation of prostate. J Endourol. 2004;18(6):519–24.
7. Talwar GL, King BJ, Mutaguchi K, Goya N, Savoca G, Saemi AM, et al. Injection treatment of enlarged prostate. Br J Surg. 1966;53(5):421–7.
8. Zvara P, Karpman E, Stoppacher R, Esenler AC, Plante MK. Ablation of canine prostate using transurethral intraprostatic absolute ethanol injection. Urology. 1999;54(3):411–5.
9. Gutierrez J, Saita A, Velez E. Histological changes of the prostate gland after transurethral ethanol ablation. Eur Urol Suppl [Internet]. 2002; 1(1):130. Available from: http://linkinghub.elsevier.com/retrieve/pii/S1569905602805024
10. Plante MK, Gross AL, Kliment Jr J, Kida M, Zvara P. Intraprostatic ethanol chemoablation via transurethral and transperineal injection. BJU Int. 2003; 91(1):94–8.

11. Li Y, Zhao Q, Dong L. Efficacy and safety of ultrasound-guided transrectal ethanol injection for the treatment of benign prostatic hyperplasia in patients with high-risk comorbidities: a long-term study at a single tertiary care institution. Urology. 2014;83(3):586–91.
12. Littrup PJ, Lee F, Borlaza GS, Sacknoff EJ, Torp-Pedersen S, Gray JM. Percutaneous ablation of canine prostate using transrectal ultrasound guidance. Absolute ethanol and Nd: YAG laser. Invest Radiol. 1988;23(10):734–9.
13. Levy DA, Cromeens DM, Evans R, Stephens LC, von Eschenbach AC, Pisters LL. Transrectal ultrasound-guided intraprostatic injection of absolute ethanol with and without carmustine: a feasibility study in the canine model. Urology. 1999;53(6):1245–51.
14. Plante MK, Larson BT, Gautam G, Gross AL, Larson BT, Arora N, et al. Diffusion properties of transurethral intraprostatic injection. BJU Int. 2004;94(9):1384–8.
15. Savoca G, De Stefani S, Gattuccio I, Paolinelli D, Stacul F, Belgrano E. Percutaneous ethanol injection of the prostate as minimally invasive treatment for benign prostatic hyperplasia: preliminary report. Eur Urol. 2001;40(5):504–8.
16. Chiang POH, Chuang YC, Huang CC, Chiang CP. Pilot study of transperineal injection of dehydrated ethanol in the treatment of prostatic obstruction. Urology. 2003;61(4):797–801.
17. Goya N, Ishikawa N, Ito F, Ryoji O, Tokumoto T, Toma H, et al. Ethanol injection therapy of the prostate for benign prostatic hyperplasia: preliminary report on application of a new technique. J Urol. 1999;162(2):383–6.
18. Ditrolio J, Patel P, Watson RA, Irwin RJ. Chemo-ablation of the prostate with dehydrated alcohol for the treatment of prostatic obstruction. J Urol. 2002;167(5):2100–3; discussion 2103–4.
19. Plante MK, Bunnell ML, Trotter SJ, Jackson TL, Esenler AC, Zvara P. Transurethral prostatic tissue ablation via a single needle delivery system: initial experience with radio-frequency energy and ethanol. Prostate Cancer Prostatic Dis. 2002;5(3):183–8.
20. King BJ, Plante MK, Kida M, Mann-Gow TK, Odland R, Zvara P. Comparison of intraprostatic ethanol diffusion using a microporous hollow fiber catheter versus a standard needle. J Urol. 2012;187(5): 1898–902.
21. Goya N, Ishikawa N, Ito F, Kobayashi C, Tomizawa Y, Toma H. Transurethral ethanol injection therapy for prostatic hyperplasia: 3-year results. J Urol. 2004;172(3):1017–20.
22. Grise P, Plante M, Palmer J, Martinez-Sagarra J, Hernandez C, Schettini M, et al. Evaluation of the transurethral ethanol ablation of the prostate (TEAP) for symptomatic benign prostatic hyperplasia (BPH): a European multi-center evaluation. Eur Urol. 2004;46(4):496–501; discussion 501–2.
23. Plante MK, Marks LS, Anderson R, Amling C, Rukstalis D, Badlani G, et al. Phase I/II examination of transurethral ethanol ablation of the prostate for the treatment of symptomatic benign prostatic hyperplasia. J Urol. 2007;177(3):1030–5; discussion 1035.
24. Badlani G. A randomized trial comparing transurethral ethanol ablation of the prostate (EAP) treatment and TURP for bladder outlet obstruction (BOO). J Urol. 2003;169(4):391. Williams and Wilkins Co.
25. Mutaguchi K, Matsubara A, Kajiwara M, Hanada M, Mizoguchi H, Ohara S, et al. Transurethral ethanol injection for prostatic obstruction: an excellent treatment strategy for persistent urinary retention. Urology. 2006;68(2):307–11.
26. Larson BT, Netto N, Huidobro C, de Lima ML, Matheus W, Acevedo C, et al. Intraprostatic injection of alcohol gel for the treatment of benign prostatic hyperplasia: preliminary clinical results. Scientific World J. 2006;6:2474–80.
27. Sakr M, Eid A, Shoukry M, Fayed A. Transurethral ethanol injection therapy of benign prostatic hyperplasia: four-year follow-up. Int J Urol. 2009;16(2):196–201.
28. El-Husseiny T, Buchholz N. Transurethral ethanol ablation of the prostate for symptomatic benign prostatic hyperplasia: long-term follow-up. J Endourol. 2011;25(3):477–80.
29. Arslan M, Oztürk A, Goger YE, Aslan E, Kilinc M. Primary results of transurethral prostate ethanol injection. Int Urol Nephrol. April 2014 [E-pub ahead of print]
30. Bschleipfer T, Bach T, Gratzke C, Madersbacher S, Oelke M. Intraprostatic injection therapy in patients with benign prostatic syndrome. Urologe A. 2013;52(3):354–8.
31. Plante MK. Complications associated with transurethral ethanol ablation of the prostate for the treatment of benign prostatic hyperplasia: a worldwide experience. J Urol. 2003;169(4):392. Williams and Wilkins Co.
32. Ikari O, Leitão VA, D'ancona CAL, Matheus WE, Rodrigues NN. Intravesical calculus secondary to ethanol gel injection into the prostate. Urology. 2005;65(5):1002.
33. Levy DA, Levy DA, Cromeens DM, Cromeens DM, Evans R, Evans R, et al. American Urological Association Guideline: Management of Benign Prostatic Hyperplasia (BPH). Urology [Internet]. 2012; 5;53(6):1245–51. Available from: http://eutils.ncbi.nlm.nih.gov/entrez/eutils/elink.fcgi?dbfrom=pubmed&id=10367863&retmode=ref&cmd=prlinks
34. Oelke M, Bachmann A, Descazeaud A, Emberton M, Gravas S, Michel MC, et al. EAU guidelines on the treatment and follow-up of non-neurogenic male lower urinary tract symptoms including benign prostatic obstruction. Eur Urol. 2013;64:118–40.
35. Mangera A, Zvara P, Plante MK, Plante MK, Kaplan SA, Littrup PJ, et al. Contemporary management of lower urinary tract disease with botulinum toxin A: a systematic review of botox (onabotulinumtoxinA) and dysport (abobotulinumtoxinA). Eur Urol. 2011;60(4):784–95.

36. Marberger M, Faruque MS, Chartier-Kastler E, Faruque MS, Egerdie B, Alam MK, et al. A randomized double-blind placebo-controlled phase 2 dose-ranging study of onabotulinumtoxinA in men with benign prostatic hyperplasia. Eur Urol. 2013;63(3):496–503.

37. Elhilali MM, Pommerville P, Yocum RC, Merchant R, Roehrborn CG, Denmeade SR. Prospective, randomized, double-blind, vehicle controlled, multicenter phase IIb clinical trial of the pore forming protein PRX302 for targeted treatment of symptomatic benign prostatic hyperplasia. J Urol. 2013;189(4):1421–6.

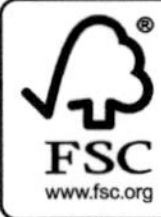

MIX
Papier aus verantwortungsvollen Quellen
Paper from responsible sources
FSC® C105338

If you have any concerns about our products,
you can contact us on
ProductSafety@springernature.com

In case Publisher is established outside the EU,
the EU authorized representative is:
Springer Nature Customer Service Center GmbH
Europaplatz 3, 69115 Heidelberg, Germany

Printed by Libri Plureos GmbH
in Hamburg, Germany